American Heart Association®

Fighting Heart Disease and Stroke

ACLS Provider Manual

Editor

Richard O. Cummins, MD, MPH, MSc,
ECC Senior Science Editor

Major Contributors

John M. Field, MD
ACLS Science Editor

Mary Fran Hazinski, RN, MSN
ECC Senior Science Editor

Special Contributors

Charles F. Babbs, MD, PhD
Paul Berlin, MS, EMT-P
John E. Billi, MD
Keith Chapman, EMT-P
Louis Gonzales, BS, NREMT-P
Robert W. Hickey, MD
Richard E. Kerber, MD
Karl B. Kern, MD
Rashmi U. Kothari, MD
Peter J. Kudenchuk, MD
Murray Lorance, NREMT
Thomas G. Martin, MD, MPH
Steve Miller, MD
Deems Okamoto, MD
Janice Ritchie Saia, RN
Charles Sand, MD
Petter A. Steen, MD

ISBN 0-87493-327-7

ACLS Subcommittee 1994-1997

Arthur B. Sanders, MD, MHA, Chair
Richard O. Cummins, MD, MPH, MSc,
  Immediate Past Chair, 1994-95
Tom P. Aufderheide, MD
John E. Billi, MD
Jay Deshpande, MD
John M. Field, MD
Henry R. Halperin, MD
Karl B. Kern, MD
Rashmi U. Kothari, MD
Peter J. Kudenchuk, MD
Katherine A. Littrell, RN, PhD
Mary E. Mancini, RN, MSN
Norman A. Paradis, MD
Corey Slovis, MD

ACLS Subcommittee 1997-2000

Karl B. Kern, MD, Chair
Arthur B. Sanders, MD, MHA,
  Immediate Past Chair, 1997-1998
Charles F. Babbs, MD, PhD
John E. Billi, MD
Jay Deshpande, MD
John M. Field, MD
Henry R. Halperin, MD
Rashmi U. Kothari, MD
Peter J. Kudenchuk, MD
Katherine A. Littrell, RN, PhD
Mary E. Mancini, RN, MSN
Thomas G. Martin, MD, MPH
Norman A. Paradis, MD
Mary Ann Peberdy, MD
Emanuel Rivers, MD
Terry L. Vanden Hoek, MD

ACLS Subcommittee 2000-2001

Henry R. Halperin, MD, Chair
Karl B. Kern, MD,
  Immediate Past Chair, 2000-2001
Charles F. Babbs, MD, PhD
Dolores Kappel, RN
Rashmi U. Kothari, MD
Robert O'Connor, MD
Mary Ann Peberdy, MD
Terry L. Vanden Hoek, MD
Max Harry Weil, MD, PhD

Contents

Chapter 3
The Advanced ACLS Skills

Chapter 4
The Human Dimension of CPR and ACLS: Human, Ethical, and Legal Issues

Chapter 5
Final, Take-Home ACLS Concepts 47

Preface

During a rare quiet time in the ED one night I walk past the ED nursing station. Leaning over the write-up counter, chin cradled on her palm, eyes glazed and unblinking, stands a nurse. A small dollop of saliva has collected at the corner of her mouth, and for a moment I consider calling a code. And then I see, lying open on the counter before her, the explanation for her near-catatonic state—the 1994 *ACLS Textbook,* opened to *Pharmacology II* or the *sodium-potassium pump* or some other enthralling section. This is a good nurse, a clinically excellent professional, a true "code partner." I would rather work with her during a code than with more than 90% of the hospital residents. She annually saves countless patients from the naïve and inappropriate orders of new house staff by her quiet question, intoned through clenched teeth, "Are you *sure* you want to order that drug, doctor?"

"Cecile! What's wrong?" I ask. "I was about to order a stat arterial blood gas on you! You look like a GCS 7 or 8!" She raises her head and looks around. Comprehension slowly plays across her face. "Oh, nothing's wrong. I was just trying to finish reading the *ACLS Textbook.* I have to renew my ACLS card at a provider course tomorrow."

The idea for this new 2001 *ACLS Provider Manual* resulted directly from observing Cecile's sad experience and hearing from many other ACLS instructors, providers, and provider candidates all across the country—trying to plow through the *ACLS Textbook* as the best way to prepare for the ACLS Provider Course. Let's admit it: except for a few resuscitation mavens, reading previous editions of the *ACLS Textbook* was laborious. Although it is an excellent, scholarly, evidence-filled tome, it is not John Grisham. The *ACLS Textbook* (titled *ACLS—The Reference Textbook* in the 2003 edition) presents the science behind our resuscitation guidelines and conveys critical information to enhance our understanding. It does not, however, provide efficient support for time-poor healthcare professionals trying to prepare for the clinically oriented, case-based ACLS Provider Course. The 77-page Chapter 1, "Essentials of ACLS," proved to be a great success with adult learners because it attempted to walk the reader through each of the ACLS algorithms in a practical, clinically oriented style. There was a widespread sense, however, that ACLS learners needed more than just the "Essentials" chapter.

The traditional subject-based focus of the ACLS Provider Course changed to a case-based orientation in 1994. We took this step to align the ACLS training program with what experts in education were teaching us about adult, professional learning. For adult learners to learn, they need courses that were practical, relevant to their work, and consistent with their learning objectives. Healthcare professionals seek out ACLS courses to get better at meeting their daily professional responsibilities—they want to do the best job they possibly can during cardiopulmonary emergencies. Case-based ACLS training allows provider candidates to experience the same clinical challenges they face in their professional lives.

To support the new case-based orientation of the ACLS Provider Course, we prepared the 1994 *ACLS Instructor's Manual* for instructors and course directors. This manual contained numerous new features that proved popular with ACLS instructors. For each core case the instructor manual provided sample scenarios for the 4 most common settings for cardiopulmonary emergencies: the out-of-hospital EMS environment; the Emergency Department; in-hospital critical care areas such as intensive care and coronary care units; and nonspecialized in-hospital locations, such as general medical and surgical floors, the outpatient clinics, and diagnostic service areas such as radiology. The *ACLS Instructor's Manual* supplied instructors with a list of critical actions that needed to be implemented for a good outcome, a list of unacceptable or harmful actions that would prevent a positive outcome, and a detailed list of the most important teaching points to convey in each case.

Within a few short months we began to hear intriguing comments from people who had experienced a case-based ACLS Provider Course and who had advanced further to the ACLS instructor level. Upon viewing the 1994 *ACLS Instructor's Manual* for the first time, these providers-now-instructors often were struck by a sense that many sections of the instructor manual would have been immensely helpful to them as they prepared for the ACLS Provider Course. In particular, they advised us that ACLS providers should know in advance the actions and thought patterns expected by ACLS instructors of provider candidates. If with each case ACLS instructors were looking for provider candidates to take certain critical actions and avoid specific unacceptable actions, then ACLS providers should know these actions beforehand. Such advance review and repetition could only enhance their educational experience.

Thus the format and contents of this new *ACLS Provider Manual* began to take shape in the late 1990s. We needed a case-based ACLS provider manual that matched our case-based ACLS Provider Course. We needed to lead the provider candidates on "a walk through the algorithm" for each of the 10 core cases. We needed to share in advance the recommended critical actions list and the unacceptable actions list that the instructors were going to follow in the course. Finally the *ACLS Provider Manual* still had to teach the fundamentals as a core part of the ACLS Provider Course.

So what is this *ACLS Provider Manual* that you now have in your hands? And what are the best ways to use this manual as you prepare for your first ACLS Provider Course? At first you will probably exclaim "Some *manual!*" as you heft this fairly weighty publication from the shelf. But this book does fulfill the defining elements of a manual—"a softcover book that attempts to provide complete coverage of a major topic, but in a broad, overview manner, lacking the depth of a true textbook, where the materials are arranged in a practical way to allow ready access to specific topics."

In Part I we present 5 chapters that cover the foundation of ACLS: the *systematic ACLS Approach* that you should apply to every cardiopulmonary emergency you face; the *advanced skills of ACLS* that you will need to manage the ACLS core cases, and coverage of the important, and often neglected, *human dimensions of CPR and ACLS.*

In Part II we present the 10 core cases of ACLS. This material contains much of the popular "Essentials of ACLS" chapter of the *ACLS Textbook* throughout the 1990s. With some variation, each case follows this outline:

- A review of what's new in the *ECC Guidelines 2000,* a valuable distillation of all the additions or changes that affect that particular case
- A description of the case, defining the topics covered during case management
- Sample case scenarios to illustrate the type of cases managed in the 4 common scenarios: out-of-hospital emergencies, Emergency Department cases, in-hospital critical care units, and nonspecialized in-hospital locations
- A statement of the learning objectives of the case, including the specific new skills, drugs, and rhythms to learn
- The well-received "walk through the algorithm" using the technique of annotated algorithms that we introduced in the 1997 *ACLS Textbook* chapters on acute coronary syndromes and acute ischemic stroke.
- An innovation follows—the Critical Actions Checklist for assessment and management. Each step in the systematic approach to ACLS is really a 2-step process of assessment and management, and the checklist provides the details for both what is assessed and how to manage the results of that assessment.
- From the *ACLS Instructor's Manual,* we next list the Unacceptable Actions (common errors, perils, and pitfalls). Both ACLS providers and instructors have found these lists to be particularly helpful, for the last thing any clinician wants to do is to make the patient worse.
- Each case ends with the Workbook Review. These multiple-choice, single-answer questions will help the reader review the major learning objectives for that particular case. The right answer and the distractor answers are annotated in Appendix 2, with a careful explanation of why the right answer was right and the wrong answers were wrong.
- To help interested ACLS providers, the Read More About It section provides cross-references to the most relevant pages in the *ECC Handbook* and the *ECC Guidelines 2000.*

The appendices are an unusually large page count because we consider them of critical importance to ACLS learners. The section "Basic Skills of ACLS" covers basic adult CPR and operation of an AED. In the past ACLS provider courses have neglected these areas based on 1 of 2 assumptions: either ACLS provider candidates already knew how to perform CPR and use a "real" defibrillator or that time spent learning CPR and AED operation could be better spent on learning more about drugs, rhythms, and advanced airway tools. These are both false assumptions: most ACLS provider candidates do not perform satisfactory CPR when they are first evaluated in an ACLS course, and as extensively described in the *ECC Guidelines 2000,* nothing has a greater impact on survival from sudden cardiac arrest than early, good CPR and early defibrillation. As the *ECC Guidelines 2000* and the 2003 *ACLS Reference Textbook* point out in heartbreaking detail, there is little evidence that pressor agents and antiarrhythmic agents make any difference in successful resuscitation, and the gold standard for airway control, the tracheal tube, is proving to be a double-edged sword when wielded by ACLS providers of marginal skill.

This new *ACLS Provider Manual* has a powerful learning tool: the Workbook Review. This is the extensive compilation of the annotated workbook questions from each chapter. This format of exam questions, followed by annotated right and wrong answers, has been documented as a successful method for improving the review of a specialty topic. This method has been widely adopted for board certification courses in emergency medicine, internal medicine, and family medicine. Many experienced ACLS providers will find that working their way through the workbook alone will provide a helpful review of ACLS.

Finally, we must strongly recommend that you purchase a personal copy of the *ACLS Reference Textbook* or have ready access to one wherever you work professionally. The *ACLS Provider Manual* does not replace the *ACLS Reference Textbook,* which provides much more in-depth, comprehensive coverage of all aspects of advanced cardiopulmonary life support. The *ACLS Provider Manual* is more an introduction and supplement to the entire domain of advanced resuscitation; the *ACLS Reference Textbook* is **the** ACLS textbook. The editor of our new *ACLS Reference Textbook* has done a superb rewrite of the 1994 and 1997 editions, focusing on a clear presentation of the science behind resuscitation. Furthermore, about one third of the *ACLS Reference Textbook* is devoted to the topics covered in the new ACLS for the Experienced Provider Course.

We encourage all ACLS providers to look upon ACLS training as a 2-part experience, starting with the ACLS Provider Course, followed 2 years later by the ACLS for Experienced Provider Course. Not only will that sequence provide the most in-depth coverage of ACLS knowledge and skills, it will also provide a stimulating way to renew your ACLS provider status and allow you to really get full benefit from purchase of your personal copy of the *ACLS Reference Textbook.*

Acknowledgments

The *ACLS Provider Manual* is the result of the enthusiasm, intellect, knowledge, experience, and plain hard work of many people. The 2 people most responsible for the content of this book were Mary Fran Hazinski, RN, MSN, ECC senior science editor, and John Field, MD, associate editor of the *ACLS Reference Textbook.* Their contributions have been immense and invaluable.

Jack Billi, MD, vice chair of the national ECC Committee, is the educational and conceptual father of the case-based ACLS course. He first articulated the need for a case-based textbook to support the course.

Many members of the ACLS Subcommittee provided helpful reviews of this material in order to make it as scientifically and clinically accurate as possible.

Ted Borek, former vice president of ECC Programs at the American Heart Association, and Mike Bell, acting vice president of ECC, consistently provided encouragement and support as well as financial resources for both the concept and development of a provider manual.

David Barnes, account team manager in AHA design and media services, has coordinated the production of this provider manual and all the other ECC products with dedication and skill.

Mary Ann McNeely, director of product development, assembled and supported, prodded and praised not only the editor but also an excellent editorial team of Starr Wheelan, Jackie Haigney, Kara Robinson, Julie Noe, and Sarah Johnson. The manual is just one of a seemingly endless array of high quality ECC products that this team has been turning out month after month without pause.

Finally, there is F. G. Stoddard, ECC editor in chief. The knowledge, talent, skill, personality, and just plain hardworking goodness of this man percolates through every ECC product, but especially through this *ACLS Provider Manual.* If anyone is ever going to merit the tribute "irreplaceable," it is F. G. Thank you, pardner.

Richard O. Cummins, MD

Note on Medication Doses

Emergency Cardiovascular Care is a dynamic science. Advances in treatment and drug therapies occur rapidly. Readers are advised to check for changes in recommended dose, indications, and contraindications in the following sources: *Currents in Emergency Cardiovascular Care,* the *ECC Handbook of Emergency Cardiovascular Care for Healthcare Providers,* and the package insert product information sheet for each drug.

Introduction to the ACLS Provider Course

What to Expect in the ACLS Provider Course

During this course you will learn by observing, discussing, and doing. ACLS instructors will help you achieve the course objectives using the following approaches.

Manage 10 Core Cases Through Small-Group Case-Based Teaching

The ACLS Provider Course uses case-based teaching. Your instructors will expect you to learn the critical assessment-management actions for 10 core cases by conducting the Primary and Secondary ABCD Surveys and implementing the algorithms. You must recognize the need for specific critical actions and be able to carry them out in a timely manner.

You will learn to manage these 10 core cases during small group discussions and occasional larger group sessions. Since 1994 small group discussion has been the main format used in all ACLS provider courses. In each case you will review 3 rescuer roles: (1) lone rescuer, (2) resuscitation team member, and (3) resuscitation team leader. Part 2 of this manual will walk you through the 10 core cases and their successful management.

The cases cover respiratory emergency, 4 types of cardiac arrest (simple ventricular fibrillation/ventricular tachycardia [VF/VT], complex VF/VT, pulseless electrical activity [PEA], and asystole), 4 types of prearrest emergencies (bradycardia, stable tachycardia, unstable tachycardia, and acute coronary syndromes), and stroke. Generally the cases follow a specific sequence with each case reinforcing knowledge and skills learned in the preceding cases: respiratory arrest, simple VF, complex VF, PEA, asystole, acute coronary syndromes, tachycardias, and ischemic stroke.

Successful case management both during the course and in professional situations requires constant thinking and analysis. Some of these cases require interventions that ACLS providers have never used or interventions that are—by licensing regulations—outside their scope of practice. Do not worry. Successful completion requires that you see and understand, not that you must see and do. The course gives you a framework on which to build your knowledge, skills, confidence, and expertise. With self-directed study, renewal training, and a lifelong approach to case-based learning, you will be able to meet the challenges of cardiovascular/cardiopulmonary emergencies.

Learn and Practice: Key Skills in BLS and ACLS

In the ACLS Provider Course you will receive guided training and hands-on practice in the key skills of BLS and ACLS:

Key BLS Skills

- Adult CPR
- Basic airway management, including the use of adjuncts for delivery of oxygen, barrier devices, oropharyngeal airways, nasopharyngeal airways, pocket face masks, and suction devices
- Use of an automated external defibrillator (AED)

Key ACLS Skills

- Use of conventional defibrillator/monitors for defibrillation and cardioversion
- Use of transcutaneous pacing devices
- Advanced airway management, including the use of the Combitube, laryngeal mask airway, and tracheal tube
- Use of qualitative and quantitative end-tidal CO_2 measurement devices
- Use of esophageal detector devices
- Application and use of commercial tracheal tube holders and a generic technique based on adhesive tape, umbilical ties, and benzoin[1]
- Recognition of cardiac arrest rhythms and the most common bradycardias and tachycardias

[1]Many hospitals and healthcare specialties such as anesthesiology, emergency medicine, and respiratory therapy have developed simple tape-and-tie procedures that are documented, standardized, and taught effectively. The use of these approaches is acceptable.

- Recognition of the 12-lead ECG signs of acute injury and ischemia
- Initiation of intravenous (IV) access
- Administration of medications by the intravenous and endotracheal routes

Most healthcare providers who attend the ACLS Provider Course are already employed in positions that require these skills. In some courses, however, learners may have little or no background in ACLS skills. In such courses the course director can provide specific skills stations for learners to focus on skills they have not yet mastered.

Skills Evaluation: CPR, Airway, and AED

The 3 skills listed above are taught, practiced, and evaluated during case management in small groups or during separate skills stations. Learners are encouraged to practice and review as often as needed.

Successful completion of the ACLS Provider Course requires all ACLS learners to demonstrate satisfactory hands-on skills in adult 1- and 2-rescuer CPR, use of the noninvasive airway adjuncts listed above, and application and operation of an AED. Appendix 1 of this manual contains the Heartsaver AED skills that instructors follow during this evaluation. There is only one formal examination of skills in the course: the Heartsaver AED examination station.

Class Lectures

The course director may prefer to present some learning objectives during a large group lecture. For example, a single lecture to the entire class may address topics such as the evaluation of 12-lead ECGs for injury and ischemia or the criteria for fibrinolytic therapy.

Precourse Written Examination

Before the course you will receive a multiple-choice written examination of 30 to 40 questions to help you assess your precourse strengths and weaknesses and give you areas for precourse review. At the beginning of the course you will be given an annotated answer sheet that explains the rationale for both correct and incorrect answers to the exam. Learners will be given some time to review and discuss the annotated answers.

Postcourse Written Examination

At the end of the course you will be given another written examination. After you complete and grade the examination, the instructor will distribute an annotated answer sheet for review and discussion.

Learning Objectives of ACLS Provider Training

At the end of the ACLS Provider Course the successful learner will know how to manage cardiorespiratory emergencies using the *systematic* ACLS Approach. Resuscitation team members will know *what to do* and *when to do it,* minimizing the confusion sometimes observed in such situations. Learning and practicing the ACLS Approach helps learners feel more comfortable about their role and about facing future resuscitation challenges.

Core Course Objective: Manage First 10 Minutes of a Sudden, Witnessed VF/Pulseless VT Arrest

In general, defining the primary objective for any ECC course requires answering the following question: *upon successful completion of this course, what are the most important skills a provider should be able to perform?* The primary objective of the ACLS course is to provide you with the knowledge and skills to evaluate and manage a sudden, witnessed VF/VT arrest in an adult.

This is **not** a simple matter! The ACLS provider must be able to make multiple decisions about assessment and management quickly and under pressure. After completing the course an ACLS provider should be able to manage the following core scenario with confidence.

Managing this critical first 10 minutes of a witnessed VF arrest requires these skills:

- Basic life support (CPR)
- Operation of an AED (in nonspecialized care units)

The Core VF Scenario

You are a healthcare provider who must evaluate a patient for an acute cardiovascular/cardiopulmonary problem (heart irregularity, possible acute coronary syndrome, possible acute stroke). With little warning the patient collapses. As the only witness you must manage the patient for several minutes. Begin the management of this patient now.

- Start with the Primary ABCD steps of CPR; then get, attach, and use an AED. The AED detects VF and delivers several shocks. The last shock results in asystole.
- After several minutes other ACLS providers arrive. You direct these responders to perform specific actions in the Secondary ABCD Survey, including advanced airway management, IV access, administration of rhythm-appropriate medications, and further defibrillation, cardioversion, and transcutaneous pacing when needed.
- The patient's rhythm changes from asystole to pulseless electrical activity (PEA) to pulseless VT. You must treat each rhythm variation according to the appropriate *ECC Guidelines 2000* ACLS algorithm.
- Five to 10 minutes after collapsing, the patient regains spontaneous circulation. You continue to manage the case appropriately for several minutes during the immediate postresuscitation period.

- Operation of a conventional defibrillator (in specialized care units)
- Transcutaneous pacing
- Advanced airway management, including secondary confirmation of correct device placement and prevention of tube dislodgment
- Vascular access
- Choice of rhythm-appropriate medications consistent with the ACLS algorithms

What Do I Have to Know to Pass?

The learner in the ACLS Provider Course has achieved the *core learning objectives* when she or he successfully demonstrates management—appropriate for her or his professional role—of the first 10 minutes of VF arrest. At a minimum this successful management is determined by performance during case scenarios and specifically by

1. Successful demonstration of adult CPR skills and use of the AED
2. Successful management of the 10 core cases consistent with the learning objectives for each core case outlined in the critical evaluation checklists
3. Achievement of a satisfactory score on the written examination

Leadership Objectives for ACLS Providers

At some point after the ACLS Provider Course the ACLS provider will need to direct others during a resuscitation attempt. The informal phrase "running a code" refers to directing others during resuscitative efforts. The leadership objective for a healthcare provider taking his or her first ACLS Provider Course is modest: assign tasks to responders as they arrive on the scene. Long-term leadership objectives for the code leader include the following:

- Direct bystanders and other rescuers who arrive at the scene.
- Know about advance directives and how to respond to them and be willing to assume responsibility for deciding whether to follow the advance directive.
- Know the indications for *not* starting resuscitative efforts and when to stop them.
- In a respectful, effective manner inform the patient's family or loved ones about the resuscitation attempt.
- Know how and when to conduct a critical incident stress debriefing about the resuscitation attempt.
- Know the ACLS Approach and follow it as much as possible during resuscitative efforts.
- Know how to implement the *ECC Guidelines 2000* recommendation to facilitate family presence during resuscitative efforts.

Although the ability to run a code is a valuable skill for all ACLS providers, it is not a core objective of the initial ACLS Provider Course.

Precourse Skills

Basic life support is the foundation of ACLS. You must know BLS before you can take an ACLS course. The ACLS course curriculum assumes that you have had some professional training in a healthcare-related profession such as medicine, nursing, respiratory therapy, or emergency medical services. You must understand basic human anatomy and pathophysiology and possess a working knowledge of taking a patient's history, performing a physical examination, performing basic assessment, and providing treatment. Training in ACLS offers an opportunity to combine previous training and experience with new knowledge and skills. You will acquire psychomotor skills such as intubation, clinical skills such as ECG interpretation, and leadership skills to help you impose calm, order, and logic on an often complex challenge.

Support Materials for the ACLS Provider Course

The ECC Programs of the American Heart Association (AHA) support the ACLS Provider Course with several publications.

This manual will help you prepare for the case-based (not subject-based) ACLS Provider Course. This manual is not an in-depth textbook; for that you are referred to the textbook *ACLS—The Reference Textbook* (see below).

The *Handbook of Emergency Cardiovascular Care for Healthcare Providers* serves as a quick reference and provides an opportunity for continued learning. This pocket handbook contains all the ACLS algorithms and provides information about the medications and interventions you need to know to manage the core cases.

The *ACLS Reference Textbook* is a subject-based, in-depth, scholarly review of the full range of resuscitation subjects. A personal copy of the textbook is a useful learning resource for the ACLS Provider Course. Of note, the ACLS textbook provides economic value because it also serves as the course textbook for the new ACLS Course for Experienced Providers.

The ACLS Approach to Cardiovascular and Cardiopulmonary Emergencies

The ACLS Approach originated as a simple memory aid to remind ACLS providers of a sequence of 8 actions that must be performed during a resuscitation attempt. These actions form the Primary ABCD Survey and the Secondary ABCD Survey. With a little elaboration, these 8 steps provide a logical approach to most cardiovascular and cardiopulmonary emergencies. Routine use of the Primary and Secondary Surveys for all patients ensures that providers will check for an adequate airway, breathing (ventilation), and circulation, including defibrillation if necessary. The need for more advanced interventions is quickly apparent with this approach; at the same time providers are reminded to consider an initial diagnosis. Further treatment is guided by the appropriate ACLS algorithm and repeated attention to the Primary and Secondary ABCD Surveys.

The ACLS Approach is a simple yet powerful tool to help ACLS providers recognize and anticipate critical needs of the victim and provide effective leadership or contribute as a valuable team member. The 2 ABCD surveys are familiar to all physicians, nurses, and emergency personnel who practice and teach emergency and critical care medicine. The surveys identify the sequence of tasks to follow when managing cardiorespiratory emergencies.

The Primary ABCD Survey

You should consider each step in the Primary ABCD Survey as a cycle of ***assess*** and ***manage***. This cycle pattern ensures that in the heat of battle you will clinically *assess* critical features before starting to *manage* the emergency. For example, with Step D you *assess* the rhythm (VF), then you *manage* the rhythm (defibrillation). In practically all emergencies, when your assessment identifies a life-threatening problem you must first ***stop!—go no further!***—manage and solve that problem before moving to the next assess-manage cycle. An upper airway obstructed by a foreign body provides an excellent example of this "go no further" principle. If the blocked airway is discovered in the Step B assessment of the Primary Survey, the blocked airway must be managed in Step B.

ACLS providers can also apply the ACLS Approach to patients who are not yet in cardiac arrest but are at *high risk* of the heart stopping. In addition, instructors and providers have learned the value of reviewing the Primary and Secondary ABCDs at all major decision points during a difficult resuscitation.

The Primary ABCD Survey

Focus on basic CPR and defibrillation

- **A**irway: open the airway
- **B**reathing: provide positive-pressure ventilations
- **C**irculation: give chest compressions
- **D**efibrillation: shock VF/pulseless VT

The Primary Survey reviews the familiar steps of BLS, including CPR and defibrillation. In the preliminary steps you assess the victim's responsiveness, call for help, and position the victim and yourself. You then conduct a Primary Survey to assess and manage the need for an open **A**irway, manage and provide **B**reathing, and assess and provide **C**irculation. You assess for VF or pulseless tachycardia, and if one of these is present, you provide **D**efibrillation shocks.

The Secondary ABCD Survey

The Secondary Survey focuses on rapid assessment and advanced treatment to restore and maintain spontaneous breathing and circulation. Because the Secondary Survey includes advanced medical interventions, healthcare providers are required to have advanced skills. The team leader must confirm that the Secondary Survey is carried out. As in the Primary Survey, **A, B,** and **C** refer to *Airway, Breathing,* and *Circulation,* although you will open the airway, secure breathing, and provide intravenous medications with more advanced skills and devices.

The **D** of the Secondary Survey, however, does not refer to assessment for VF and defibrillation as it does in the Primary Survey. The **D** of the Secondary Survey directs you to construct a **Differential Diagnosis**—to answer the question *"What caused this cardiac arrest?"* or *"Why has the patient not responded to this treatment?"*

The Secondary ABCD Survey

Focus on advanced assessments and treatments

- **A**irway: provide advanced airway management (tracheal intubation, laryngeal mask airway, Combitube)
- **B**reathing: check for adequate oxygenation and ventilation, including
  - — Primary confirmation (physical examination) of proper placement of the airway device
  - — Secondary confirmation (end-tidal CO_2 detectors, esophageal detector devices) of proper device placement
  - — Continuous or intermittent monitoring of CO_2 and oxygen levels
  - — Active effort to prevent tracheal tube dislodgment, using commercial tube holders rather than the traditional tape-and-tie techniques
- **C**irculation: obtain IV access, determine rhythm, give appropriate agents
- **D**ifferential **D**iagnosis: search for, find, and treat reversible causes

The ACLS Algorithms: Effective Support Tools

The familiar perspective of the *rhythm-assessment* or *algorithm approach* has proved successful in teaching and learning. The algorithms direct the management of patients on the basis of 1 of 3 arrest rhythms—VF/VT, PEA, or asystole—and 1 of 2 nonarrest rhythms—bradycardia or tachycardia (stable or unstable). The algorithms begin with the ECC Comprehensive Algorithm, which directs the rescuer simply to identify the cardiac rhythm of the patient, choose the algorithm that goes with that rhythm, and manage the case accordingly. Each algorithm is different and requires memorization of the treatments and their sequence.

ACLS providers should think of the algorithms as support tools for the ACLS Approach. The algorithms are like pull-down computer menus. When you get to **C** in the Secondary ABCD Survey, for example, you pull down the "menu," which states

- Gain access to the circulation
- Attach the cardiac monitor (if not already done)
- Identify the rhythm
- Give rhythm-appropriate medications

You do not need to memorize the details of all the drugs and doses in the algorithms and their sequences of use. When working clinically you should always have the algorithms immediately available. They are best displayed for quick reference in the *ECC Handbook*.

The Thinking Cook

An algorithm presents a way to treat a broad range of patients. By their very nature, however, algorithms oversimplify. The effective ACLS provider follows algorithms wisely, not blindly. Some patients may require extra care not specified in the algorithms. The AHA accepts and encourages flexibility when clinically appropriate. Algorithms do not replace clinical understanding, nor should they be considered endorsements, requirements, or "standards of care" in a legal sense. You will not find everything you need to know in the algorithms, but they are good memory aids. The algorithms list many interventions and actions as "considerations" to help providers think. Although the algorithms provide a good "cookbook," the patient always requires a "thinking cook."

A Powerful Combination: The ACLS Approach and the ACLS Algorithms

The ACLS Approach, in combination with the easily learned Primary and Secondary ABCD Surveys, conveys a simple conceptual model that ACLS providers can apply to all cardiorespiratory emergencies. The algorithms function as *memory aids*. This combination of the ACLS Approach and the algorithms takes advantage of the strengths of each approach. The surveys provide a rational, disciplined approach to assessment and treatment of the *patient*, not just treatment of the cardiac rhythm.

The algorithms are supplemental educational tools that summarize important points in the management of cardiorespiratory emergencies. The visual display of the algorithms provides clues to help you remember the important points.

A Kinder, Gentler ACLS Experience: Ending the Anxiety of ACLS Training

Before 1994 the ACLS course was often described by course participants as an intimidating, inflexible, and negative learning experience. Although this description was inaccurate in most locations, actions that would merit such a reputation did occur in some courses. Instructor behavior that creates a negative learning experience has always been roundly condemned by the AHA and ECC Programs. Beginning in 1992 ECC Program leaders instituted strong measures to ensure a positive adult learning experience in ACLS training. Many adult education experts credit the 1994 transition from subject-based courses to case-based courses with transforming ACLS training.

There is no defense for intimidation and negative reinforcement in adult professional education and training. Healthcare professionals, however, often have a low threshold for anxiety and intimidation when challenged to display their knowledge and skills. "They do it to themselves," observed one experienced ACLS instructor. Faced with a first ACLS course, some participants become anxious and begin to doubt their own abilities. The amount of information to learn and the number of skills to practice seem overwhelming. Participants sometimes become preoccupied with such questions as "How will I recognize all the rhythms that demand immediate treatment?" or "How can I remember which medications are used for which rhythm?" During case management some first-time learners may focus on a particularly intimidating skill such as intubation or starting a peripheral IV line but neglect to gain the broader perspective.

Some apprehension about a professional training course is reasonable. There is much to learn and practice. The scenarios in the course ask participants to face life-and-death issues. Often learners must perform before their peers. This new ACLS Provider Course has continued the trend in the 1990s to identify and eliminate any aspects of ACLS training that provoke inappropriate anxiety or interfere with efficient learning.

Summary and Review

This chapter describes the educational objectives for the ACLS Provider Course. ACLS provider candidates can identify areas of knowledge and skills that may need more attention and review. Chapter 1 introduces the ACLS Approach and recommends the use of the Primary and Secondary ABCD Surveys throughout the course and in actual emergencies. Review the following summary of the ACLS Approach. This sequence, with all the assess-and-manage variations, will soon become second nature to you, the new ACLS provider.

Recognize the Need to Respond

- *Assess* victim responsiveness.
- Shout for help or phone 911.
- Position the victim.
- Position yourself as the rescuer.

Conduct the Primary ABCD Survey

You need only your gloved hands, a mask for ventilations, and an AED for defibrillation. The Primary ABCD Survey guides you to assess and manage all life-threatening conditions:

- *Assess and manage* the **A**irway with noninvasive techniques.
- *Assess and manage* **B**reathing with positive-pressure ventilations.
- *Assess and manage* **C**irculation by performing CPR until the AED arrives.
- *Assess and manage* any need for **D**efibrillation by assessing the cardiac rhythm for VF/VT and providing defibrillatory shocks as needed in a safe and effective manner.

Conduct the Secondary ABCD Survey

Assess and manage the patient using *advanced* and *invasive* techniques. If possible, restore spontaneous respiration and circulation. Continue to assess and manage the patient until he or she is transferred to the next level of appropriate professional care. In brief, ***resuscitate, stabilize,*** and ***transfer*** to higher-level care.

- *Assess and manage* the **A**irway. When indicated, use advanced airway devices to manage a compromised airway.
- *Assess and manage* **B**reathing. Confirm proper airway device placement by physical examination criteria, measurement of CO_2 exhalation, and detection of esophageal placement. Properly secure the airway device to prevent dislodgment. *Assess* the adequacy of oxygenation and ventilation by clinical criteria (chest rise), oxygen saturation, and capnometry or capnography. Correct any problems detected.
- *Assess* and *manage* **C**irculation and delivery of medication by
  - — Starting a peripheral IV line
  - — Attaching monitor leads and monitoring for rhythm irregularities and onset of cardiac arrest rhythms (VF, pulseless VT, asystole, and PEA)
  - — Providing appropriate medications for the rhythm (eg, amiodarone, lidocaine, procainamide, magnesium) and vital signs (eg, epinephrine, vasopressin, atropine, dopamine, dobutamine)
- *Assess and manage* the **D**ifferential **D**iagnosis that you develop as you search for, find, and treat reversible causes.

Know and Apply the Cardiac Arrest Algorithms

- Comprehensive ECC algorithm
- VF/pulseless VT
- Asystole
- PEA
- Use of AEDs

Know and Apply the "Periarrest" Algorithms

- Bradycardias
- Tachycardias (unstable)
- Tachycardias: the overview algorithm and the table on atrial fibrillation/flutter
- Tachycardias: the 2 algorithms on narrow- and wide-complex tachycardias
- Acute coronary syndromes
- Acute ischemic stroke

Run the Code: Know How to Direct Others During a Resuscitation Attempt

- Use the Primary and Secondary ABCD Surveys when a witness to the arrest and when arriving after the code has started.
- Direct bystanders and other rescuers who arrive on the scene.
- Check for advance directives, especially when clinical evidence strongly indicates a resuscitation attempt is not indicated.
- Consider the presence of the patient's family and loved ones during resuscitation attempts.
- Learn the local regulations about death certification when out-of-hospital resuscitative efforts fail and there are clinical indications to end resuscitative efforts.
- Know the indications for when *not* to start resuscitative efforts and when to stop them.
- Know respectful, effective techniques for telling the patient's family or loved ones about the outcome of resuscitative efforts.
- Know the recommended steps to use to conduct a critical incident stress debriefing of the resuscitation attempt.

The Systematic ACLS Approach

This chapter uses the systematic ACLS Approach to expand the ACLS provider's conceptual framework about cardiopulmonary emergencies. Use the ACLS Approach introduced in Chapter 1 to guide your actions and your thinking. Use it at the start of a resuscitation attempt, use it when you are the leader, use it when you join a resuscitation attempt in progress, and use it whenever a resuscitation is not going well.

Origins of the ACLS Approach

ACLS training originated in Nebraska in the early 1970s. Its purpose was to bring order and organization to the treatment of in-hospital cardiac arrest. Severe life-and-death emergencies demand the presence of trained, experienced professionals working in close coordination. Before ACLS training the in-hospital response to cardiac arrest was often a scene of chaos and confusion.

In ACLS it may be many years before you progress from doing chest compressions and carrying blood gases to the laboratory to running the code and making the major decisions about therapy. Codes, however, do not just happen: they evolve with a dynamic history that runs a unique and unpredictable course. The greater the number of people who are trained in ACLS and know what's supposed to happen next, the better the response to routine events as well as the twists and turns that occur in every resuscitation attempt.

Resuscitation attempts are complex emotional and professional challenges. The more your thinking becomes automatic, like that of aircraft pilots following preflight checklists, the better you will respond. Knowing the ACLS Approach allows you to see and understand how the response is proceeding, what roles are played by different responders, what roles seem to go unfilled, and what scenes happen next. You will also learn to recognize your role and to see when you must step in to lend support or correct an error.

Learning Objectives

At the end of this chapter you should be able to

1. Describe the 8 steps of the ACLS Approach.
2. For each step of the ACLS Approach describe 2 acts of assessment and management that occur with each step.
3. Describe how you can apply this approach to almost all cardiovascular emergencies.

Easy Ways to Recall 8 Things to Look for in an Emergency

Every time you evaluate a critically ill patient, respond to serious complaints, or approach the scene of a possible cardiopulmonary emergency, begin by going down the checklist of the ACLS Approach. The Table below presents the basic steps of the Primary and Secondary ABCD Surveys as presented in Chapter 1. In addition, the Table lists the matching clinical questions that an ACLS provider must ask as he or she conducts the 2 ABCD surveys. Note that the list of clinical questions to review is more sophisticated than the basic steps. The answers to these questions require the clinical assessment and reasoning that can only be provided by more experienced healthcare professionals.

The Primary and Secondary ABCD Survey steps are like the pull-down menus on computer screens. With growing clinical experience ACLS providers learn to add more and more information to personal pull-down menus. The table on the next page shows how more and more information can be "hooked" to each step within the simple 8-step framework.

ACLS professionals have learned that the ***Secondary D: Differential Diagnosis*** step is the step that will expand the most. The

Primary Survey: ABCD *(Basic Steps From Chapter 1)*	**Primary ABCD Survey** *(ACLS Questions to Ask)*
Airway: open the airway *Breathing:* provide positive-pressure ventilations *Circulation:* give chest compressions *Defibrillation:* shock VF/pulseless VT	*Airway:* Is the airway open? *Breathing:* Is the victim moving air adequately? *Breathing:* If not, is someone providing proper artificial ventilations? *Circulation:* Is there a pulse? If not, is CPR being performed effectively? *Defibrillation:* If no pulse, has someone checked whether rhythm is VF? Is a defibrillator on the way? Is it ready to deliver a shock?
Secondary Survey: ABCD *(Basic Steps From Chapter 1)*	**Secondary ABCD Survey** *(ACLS Questions to Ask)*
Airway: provide advanced airway management (tracheal intubation, laryngeal mask airway, Combitube) *Breathing:* confirm tube placement primarily (physical examination), secondarily (check end-tidal CO_2 and esophageal placement), check for adequate oxygenation and ventilation *Circulation:* obtain IV access, determine rhythm, give medications appropriate for rhythm and vital signs *Differential Diagnosis:* search for, find, and treat reversible causes	*Airway:* Is advanced airway needed now? If yes, intubate victim with laryngeal mask airway, Combitube, or tracheal tube *Breathing:* Primary confirmation (physical examination) of proper placement of airway device *Breathing:* Secondary confirmation (end-tidal CO_2 detectors, esophageal detector devices) of proper device placement *Breathing:* Adequate oxygenation and ventilation? Is it possible to provide continuous/intermittent monitoring of CO_2 and oxygen levels? *Breathing:* Is tube secured to prevent dislodgment? Is commercial tube holder being used or tape-and-tie techniques? Is proper tube placement reconfirmed frequently? *Circulation:* What was initial cardiac rhythm? What is current cardiac rhythm? *Circulation:* Has someone obtained access to the venous circulation? Can fluids and medication now be given? Have all medications and interventions been provided as indicated for this rhythm and the overall clinical condition? *Differential Diagnosis:* ***Now . . . what is wrong with this patient?*** Why did adequate respirations and heartbeat stop? Why did this patient go into an arrest? What do we see, hear, smell, know or can quickly learn that might help us identify a reversible cause of this arrest?

patient who is brought in by medics and is in cardiac arrest with a bizarre, broad-complex tachycardia and no history can represent a major treatment challenge. Some ACLS providers would remember the principle that "unstable tachycardias" should be immediately cardioverted or defibrillated. When other responders note a mass in the left arm that pulsates with compressions, the inexperienced ACLS provider might remain puzzled or fail to see a connection between a pulsatile mass in the arm and the fact that the patient is in full refractory cardiac arrest. That provider might call for immediate cardioversion or defibrillation. The more experienced ACLS professional, however, will recognize that the pulsatile mass is actually an atrioventricular hemodialysis shunt, providing a clue that the patient has chronic renal failure and is on hemodialysis. Renal dialysis patients are prone to electrolyte problems, and the experienced ACLS provider knows that severe hyperkalemia causes life-threatening arrhythmias that require specific, immediate treatment. That treatment (see the *ECC Handbook* or the *ACLS Reference Textbook*) does not include cardioversion and defibrillation, which could lead to severe complications and even death.

This obvious need to expand and deepen the **D** step of the Secondary ABCD Survey was one of the important factors leading to the development of the new *ACLS for Experienced Providers Course* in 1999. The ACLS-EP Course is actually the second part of the more comprehensive ACLS package now recommended by the American Heart Association ECC Program. The ACLS Provider Course is the first part of the ACLS package.

The ACLS-EP Course greatly expands the knowledge base of ACLS providers, presenting more information about the need for diagnosis-specific treatment of cardiac arrest. Electrolyte abnormalities, prescribed or illicit drug overdoses, allergic and pseudoanaphylactoid reactions, and hypothermia are all examples of diagnoses that can cause cardiopulmonary collapse. These emergencies, however, also require specific treatment. The ACLS provider who falls back on the "guess-the-rhythm-guess-the-drug" approach that follows simple algorithm memorization does not serve the patient well.

The ACLS Approach to a Life-Threatening Problem: "Assess, Manage, Go No Further"

ACLS providers recognize that the term the *ACLS Approach* refers to the combined Primary and Secondary ABCD Surveys. The term *approach* is used simply to provide a label for what is in essence a memory aid to assist learning. Effective resuscitation requires 8 separate actions, performed in sequence. Though far from perfect, no other memory aid has been as effective as "ABCD/ABCD," especially when anchored to a sequencing tool as powerful as the alphabet.*

- The ACLS Approach provides help with *all* cardiac emergencies.
- The 8 steps of the ACLS Approach are always appropriate; they are in the correct order, according to priority.
- Each step requires 2 actions: *assess* and *manage*. With the paired actions of *assess* and *manage*, rescuers never lose sight of the need to both evaluate and treat the patient.
- The ACLS Approach teaches that whenever an assessment step reveals a life-threatening problem, *go no further* until that problem is solved. The obstructed airway is a common clinical problem that dramatically illustrates this point. Rescuers who fail to open a victim's airway or to provide proper ventilations *must not* proceed to chest compressions, defibrillation, or medications. ***They must open the airway.*** To do otherwise condemns the patient to certain death.

The ACLS Approach has been integrated into the 4 cardiac arrest algorithms: Comprehensive ECC, VF/Pulseless VT, PEA, and Asystole. Individuals have personal methods of learning, and the alphabetical list used in ACLS courses may not be helpful for every style of learning. The value of the Primary and Secondary ABCD Surveys, a memory aid taught and followed in all ACLS provider courses, comes from the fact that everyone, in every setting, from critical care units to airplane galleys, from emergency departments to gaming casinos, knows, understands, and follows the same protocol. All ACLS providers can enter that universal 1-act play—a resuscitation attempt—the world over and never miss a cue.

*In the mnemonic hierarchy the best mnemonics use signal letters to spell a word or phrase related to the topic or treatment. Thus, the mnemonic "vowels-tips" ("A-E-I-O-U-T-I-P-S"), which lists the major causes of altered mental status, is inferior to the mnemonic "C-R-A-S-H-T-E-S-T," which represents the components of the physical examination of a victim of multisystem trauma.

A Walk Through the Comprehensive ECC Algorithm

The Comprehensive ECC Algorithm (Figure 1) depicts a sequence of steps to be followed by ACLS providers. This sequence can be applied in a high percentage of cardiovascular emergencies.

Recognition of an Emergency: Initial Responses

Rescuer Safety

Before initiating the ACLS Approach with the Primary ABCD Survey, emergency responders must remember *rescuer safety*. A major principle of emergency medicine, especially in the out-of-hospital setting, is *never create a second victim: the rescuer*. Rescuer safety requires attention to location, traffic, weather, and dangerous objects or conditions in the immediate environment (eg, electric power lines, lightning). Rescuer safety requires compliance with precautions for infectious disease, including the use of pocket masks, gloves, and protective clothing. In many areas of emergency medicine this principle of rescuer safety is sacred: major injuries—even death—are unacceptable. Of course some areas of emergency search and rescue involve danger, but the professionals who play those roles are highly trained, well equipped, and superbly supported. The principle of rescuer safety simply means a rescuer should never place himself or herself in significant danger for the sake of a victim in extreme cardiopulmonary arrest.

Initial Responses

The initial responses also include

- Assess responsiveness.
- Call fast.
- Appropriately position the victim.
- Appropriately position yourself as the rescuer.

FIGURE 1. Comprehensive ECC Algorithm.

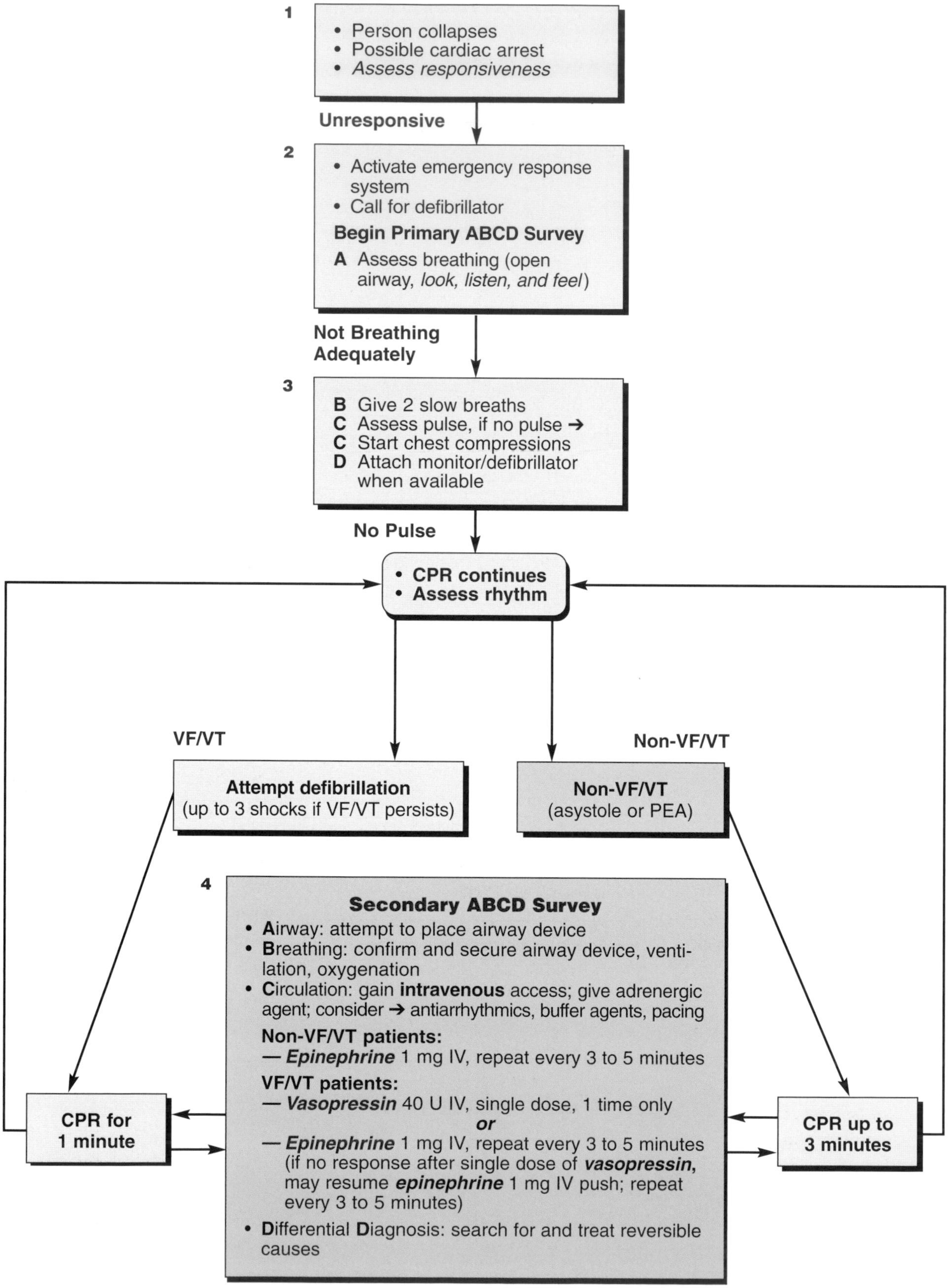

- Person collapses
- Possible cardiac arrest
- *Assess responsiveness*

Box 1.

Assess Responsiveness

"Man down—unconscious, unresponsive" is a familiar and riveting call in emergency care. Always assume that the victim is in cardiac or respiratory arrest or both until proved otherwise.

- Establish unresponsiveness with the traditional "shake and shout" step: tap or gently shake the victim and shout "Are you OK?"
- A shake can aggravate traumatic injuries in victims with possible cervical trauma. In such a case, "touch and talk" is a better approach.
- These techniques distinguish the person who is asleep or who has a depressed level of consciousness from one who is clinically comatose.

Once a rescuer/responder verifies unresponsiveness, immediately shout for help (see Box 2: activate emergency response system). In the hospital or Emergency Department this may simply involve stepping quickly to the doorway and shouting *"I need help right now in Room 3A!"*

- Tell the person who responds to the call to activate the in-hospital paging operator or other designated operator. Outside the hospital the person will usually dial 911 to activate the local emergency response system, although in some locations it is still necessary to dial a 7-digit number.
- If traveling outside the United States remember that 911 is not a universal code; it is used only in Canada and the Dominican Republic. Other countries, however, do have easily remembered 2- to 4-digit numbers that activate the emergency system. See the *ECC Guidelines 2000,* page 360, Table 3: "Emergency Response Numbers," for a list of the 911 equivalent for more than 60 countries.
- Remember: once you verify unresponsiveness, your next priority is to *call for help*. Advanced care, in the form of electrical defibrillation, advanced airway management, and IV medications, must be on the way to the patient as soon as possible.

Appropriate Positions for Victim and Rescuer

Position the Victim: Possible Cervical Spine Trauma?

The cardiac arrest victim should be flat on his or her back on a firm, stable surface. If you need to move the victim onto his or her back, first consider the possibility of a cervical spinal injury. Did the victim fall from a height? Or collapse with great force? Or dive head first? Or experience a motor vehicle crash?

Position Yourself as Rescuer

The most efficient position for a lone rescuer is to kneel beside the victim at the level of the victim's shoulders. This position requires the least amount of body movement when switching from giving expired air ventilations back to compressing the victim's chest. When the victim is in bed, place firm support under the chest before starting CPR. Hospitals should have a firm board available for this purpose.

The Primary ABCD Survey in the Comprehensive ECC Algorithm

- Activate emergency response system
- Call for defibrillator

Begin Primary ABCD Survey

A Assess breathing (open airway, *look, listen, and feel*)

Box 2.

Note that Boxes 2 and 3 present the first steps of the Primary ABCD Survey. This illustrates the close relationship between the Comprehensive ECC Algorithm and the Primary and Secondary Surveys.

A: Assess the Airway

Begin with an assessment of the airway, first opening the airway and checking for spontaneous breathing. The 2 basic techniques for opening the airway are the head tilt–chin lift maneuver and the jaw-thrust maneuver.

Head Tilt–Chin Lift

This maneuver pulls the base of the tongue away from the back of the throat, thus maintaining a more open airway.

- Open the mouth, inspect the upper airway for foreign objects, vomitus, or blood. If a foreign object is present, remove it with your fingers covered with a piece of cloth. If there is no possibility of a cervical spine injury, remove material obstructing the airway by turning the patient on his or her side.
- Place the edge of one hand on the victim's forehead. Begin to gently tilt the head back. At the same time place 2 fingers of the other hand under the chin and lift upward, tilting the head back.

Jaw-Thrust Maneuver

In addition to the head tilt–chin lift maneuver of basic CPR, all emergency personnel should learn the jaw-thrust technique. The jaw thrust maintains the neutral position of the cervical spine while resuscitative efforts continue. Use the jaw thrust when you encounter patients with the combination of possible cervical spine injuries and respiratory compromise or victims of trauma.

- To begin, stand or kneel at the top of the patient's head. Place your hands on the sides of the patient's face.
- Lean your elbows on the stretcher or the backboard for greatest comfort.
- Grasp the mandible of the jaw with your fingertips and lift forward.

Challenging Scenarios: The Lone Rescuer

The following scenarios illustrate some of the challenges and recommended actions for the lone rescuer.

Scenario 1: The Lone Rescuer

Questions and Challenges

What should you do if no one hears you call for help? Should you start CPR with chest compressions after opening the airway and giving 2 rescue breaths? Do you leave the victim unattended for as long as it takes to activate the emergency response system? For lay rescuers trained only in CPR, the AHA recommendation is simple—*phone first.* The health professional with ACLS training, however, can exercise some judgment.

- The dilemma is whether the victim has experienced respiratory compromise from an obstructed airway, a stroke or central nervous system event, a coma, a drug overdose, a postictal state after a seizure, or any number of other causes of respiratory arrest.
- When the rescuer suspects an obstructed airway, he or she should perform the **A**irway and **B**reathing steps first. For example, if you see a healthy adult rise from his chair in a restaurant, take a few steps, and then collapse, you should first evaluate the victim for an obstructed airway.

Scenario 2: The Lone Rescuer With an AED

Questions and Challenges

An adult, breathing normally, may suddenly grasp his or her chest in severe pain and collapse in front of witnesses. What do you do?

- Until proved otherwise, this person is experiencing a lethal arrhythmia such as VF. He or she needs immediate defibrillation.
- Every minute of delay in getting the defibrillator to this person decreases the chance of survival. A delay includes the time needed to perform the traditional 1 minute of CPR previously recommended for the lone rescuer.

Appendix 1 of this book provides detailed recommendations for the lone rescuer with access to an AED. This is the central scenario taught in the AHA Heartsaver AED Course. The authors carefully crafted the treatment protocols for the worst-case scenario, in which only 1 rescuer responds. In general the Heartsaver AED Course teaches that 1 rescuer should serve as the resuscitation director, doing both CPR and defibrillation if necessary. This approach greatly simplifies the lone-rescuer protocol. In summary the recommended sequence of actions is

Assess responsiveness—call 911—get the AED.

Return to the victim.

A: Open the airway.

B: Give 2 breaths.

C: Confirm pulselessness; confirm absence of signs of life.

D: Operate the AED; use the 4-step AED protocol:

1. POWER ON
2. ATTACH pads to patient
3. ANALYZE
4. SHOCK (if indicated)

Note that this sequence omits chest compressions until after the rescuer has used the AED to shock VF. The pulseless state is the indication for attaching an AED and assessing for VF.

The *ECC Guidelines 2000* considered interesting new evidence about a predefibrillation period of prescribed CPR to increase the probability that the postshock rhythm would be perfusing rather than asystole. If victims of out-of-hospital cardiac arrest have not received bystander CPR before the arrival of the defibrillator, a period of preshock CPR could enhance the value of the shocks. At the end of the year 2000 there was insufficient evidence to recommend any approach other than shock as soon as possible and perform CPR at all other times.

Scenario 3: Lone Rescuer, No Access to AED, Helper, or Telephone

Questions and Challenges

Another decision-making element is the time required to activate the emergency response system in either the hospital or community. A 1- to 2-minute delay in CPR to activate the EMS system is acceptable when a victim is in VF, but this assumes that the rescuer returns at once and begins the ABCs of CPR. Consider this scenario, however: your jogging partner collapses on an isolated running trail. It is a 15-minute run to the nearest telephone. A 30-minute round trip to a telephone leaves the victim an intolerably long time without the benefits of CPR. CPR only, however, will be of little help if your partner is in VF (in this scenario the probability of VF is 80% to 90%).

- Before the *1992 ECC Guidelines* the rescuer would continue CPR until exhausted. A fit rescuer can continue CPR well over 60 minutes before becoming exhausted; however, full neurological recovery of the victim after more than 60 minutes of CPR almost never occurs.
- *Recommendation:* the trained health professional in a remote situation should first ensure an open airway, provide several precordial thumps, and then start CPR. For a victim in a nonshockable rhythm, a small but real chance exists that CPR alone can restore spontaneous heartbeat.
- If no signs of life appear after 15 minutes, stop CPR. The victim has died; there is no possibility of meaningful survival.
- The following rare special circumstances are the exception to the 15-minute rule: cold-water drowning, hypothermia, certain drug overdoses. These conditions can be resolved with continued CPR.
- The key phrase here is "no signs of life"—no pulse, no gasping respirations, no maintenance of body temperature, with progressive mottling of the skin, increased dependent livido, and persistently fixed and dilated pupils.

Assess the Open Airway With "Look, Listen, and Feel"

Assessment of the patient's ability to move air is made quickly when the rescuer opens the airway with the head tilt–chin lift maneuver and then "looks, listens, and feels" for air movement.

- To look, listen, and feel, place your ear so that it almost touches the victim's mouth while you look toward the victim's chest.
- Listen and feel for breathing with your ear; simultaneously watch the victim's chest for respiratory movements.
- You may find that the victim has resumed breathing after you open the airway.
- Continued maintenance of an open airway may be the only rescue action required at this point.

Airway Management Problems in Cardiac Arrest

When you confirm breathlessness with this basic CPR step, you enter the complex arena of airway management problems in cardiac arrest. When you become the ACLS team leader, you are responsible for all aspects of airway management throughout the resuscitation attempt. Once breathlessness is confirmed, ask yourself the following questions:

- Is the air not moving because of an obstructed airway?
- How do I check for an obstructed airway?
- If the airway is obstructed, how do I clear it?
- If ventilations are needed, what ventilatory adjunct should I use?
- Are the rate and volume of ventilations correct?
- Are the ventilations effective?

B: Assess/Manage Breathing

Take Barrier Device Precautions

The professional emergency rescuer should always carry some form of ventilation barrier device. In the hospital pocket face masks (preferably with a 1-way valve) should be available at a ratio of 1 mask per bed in all patient care areas. Pocket face masks can be placed in a wall-mounted holder at the head of the bed and should also be available on all code carts.

- If an oropharyngeal airway is immediately available, insert it and begin ventilations with a pocket face mask.
- Provide 2 slow rescue ventilations, each lasting 2 to 4 seconds. Maintain the proper tilt of the patient's head to allow exhalation of breaths.
- Allow adequate time (1 to 2 seconds per ventilation) for the ventilation to be exhaled.
- Ventilations with this slow inspiratory flow rate are critical. The slow flow keeps the air pressure inside the esophagus low so you do not exceed the pressure that keeps the esophageal-gastric junction closed. This decreases the chance of gastric inflation, regurgitation, and aspiration.

Be Observant

At this point you must make several important observations:

- Did the air of the first breath go in?
- Did the chest rise?
- Could you hear the sound of air escaping during passive exhalation?

Look for a Possible Obstructed Airway

If air did not enter easily and the chest did not rise, then you must take steps to certify an obstructed airway.

- The best first step is to repeat the head tilt–chin lift maneuver quickly. Repeat 2 slow breaths. If you cannot detect air going in and coming out, the victim has an obstructed airway.
- Now follow the protocols for an obstructed airway in the unresponsive victim. Remember that the next step, closed-chest compressions, will be completely ineffective if the patient cannot be successfully ventilated.

C: Circulation Assessment: Check for a Pulse

Check for a pulse at the carotid artery on the side closer to you.

- Check the pulse for 5 to 10 seconds because the pulse may be present but difficult to detect if it is slow, irregular, weak, or rapid.
- If you feel no pulse, you have confirmed a full cardiac arrest: all criteria for cardiac arrest are present—the victim is unresponsive, is not breathing, and has no pulse.
- Faced with a victim who is unconscious, unresponsive, not breathing, and without a pulse, you must start chest compressions and provide ventilation at once.
- If you did not activate the code team, do so at once before starting CPR.

C: Treat "No Circulation" With Closed-Chest Compressions

You should know the techniques for CPR from your BLS training. (See Appendix 1 for a review of basic CPR and how to integrate CPR performance with use of an AED.)

- As an ACLS provider you must know CPR so you will be ready for the inevitable day when you arrive first at the scene of a cardiac arrest.
- You must also know CPR so that you can supervise and monitor the performance of others.

D: Hunt for VF/VT and Defibrillate if VF Is Identified

The initial *call for help* or *phone fast* after assessing unresponsiveness should result in someone arriving with a defibrillator, depending on the setting: in-hospital code response team, outpatient clinic on-site emergency code cart, out-of-hospital EMS unit, or out-of-hospital early access defibrillation program. As soon as a defibrillator arrives (either an AED or conventional monitor/defibrillator), power on the device, attach the monitor or defibrillation pads to the patient, and *hunt for VF/VT*. If you identify VF or VT, deliver defibrillatory shocks. Follow the treatment protocols for either the AED (Case 2) or the conventional monitor/defibrillator. The 2 treatment protocols are

Universal AED Protocol for VF

1. **POWER ON** the AED first.
2. **ATTACH** AED electrode pads to the victim's bare chest.
3. "Clear" victim and allow AED to **ANALYZE** rhythm.
4. "Clear" victim and **SHOCK** up to 3 times if advised.
5. After 3 shocks or after any *"no shock indicated"* messages:
   - **Check pulse.**
   - If no pulse, **perform CPR** for 1 minute.
   - **Repeat cycles** of 3 shocks and 1 minute of CPR until *"no shock indicated"* message is displayed.

Protocol for VF: Conventional Defibrillator/Monitor

1. **POWER ON** both monitor and defibrillator (could require 1 or 2 controls).
2. **ATTACH** 3-lead monitor cable, display rhythm through quick-look sternal-apex paddles.
3. "Clear" victim and **ASSESS** for a shockable rhythm by viewing monitor display.
4. **CHARGE** to 200 J, 300 J, or 360 J monophasic or clinically equivalent biphasic for shocks 1, 2, and 3.
5. "Clear" victim and **SHOCK** up to 3 times if a shockable rhythm is present, following the same *assess, charge, shock* sequence.
6. After 3 shocks or after any non-VF/VT rhythm on monitor:
   - **Check pulse.**
   - If no pulse, **perform CPR** and at the same time prepare to begin the **Secondary ABCD Survey.**

The Secondary ABCD Survey

The victim may remain in cardiac/respiratory arrest after CPR and delivery of shocks if the rhythm was shockable. Move quickly to the steps of the Secondary ABCD Survey. These steps are covered in the Comprehensive ECC algorithm, Box 4.

Secondary ABCD Survey: The Roles of Resuscitation Team Members

Resuscitation team members perform the Secondary ABCD Survey. These teams are composed of trained ACLS providers prepared and equipped to perform the steps of the ACLS Approach. Always define the roles of each team member *before* the team needs to respond.

- When the team arrives at a resuscitation emergency, all team members should begin their assigned tasks together, not in sequence.

Box 4

Secondary ABCD Survey

- **A**irway: attempt to place airway device
- **B**reathing: confirm and secure airway device, ventilation, oxygenation
- **C**irculation: gain **intravenous** access; give adrenergic agent; consider → anti-arrhythmics, buffer agents, pacing

Non-VF/VT patients:
— ***Epinephrine*** 1 mg IV, repeat every 3 to 5 minutes

VF/VT patients:
— ***Vasopressin*** 40 U IV, single dose, 1 time only

or

— ***Epinephrine*** 1 mg IV, repeat every 3 to 5 minutes
(if no response after single dose of ***vasopressin***, may resume ***epinephrine*** 1 mg IV push; repeat every 3 to 5 minutes)

- **D**ifferential **D**iagnosis: search for and treat reversible causes

Notes to Box 4

Unresponsive, not breathing; pulse present or absent → Secondary ABCD Survey

- ***Intubate*** as soon as possible
- ***Confirm*** tube placement; use 2 methods to confirm:
  — Use primary physical exam criteria ***plus***
  — Use secondary confirmation device (end-tidal CO_2; EDD)
- ***Secure*** **tracheal tube (TT):**
  — Prevent dislodgment with commercially made TT holders, which are recommended over tape-and-tie approaches
  — If patient is at risk for transport movement, cervical collar and backboard are recommended
- Confirm initial oxygenation and ventilation:
  — End-tidal CO_2 monitor
  — Oxygen saturation monitor
- Oxygen, IV, monitor, fluids → rhythm-appropriate medications
- Vital signs: Temp, BP, HR, respirations
- Consider differential diagnoses

- With proper planning the code leader should not have to direct people to perform tasks such as tracheal intubation and IV access. Each responder should know to perform the tasks without being directed.
- If there are not enough team members to perform all the Secondary Survey steps, the team leader must assume command and demand that someone start the next intervention.

At a simplistic level the Secondary ABCD Survey translates into *"tube 'em, start an IV, then try to remember which drug goes with which rhythm."* Concentration on the ABCD paradigm, however, helps emergency personnel remember to always look at the whole patient and at what is going on during the entire resuscitation attempt.

A: Airway: Insert Advanced Airway Device if Indicated

Reassess the Airway

After starting CPR and defibrillating if indicated, reassess whether the original technique for opening the airway is working. For example, if a self-inflating resuscitator bag with a face mask is used, the rate and volume of ventilations should be consistent with the AHA guidelines (see Case 1), and in the absence of regurgitation and possible aspiration tracheal intubation offers no significant advantages.

If noninvasive airway methods appear to provide sufficient ventilation, oxygenation, and protection, *definitive, invasive* airway control is not required immediately. Delays are acceptable if other critical interventions are under way, such as starting an IV line to administer fluids to a hypovolemic patient or treating severe hyperkalemia with calcium chloride.

Gain Definitive Control of the Airway: Place an Advanced Airway Device*

Here are several new recommendations from the *ECC Guidelines 2000.* The cuffed tracheal tube has been the gold standard for airway management for decades. The *ECC Guidelines 2000,* however, reviewed more than 10 years of data and recommend 2 additional advanced airway devices, *the laryngeal mask airway (LMA)* and the *Combitube.*

- Tracheal intubation provides definitive airway management because it is the only airway device that enters the trachea: there is no equivalent substitute. The LMA and the Combitube are much simpler to use because insertion does not require use of a laryngoscope or direct visualization of the vocal cords. When properly inserted their effectiveness approaches that of the tracheal tube. The LMA and Combitube have become the advanced airway devices of choice for less trained or skilled emergency providers.
- Verify that someone is preparing to insert an advanced airway device.
- If there are any delays, insert a nasal trumpet or nasopharyngeal airway if not already done.
- Apply cricoid pressure to prevent regurgitation and aspiration of gastric contents.
- Check that a suction device (powered electrically or by hand or foot) is available, operating properly, connected, and ready for use.
- Perform tracheal intubation or insert an LMA or Combitube (discussed in more detail in Chapter 3 and Case 1).

B: Breathing: Confirm Proper Tube Placement and Effective Ventilations

The keys to **B** of the Secondary ABCD Survey are to **reassess ventilations** immediately after inserting an advanced airway device and **verify placement of the tracheal tube** through the physical examination plus a secondary method of confirmation.

*Primary Confirmation**

The physical examination is used for primary confirmation of correct tube placement.

- The best verification technique is direct visual observation of the tracheal tube passing through the vocal cords.
- Confirm tube placement immediately, assessing the first breath delivered by the bag-valve unit. As the bag is squeezed, listen over the epigastrium and observe the chest wall for movement. If you hear stomach gurgling and see no chest wall expansion, you have intubated the esophagus. Stop ventilations. Remove the tracheal tube at once.
- Reattempt intubation after reoxygenation of the victim (15 to 30 seconds of bag ventilations using 100% oxygen).
- If the chest wall rises appropriately and stomach gurgling is not heard, listen to the lung fields in what is called *5-point auscultation*: left and right anterior, left and right midaxillary, and over the stomach. In the patient's medical records document where you heard breath sounds. If you have any doubt, stop ventilations through the tube.
- If there is continued doubt about correct tube placement, use the laryngoscope and look directly to see whether the tube is passing through the vocal cords.
- If the tube seems to be in place, reconfirm the tube mark at the front teeth (this was noted after inserting the tube 1 to 2 cm past the vocal cords).
- Secure the tube with a commercially made device designed for this purpose (preferred).
- Once the tube is secured, insert an oropharyngeal airway or add a bite block, or both, to prevent the patient from biting down and occluding the airway.

Secondary Confirmation

The *ECC Guidelines 2000* strongly recommend secondary confirmation in addition to the "5-points-to-listen approach." Secondary confirmation confirms correct tracheal tube placement by 1 or more methods not based on physical examination. These additional methods include

*See Chapter 3 and Case 1 for a more detailed discussion of this procedure.

qualitative end-tidal CO_2 detectors and esophageal detector devices (EDDs, either bulb or syringe type). These techniques are new to the *ECC Guidelines 2000.*

- EDDs connect to the end of the tracheal tube. If the bulb reexpands rapidly (less than 10 seconds on 2 separate attempts), the tracheal tube is probably correctly positioned in the trachea or bronchus. Slow reexpansion (more than 10 seconds) indicates probable esophageal intubation, and the tube should be removed at once.
- Qualitative end-tidal CO_2 methods display a color change to the CO_2 levels flowing through the tracheal tube.
- Some experts recommend use of these techniques in tandem: if the EDD indicates successful tube placement, stop. If the EDD indicates possible esophageal placement, use the CO_2 detector technique.
- If *ever* in doubt that you have achieved successful intubation, remove the tube at once and start over.
- Order an immediate portable chest x-ray to provide information on pulmonary conditions. The chest x-ray takes time and should never be used for confirmation; use other methods for that. Chest x-rays help determine left or right main bronchus intubation and whether the end of the tube is too low or too high.

C: Circulation

- **Assess the cardiac rhythm and rate.** Identify the rhythm and rate. There are several ways to display the rhythm for assessment:
  - Attach 3-lead monitor leads in a modified lead II pattern.
  - Attach adhesive, dual-function defibrillation-monitor pads.
  - Apply the handheld paddles of conventional monitor/defibrillators.
- **In patients with a palpable pulse, measure blood pressure.**
- **Obtain IV access.**
  - The vein of first choice is the antecubital vein of either arm. Unless there are other problems or contraindications, always try for an antecubital vein.
  - Normal saline rather than D_5W is the recommended IV fluid. Normal saline is better than dextrose for expanding the intravascular volume. The concern that normal saline might cause pulmonary edema has not proved to be a significant problem.
  - Control the volume administered by using smaller bags and volumetric units.
- **Treat with rhythm-appropriate medications.**

All cardiac arrest algorithms are universal and can be displayed in one international ACLS algorithm (see the *ECC Handbook*).

The differences in the AHA algorithms begin only at this step: medications used to treat the arrhythmia.

- Be prepared to administer a 20- to 30-mL bolus of IV fluid and elevate the arm after each IV medication. This will enhance delivery of medications to the central circulation.
- Successful ACLS providers should know the actions, indications, doses, and precautions associated with the medications used in the algorithms.
- Do not base your selection of medication solely on the rhythm. Consider the entire ABCD picture by using the Primary and Secondary ABCD Surveys together with the algorithms.

D: Determine a Differential Diagnosis

- A differential diagnosis is simply a list of possible problems, conditions, or diagnoses that may cause a patient's condition. Your goal is to see whether reversible, treatable causes appear on your list of possible diagnoses. In particular the ACLS provider looks for causes that might have a specific therapy, such as hyperkalemia-induced cardiac arrest.
- The only possibility of resuscitation often lies in searching for, finding, and treating reversible causes. Think "what

Tracheal Administration of Medications

Remember that you can administer atropine, lidocaine, or epinephrine (A-L-E) through the tracheal tube. The recommended technique for tracheal drug administration is as follows:

- Prepare 2 to 2.5 times the normal IV dose of medications.
- Prepare a syringe with 10 mL of normal saline.
- Thread a long (35 cm) through-the-needle intracatheter rapidly down the inside of the tracheal tube.
- Stop chest compressions.
- Inject the medication through the catheter.
- Flush the catheter with 10 mL of normal saline.
- Immediately attach the ventilation bag to the tracheal tube and ventilate forcefully 3 to 4 times.
- If a suitable catheter is unavailable, use a heparin lock with a 20-gauge needle inserted through the wall of the tracheal tube to aerosolize medications and deliver with ventilations.

Note: A number of commercial attachments and connectors are available to facilitate tracheal administration of medications.

caused or precipitated this arrest?" and "why has the patient not responded to treatment?"

- The **D** of the Secondary Survey reminds you to think about the differential diagnosis. Although the **D** in the Secondary Survey could represent "drugs," cardiac medications (drugs) are represented by **C** for circulation. As an aid to memory and successful resuscitation the Secondary Survey **D** serves better as a mental link to differential diagnosis.
- Review the possible causes on your differential diagnosis list. What caused the arrest? What could cause this rhythm? Each rhythm of arrest—VF/VT, asystole, PEA, severely symptomatic bradycardia, or tachycardia—has many possible causes. Review whether the team should take other actions in addition to the algorithm recommendations.
- The review of causes is especially helpful in refractory cardiac arrest, unstable postresuscitation conditions, or non-VF rhythms or for any cardiac patient who did not respond to initial actions.
- Management of these patients requires the resuscitation team to think of specific causes and possible corrective actions. For example, postshock conversion rhythms in a patient with VF/VT may reveal an underlying bradycardia (give atropine) or a transient tachycardia (give a rapid-acting β-blocker).

Summary

This keystone chapter presents the ACLS Approach, which can be used in all cardiopulmonary emergencies. The ACLS Approach divides assessment and management into 8 steps that are easily remembered as the *Primary ABCD Survey* and the *Secondary ABCD Survey.* Mentally link *assess and manage* to each of the 8 letters. With each step you must perform an assessment, and if you observe something wrong, manage it appropriately.

In the rest of this manual you will see the ACLS Approach applied to each of the core cases. Although the fit is not always exact, the approach provides a useful structure on which to build current and future ACLS knowledge.

The Advanced ACLS Skills

Overview

The 2 *basic* ACLS skills are the ability to perform CPR and operate an AED. This chapter presents the 7 advanced ACLS skills:

1. Care of the airway
2. Recognition of rhythm
3. Electrical therapy I: defibrillation
4. Electrical therapy II: cardioversion
5. Electrical therapy III: transcutaneous pacing
6. IV access to circulation
7. Selection of appropriate resuscitation medications

These advanced skills can be organized in several ways. Use the Primary and Secondary ABCD Surveys as memory aids. Note that each advanced skill fits within the secondary, or advanced, ABCD Survey:

- **Secondary A:** establish an *airway* with *1. tracheal intubation*
- **Secondary B**: provide ventilation *(breathing)* with a properly placed tracheal tube and airway adjuncts
- **Secondary C:** restore the *circulation* with 2. *defibrillation, 3. cardioversion, 4. transcutaneous pacing;* then provide *5. recognition of the rhythm;* then *6. initiation of IV access*; and finally, based on the identified rhythm, give rhythm-appropriate *7. IV medications*

Learning Objectives

At the end of this section the ACLS provider should be able to describe how to

1. ***Provide supplemental oxygen with the following adjuncts:***
   - Nasal cannula
   - Face mask
   - Face mask with oxygen reservoir
   - Venturi mask
2. ***Open the airway with the following techniques and adjuncts:***
   - Head tilt–chin lift maneuver
   - Foreign-body airway obstruction techniques: Heimlich maneuver
   - Oropharyngeal or nasopharyngeal technique
   - Direct laryngoscopy and suction devices
3. ***Maintain the open airway with the following adjuncts:***
   - Oropharyngeal airway
   - Nasopharyngeal airway
   - Laryngeal mask airway
   - Esophageal-tracheal combitube
   - Tracheal intubation
4. ***Ventilate the patient using the mouth-to-mouth/mouth-to-nose or bag-mask technique***
   - Never use the mouth-to-mouth or mouth-to-nose techniques without barrier protection. In general use *either*
     — Mouth-to-face shield or
     — Mouth-to-pocket face mask
     or
     — Bag-mask device
5. ***Provide advanced ventilation by adding bag-mask ventilation to the following advanced airway devices:***
   - Tracheal intubation
   - Laryngeal mask airway (LMA)
   - Esophageal-tracheal combitube
6. ***Provide definitive airway control with tracheal intubation using an inflatable cuffed tracheal tube***
7. ***Provide primary and secondary tracheal tube confirmation plus protection from dislodgment with the following skills:***
   - Primary confirmation of correct tube placement by physical examination
   - Secondary confirmation of correct tube placement by (a) end-tidal CO_2 sensors and (b) devices that can detect esophageal intubation
   - Prevention of inadvertent dislodgment of the airway device by using at least 1 commercial tube holder
   - Prevention of inadvertent dislodgment of the advanced airway device by using at least one local-practice tape/tie/benzoin technique

- **Secondary D:** perform a *differential diagnosis* to identify reversible causes—causes that have a specific therapy

ACLS Skill 1: Take Care of the Airway

1. Provide supplemental oxygen

Oxygen is always appropriate for patients with acute cardiac disease or pulmonary distress. It should be provided as follows:

- For patients without respiratory distress: give 2 L of oxygen per minute by nasal cannula.
- For patients with mild respiratory distress: give 5 to 6 L of oxygen per minute.
- For patients with severe respiratory distress, acute congestive heart failure, or cardiac arrest: use a system that provides a high inspired oxygen concentration (preferably 100%).
- For patients with chronic obstructive pulmonary disease (COPD), who may be dependent on hypoxia-driven ventilation: provide "low-dose" supplemental oxygen via a 24% Venturi mask. Administer oxygen with caution and monitor closely.
- Titrate oxygen up or down according to Pa_{O_2} or oxygen saturation value.
- In the most serious cases: move quickly to advanced airway devices, intubation, and 100% oxygen.

Emergency Oxygen Supplies

To allow a broad range of responders to supply supplemental oxygen, the US Food and Drug Administration (FDA) and the Occupational Safety and Health Administration (OSHA) allow the use of *emergency oxygen devices* in the workplace without prescription. These devices must have an oxygen flow rate of 6 L/min or more for at least 15 minutes. Although OSHA requires that personnel be trained before using emergency oxygen devices, adjustment of the oxygen flow rate is prohibited. A *prescription-only oxygen supply device* can be adjusted to a flow rate of less than 6 L/min for less than 15 minutes.

Recommended oxygen flow rates for ACLS providers range from 4 L/min for patients with suspected acute coronary syndromes (ACS) to 8 to 12 L/min for patients in cardiac arrest who are being ventilated with noninvasive face masks or bag-mask devices. This apparent conflict between specific oxygen flow rates for ACLS providers and a fixed flow rate of 6 L/min for BLS and first aid responders poses no problems.

When providing first aid to patients with suspected ACS, emergency responders should not be concerned about the inability of an emergency oxygen device to supply 4 L/min of supplemental oxygen. In the workplace the difference of 2 L/min is clinically insignificant.

Similarly responders who treat cardiac arrest patients by providing oxygen at the 6 L/min flow rate instead of the recommended 8 to 12 L/min are still providing safe and beneficial therapy. BLS and first aid responders are not ACLS-level providers and need not meet the range of flow rates required of ACLS personnel. The American Heart Association (AHA) attempts to base all its recommendations on the best available science but never at the exclusion of practicality and common sense. The widespread availability of emergency oxygen devices with fixed flow rates of 6 L/min is a valuable resource and should be used without concern for possible conflicts with AHA recommendations.

Devices Used to Administer Supplemental Oxygen

Whenever you provide professional care to a patient receiving supplemental oxygen, perform a rapid visual review of the oxygen delivery system in use:

- ***Oxygen supply (cylinder or piped wall oxygen)***
  - — Valve handles to open the cylinder, pressure gauge, and flow meter
  - — Tubing connecting the oxygen supply to the patient's oxygen administration device
- **Nasal cannula:** starting device; provides up to 44% oxygen
  - — A nasal cannula is a low-flow system in which the tidal volume mixes with ambient gas (room air). Inspired oxygen concentration depends on the flow rate through the cannula and the patient's tidal volume.
  - — Increasing the oxygen flow by 1 L/min (starting with 1 L/min) will increase the inspired oxygen concentration by approximately 4%:
    - ◆ 1 L/min: 21% to 24%
    - ◆ 2 L/min: 25% to 28%
    - ◆ 3 L/min: 29% to 32%
    - ◆ 4 L/min: 33% to 36%
    - ◆ 5 L/min: 37% to 40%
    - ◆ 6 L/min: 41% to 44%
- **Face mask:** Up to 60% oxygen can be supplied through the oxygen port at 6 to 10 L/min
- **Face mask with oxygen reservoir**: provides up to 90% to 100% oxygen
  - — In this system a constant flow of oxygen enters an attached reservoir. Each liter-per-minute increase in flow over 6 L/min will increase the inspired oxygen concentration by approximately 10%:
    - ◆ 6 L/min: 60% oxygen
    - ◆ 7 L/min: 70% oxygen
    - ◆ 8 L/min: 80% oxygen
    - ◆ 9 L/min: 90% oxygen
    - ◆ 10 to 15 L/min: 95% to 100% oxygen

— Use a face mask with a reservoir for
  - ◆ Patients who are seriously ill, responsive, and spontaneously breathing and require high oxygen concentrations
  - ◆ Patients who may avoid tracheal intubation if acute interventions produce a rapid clinical effect (patients with acute pulmonary edema, COPD, severe asthma)
  - ◆ Patients who have relative indications for tracheal intubation but maintain an intact gag reflex
  - ◆ Patients who have relative indications for intubation but have clenched teeth or other physical barriers to immediate intubation (eg, head injury, carbon monoxide poisoning, or near-drowning)

— These patients may have diminished levels of consciousness and may be at risk for nausea and vomiting. A tight-fitting mask always requires close monitoring. Suctioning devices should be immediately available.

- **Venturi mask: use for patients who retain carbon dioxide (CO_2)**

  Venturi masks can accurately control the proportions of inspired oxygen. Use Venturi masks in patients with chronic hypercarbia (high CO_2) and moderate to severe hypoxemia.

  High oxygen concentrations in these patients may produce respiratory depression because the increase in Pao_2 blocks the stimulant effect of hypoxemia on the respiratory centers.

  Never withhold oxygen, however, from patients who have respiratory distress simply because you suspect hypoxic ventilatory drive. Oxygen concentrations can be adjusted to 24%, 28%, 35%, and 40%. Use 24% initially and observe for respiratory depression. Use a pulse oximeter to quickly titrate to the preferred level of Pao_2; check arterial blood gas.

2. Open the airway: recognize airway obstruction

- **Head and jaw position.** The most common cause of upper airway obstruction in the unresponsive victim is loss of tone in the throat muscles. This allows the tongue to fall back and occlude the airway at the level of the pharynx and allows the epiglottis to occlude the airway at the level of the larynx (Figure 1).
- In a patient who is able to breathe, partial upper airway obstruction can be distinguished from noisy airflow during inspiration (stridor or "crowing"), cyanosis (indicates prolonged partial airway obstruction), and retractions of the suprasternal, supraclavicular, and intracostal spaces. It may be difficult to recognize airway obstruction in patients who are not attempting to breathe.
- **Basic opening techniques.** The basic opening technique is head tilt with anterior displacement of the mandible (chin lift and if necessary jaw thrust) (Figure 2).

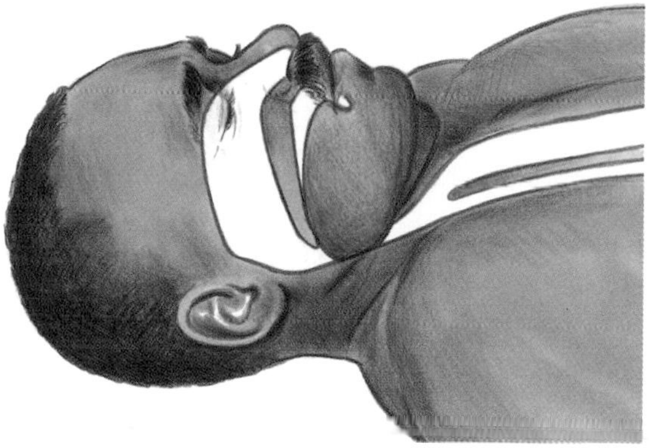

FIGURE 1. Obstruction by the tongue and epiglottis.

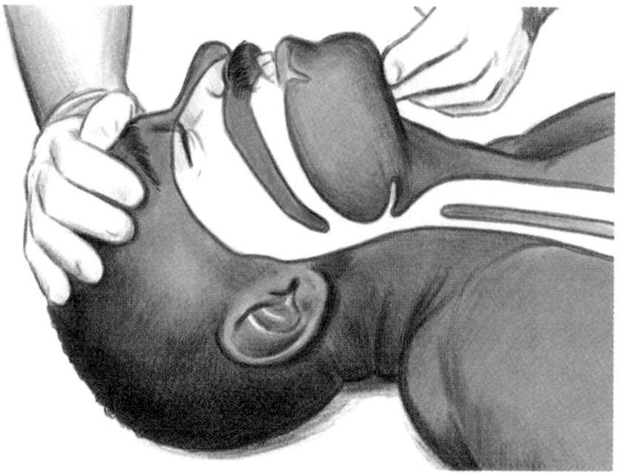

FIGURE 2. Head tilt–chin lift.

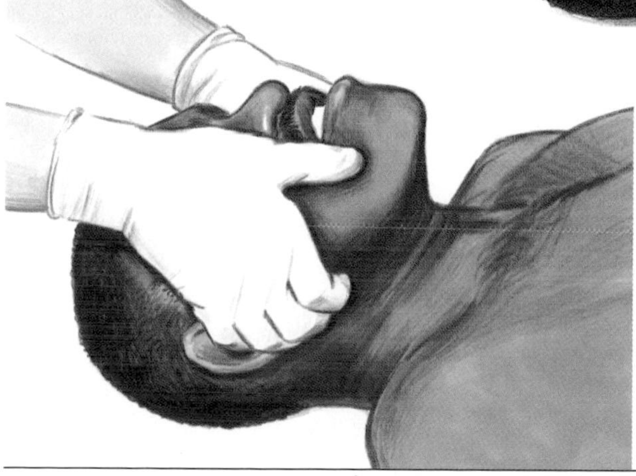

FIGURE 3. Jaw thrust without head tilt.

- In the trauma victim with suspected neck injury, use the chin lift or jaw thrust *without head tilt* (Figure 3). If the airway remains obstructed, slowly add head tilt until the airway opens. Proper airway positioning may be all that is required for patients who can breathe spontaneously. In patients with an altered level of consciousness or paralysis, insert an oropharyngeal or nasopharyngeal airway to maintain airway patency.

3. Maintain the open airway using airway adjuncts

- Assume as a first step that the airway obstruction is produced by either the tongue or relaxed throat muscles. Use the head tilt–chin lift maneuver. If this seems insufficient, insert an oropharyngeal or nasopharyngeal airway.
- Manage foreign-body airway obstruction with the BLS technique of subdiaphragmatic abdominal thrusts (the Heimlich maneuver) and the advanced technique of direct laryngoscopy to see. Use forceps or suction tools to grasp and remove the foreign body.

Oropharyngeal Airways

- Oropharyngeal airways (Figure 4) are S-shaped devices that hold the tongue away from the posterior wall of the pharynx. They are most helpful in the spontaneously breathing patient who is unconscious or semiconscious *with no cough or gag reflex* and at risk of occluding the airway via tongue and pharyngeal relaxation.
- Oropharyngeal airways keep the airway open during bag-mask ventilation when rescuers tend to unknowingly push down on the chin, blocking the airway. These devices help suction the mouth and throat and prevent the patient from biting and occluding a tracheal tube.

Technique

- Clear the mouth and pharynx of secretions, blood, or vomitus using a rigid pharyngeal catheter with suction tip.
- Place the airway so that it is turned *backward* as it enters the mouth.
- As the airway passes through the oral cavity and approaches the posterior wall of the pharynx, rotate the airway 180 degrees into the proper position.
- Another method is to move the tongue out of the way with a tongue blade depressor before inserting the airway.
- The airway is properly sized and placed when there are clear breath

FIGURE 4. Oropharyngeal airways. **A,** Four airways; **B,** One airway inserted.

A

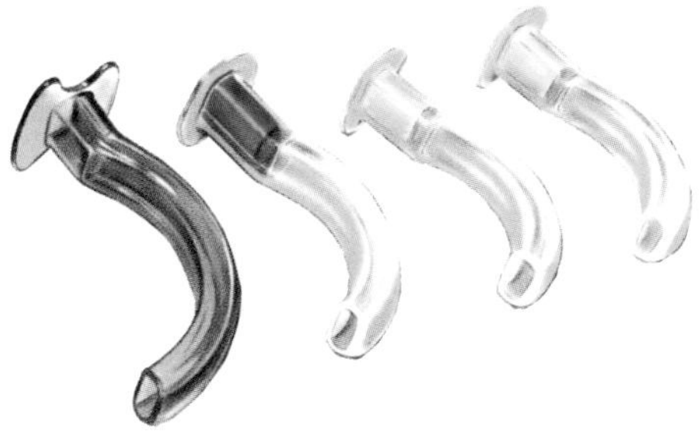

B

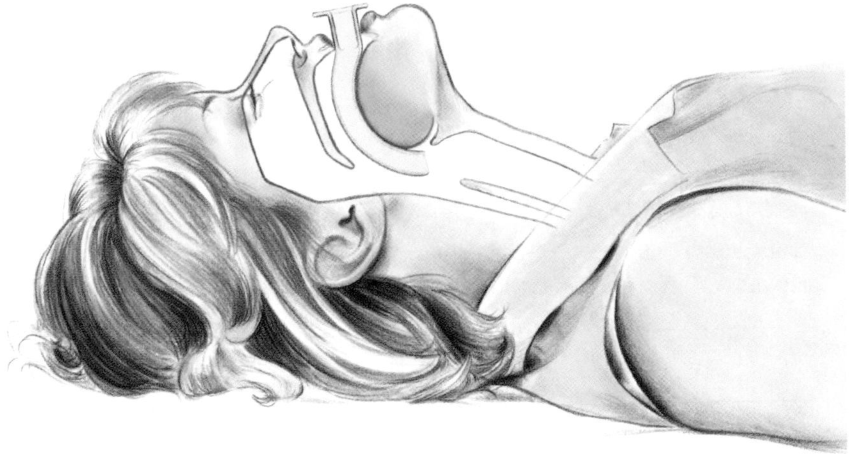

FIGURE 5. Nasopharyngeal airways. **A,** Three airways, **B,** One airway inserted.

A

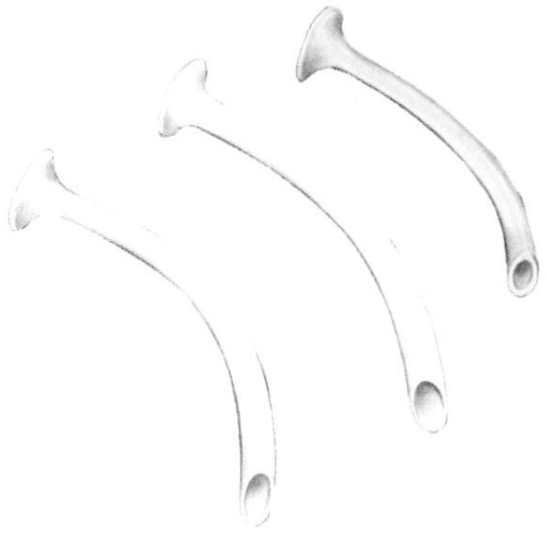

B

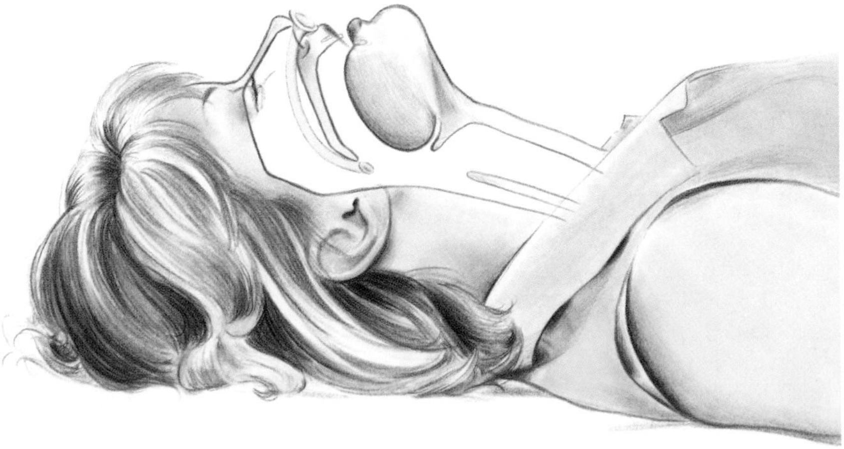

sounds on auscultation of the lungs during ventilation.

- Once the airway is in place, continue to maintain proper head position.

Hazards

- A long oropharyngeal airway may press the epiglottis against the entrance of the larynx, producing complete airway obstruction.
- If the airway is not inserted properly, it may push the tongue posteriorly, aggravating upper airway obstruction.
- To prevent trauma, the operator should make sure that the lips and tongue are not between the teeth and airway.
- The airway should be used only in the unconscious or semiconscious patient *with no cough or gag reflex* because it may stimulate vomiting and laryngospasm in the patient with a cough or gag reflex.

Nasopharyngeal Airways

- Nasopharyngeal airways (Figure 5) are uncuffed tubes made of soft rubber or plastic.
- They are used most frequently for the intoxicated or semiconscious patient who cannot tolerate an oropharyngeal airway.
- A nasopharyngeal airway is indicated when insertion of an oropharyngeal airway is technically difficult or impossible (because of strong gag reflex, trismus, massive trauma around the mouth, or wiring of the upper and lower jaws).

Technique

- The proper-sized airway is lubricated with a water-soluble lubricant or anesthetic jelly and gently inserted close to the midline along the floor of the nostril.
- Continue inserting the airway into the posterior pharynx, behind the tongue.
- If resistance is encountered, slight rotation of the tube may facilitate insertion at the angle of the nasal passage and the nasopharynx.

Hazards

- A long nasopharyngeal airway may enter the esophagus. With active ventilation, such as bag mask, the nasopharyngeal airway will cause gastric inflation and possible hypoventilation.
- Although a nasopharyngeal airway is better tolerated by semiconscious patients, its use may also precipitate laryngospasm and vomiting.
- Insertion of the airway may injure the nasal mucosa and cause bleeding, with possible aspiration of clots into the trachea. Suction may be necessary to remove blood or secretions.
- Maintain head tilt with anterior displacement of the mandible by chin lift and if necessary by jaw thrust when using this airway.

Precautions

- Always check spontaneous respirations immediately after insertion of an oropharyngeal or nasopharyngeal airway.
- If respirations are absent or inadequate, start artificial positive-pressure ventilation at once with an appropriate device.
- If adjuncts are unavailable, use mouth-to-mouth ventilation.

4. Ventilate the patient

Mouth-to-Mouth and Mouth-to-Nose Ventilation

Mouth-to-mouth ventilation is the default method of ventilation (see Appendix 1). If circumstances require a healthcare provider to provide mouth-to-mouth rescue breathing, it is because a major mistake has been made. Expired-air ventilation can provide adequate volumes of air to the victim. The only limitation is the rescuer's vital capacity and the reduced concentration of oxygen in exhaled air (approximately 17%). The average person's vital capacity, however, is several liters larger than the tidal volume of 10 to 15 L/min needed to provide adequate lung inflation.

Professional rescuers should always have a barrier device available to perform mouth-to-mouth breathing (Figure 6).

Exhaled air breathing without a barrier device is strongly discouraged. Small, portable barrier devices are widely available and should be carried by all healthcare providers.

Mouth-to-Pocket Face Mask

Well-fitting face masks are simple yet effective adjuncts for use in artificial ventilation by all trained rescuers. The new Heartsaver AED Course teaches lay rescuers to routinely use a pocket face mask. Masks must be transparent for detection of regurgitation, capable of a tight fit on the face, furnished with an oxygen inlet, and available in an average size for adults and additional sizes for infants and children.

Advantages

- Provides effective ventilation and oxygenation
- Eliminates direct contact with the victim's mouth and nose
- Makes administration of supplemental oxygen possible (in units with an oxygen port)
- Eliminates exposure to victim's exhaled gases (in units with a 1-way valve)
- Easy to teach and easy to learn
- Superior to bag-mask technique for delivering adequate tidal volume (on manikins)

Ventilation Techniques

A lone rescuer can provide effective ventilations with a pocket face mask. If a second rescuer is available, the first rescuer changes positions. If a lone rescuer has to provide both ventilations and chest compressions, he or she takes a position lateral to the victim (Figure 7). If a second rescuer is available to provide chest compressions, then the first rescuer takes a position at the top of the victim's head (Figure 8).

The *ECC Guidelines 2000* recommend the 2-rescuer technique, with 1 rescuer doing chest compressions and 1 rescuer at the head of the bed/stretcher (or on his or her knees if the victim is on the floor or ground). Here are the steps to take in a 2-rescuer scenario with one rescuer doing chest compressions at a rate of at least 100 compressions per minute and the airway/ventilation rescuer providing 2 ventilations after every 15 compressions. The rescuer providing ventilations should be at the head of the stretcher, facing the victim's feet.

1. If time permits, attach oxygen tubing to the oxygen inlet port on the mask (see Figure 9).
2. Use the pocket face mask with attached oxygen to enrich the oxygen mixture delivered to a spontaneously breathing patient.
   - Use an oxygen flow rate of 10 L/min to yield an inspired oxygen concentration of about 50%.
   - Use an oxygen flow rate of 15 L/min to provide an inspired oxygen concentration of about 80%.
3. Insert an oropharyngeal airway in all patients who can tolerate insertion without gagging.
4. Apply head tilt and place the mask on the victim's face.
5. With the thumb side of the palms of both hands, apply pressure to the sides of the mask.
6. Apply upward pressure to the mandible just in front of the ear lobes, using the thumb and thenar eminence on top of the mask (Figure 8) or circling the thumb and first finger around the top of the mask (Figure 9). Continue to maintain head tilt.
7. Keep the mouth open if no oropharyngeal airway is in place.
8. Blow in through the opening of the mask, observing the rise and fall of the chest.
9. Deliver the breaths slowly and steadily. *Note:* Without supplemental oxygen, positive-pressure ventilation must be delivered slowly and gently over at least 2 seconds. If oxygen is available, deliver a smaller tidal volume (enough to produce a visible chest rise) over a slightly shorter period of 1 to 2 seconds.
10. If the victim is in pulseless cardiac arrest with an unprotected airway (the situation with a pocket face mask), use the ratio of 15 compressions to 2 ventilations. Deliver long, slow breaths, taking at least 2 seconds to deliver each breath.
11. If the airway is protected (with insertion of a cuffed tracheal tube), continue to deliver chest compressions at a rate of approximately 100 compressions per minute *but* without a compression pause for ventilations *(asynchronous ventilations).* Deliver 1 ventilation over 2 seconds asynchronously every 5 seconds for a minute rate of 12 ventilations.
12. When available, have a third rescuer apply cricoid pressure (Figure 10). Cricoid pressure prevents gastric inflation during positive-pressure ventilation of an unprotected airway and reduces the possibility of regurgitation and aspiration.

Figure 6. Face shield.

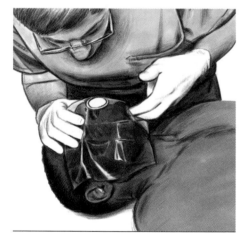

Figure 7. Pocket face mask; lateral technique.

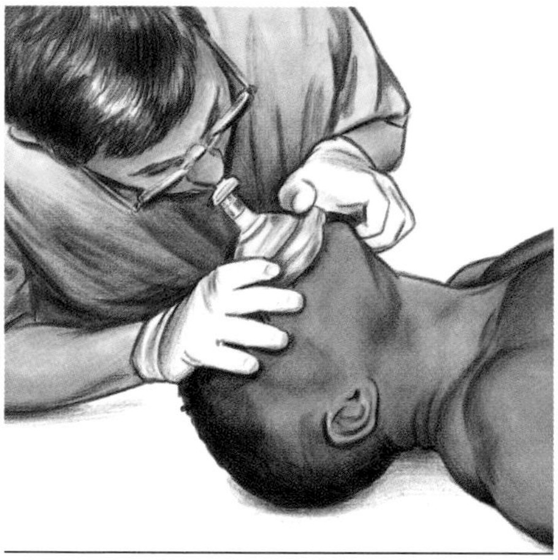

Figure 8. Pocket face mask; cephalic technique.

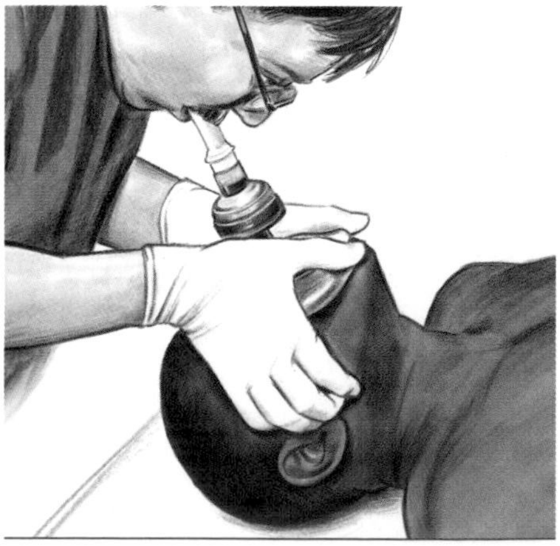

Figure 9. Pocket face mask; cephalic technique. Note the oxygen tubing attached to the oxygen port on the pocket face mask.

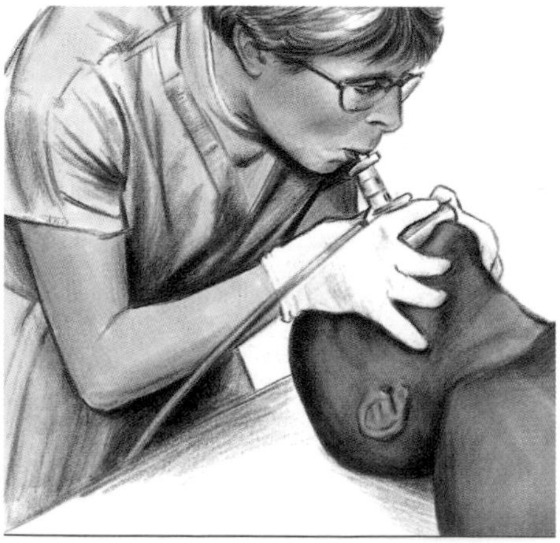

FIGURE 10. Cricoid pressure (Sellick maneuver).

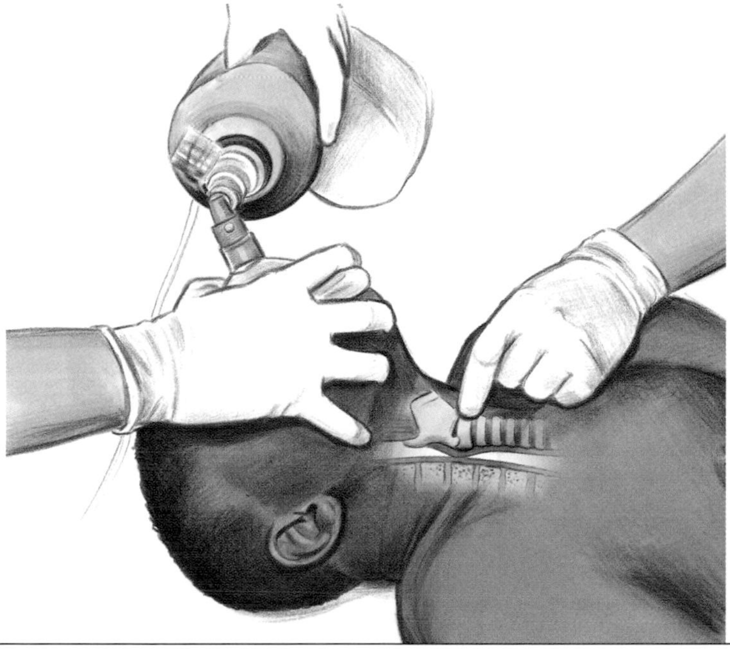

Self-Inflating Ventilation Bags: Attached to Valves, Masks, and Other Airway Adjuncts

The self-inflating ventilation bag has been a mainstay of emergency ventilation for decades. The universal connections—15 mm and 22 mm—at either end of all interconnecting airway devices allow the rescuer to connect any ventilation bag to numerous invasive and noninvasive airway adjuncts. After full manual compression the bag self-inflates in about 1 second. Different valves also can be attached to the ventilation bag through the universal 15-mm/22-mm connections. These valves provide a rich variety of features, including

- One-way valves to protect the rescuer from exhaled air
- Oxygen ports for supplemental oxygen
- Medication ports for tracheal administration of aerosolized and other medications
- Suction ports to help clear the airway
- Ports for quantitative sampling of end-tidal CO_2

The clinician can attach a variety of other adjuncts to the patient end of the valve, including a pocket face mask, oropharyngeal airway, tracheal tube, LMA, and combitube (see figure below).

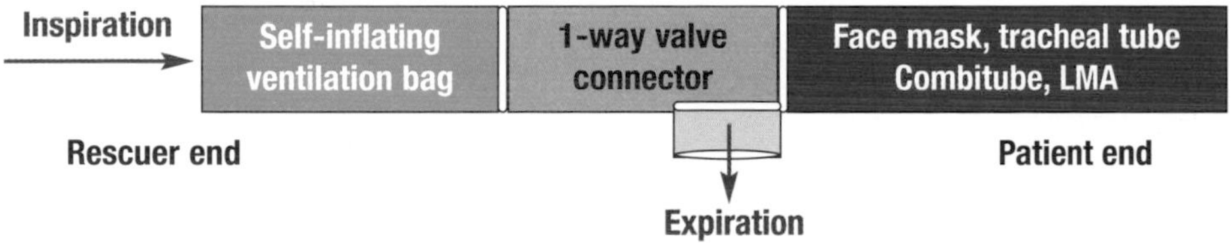

Bag-Valve Masks: Adequate Seal and Volume

An oropharyngeal airway should be inserted as soon as possible to help maintain the airway. Following are some calculations:

- The recommended tidal volume for most adults is 10 to 15 mL/kg.
- A man weighing 178 lb (80 kg) would need 800 to 1200 mL delivered with each squeeze of the bag.
- Most commercially available adult-sized bag-mask units have a 1600- to 2000-mL bag. Using a 1-handed squeeze, most rescuers can empty no more than 50% of the bag (800 mL or less).
- In addition, many rescuers cannot provide a leakproof seal between the mask and face using 1 hand. The hand holding the mask must perform 2 tasks simultaneously: form a mask-to-face seal, which requires pushing down firmly on the mask, and tilt the head back, which requires a lifting action (Figure 11).
- When rescuers attempt the 1-hand E-C technique while using a bag-mask device, the ventilation volume will not compare favorably with that provided in mouth-to-mouth or mouth-to-mask ventilation.
- For this reason many experts and clinicians recommend that 2 well-trained, experienced rescuers work together during bag-mask ventilation. One rescuer should hold the mask with 2 hands in a leakproof seal against the mouth while the other squeezes the bag slowly and gently over 2 seconds (Figure 12).

FIGURE 11. **A,** Detailed view of a bag-valve mask. **B,** Rescuer attempting 1-hand "E-C technique."

A

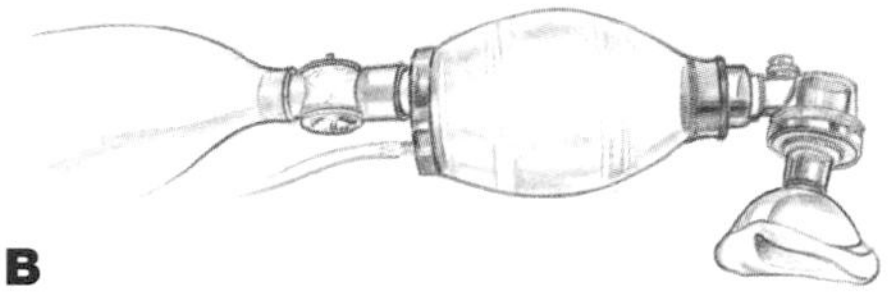

B

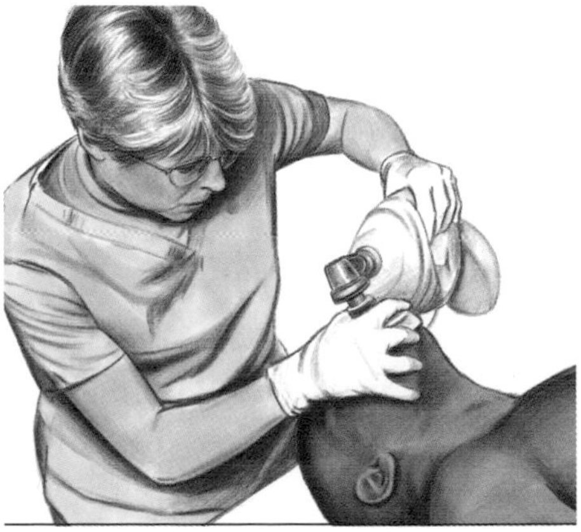

FIGURE 12. 2-rescuer use of bag-valve mask.

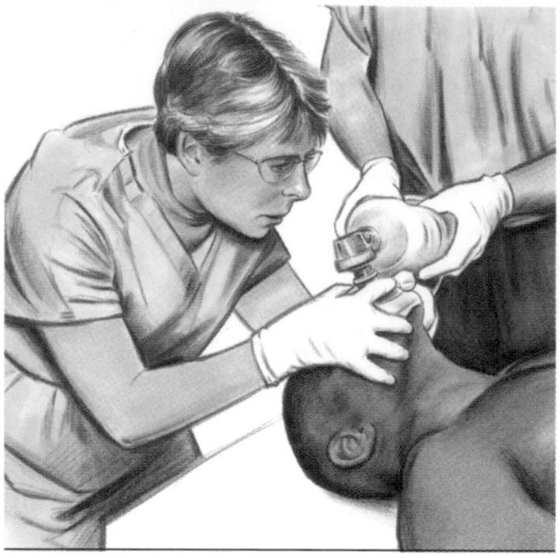

- These seal and volume problems do not occur when the bag-mask device is attached to the end of a tracheal tube, Combitube, or LMA and used to ventilate a patient with a tracheal tube in place.
- During cardiac arrest with a *protected airway,* ventilations are delivered over 1 to 2 seconds inspiratory time. After 5 seconds another ventilation is delivered. Note that these ventilations occur without reference to chest compressions, which are being performed asynchronously at a rate of at least 100 per minute.

Delivery of Long, Slow Ventilations

In the *ECC Guidelines 2000* considerable attention was given to the need to prevent gastric inflation with ventilation, thereby reducing the risk of aspiration. The phrase *long, slow ventilations* helps convey this important point: deliver prolonged breaths, taking at least 2 seconds to completely squeeze the ventilation bag while using 100% oxygen.

In a recent study of pediatric intubation by Los Angeles County paramedics, investigators instituted rigorous airway management protocols. They developed the following verbal phrase to encourage long, slow, 2-second inhalations: ***squeeze-squeeze-release.*** This phrase has become a popular memory aid and has been effective in achieving uniform slow ventilations. The figure below displays the timing for long, slow ventilations.

Timing for Long, Slow Ventilations

← "Squeeze!" →	← "Squeeze!" →	← "Release!" →
"one-one-thousand"	"two-one-thousand"	"three one-thousand"
← A single inhalation lasting 2 seconds →		1 sec → bag self-inflation
← a 3-second single ventilation cycle →		

Recommended Features of Bag Masks

The effectiveness of a bag mask depends on placement of an oropharyngeal airway, position of the patient's head, delivery rate of breaths, and use of cricoid pressure. Bag-mask units should have the following clinical features:

- A self-refilling bag that is easily cleaned and sterilized
- Connections for delivery of high concentrations of oxygen
- Capability to perform satisfactorily under all common environmental conditions and extremes of temperature
- Availability in both adult and pediatric sizes
- True nonrebreathing valve

5. Provide advanced ventilation

Tracheal Intubation

Overview

Tracheal intubation provides definitive airway management and should be performed by properly trained personnel as soon as possible during any resuscitative effort. Tracheal intubation

- Keeps the airway patent
- Ensures delivery of a high concentration of oxygen
- Ensures delivery of a selected tidal volume (10 to 15 mL/kg) to maintain adequate lung inflation
- Isolates and protects the airway from aspiration of stomach contents or other substances in the mouth, throat, or upper airway
- Permits effective suctioning of the trachea
- Provides a route for administration of several medications

Because of the advanced skill required to place a tracheal tube, tracheal intubation is a restricted medical act in the United States. Misplacement of a tracheal tube can result in severe—even fatal—complications. In most states medical practice acts determine the level of personnel allowed to perform intubation. For clinical reasons intubation should be restricted to medical/healthcare personnel who meet the following criteria:

- Personnel are well trained.
- Personnel perform intubation frequently.

or

- Personnel take renewal courses frequently.
- Tracheal tube placement is included in the scope of practice defined by governmental regulations.

Technique

The *ACLS Reference Textbook* provides detailed directions on the technique of tracheal intubation. Many ACLS providers do not perform intubation in their practice because of the professional restrictions noted above. All members of a resuscitation team, however, must understand the concept of tracheal intubation and the steps involved in successful intubation and must be able to recognize *when intubation is being done incorrectly.* This knowledge is often of more importance than knowing how to perform the actual psychomotor skill itself.

All ACLS providers must understand

- When to intubate
- How to intubate
- How to recognize when intubation is being done incorrectly
- How to verify successful tube placement
- How to prevent tube dislodgment
- How to provide subsequent ventilations and chest compressions

Indications

- Cardiac arrest with ongoing chest compressions
- Inability of a conscious patient in respiratory compromise to breathe adequately
- Inability of the patient to protect the airway (coma, areflexia, or cardiac arrest)
- Inability of the rescuer to ventilate the unresponsive patient with conventional methods

6. Provide definitive airway control

Technique Overview (See *ACLS Reference Textbook*)

- Prepare for intubation with necessary equipment.
- Ask second rescuer to apply cricoid pressure.
- Perform tracheal intubation in the standard manner as described in the *ACLS Reference Textbook.*
- Inflate cuff on tube.
- Attach ventilation bag.
- Confirm correct placement by primary (physical examination) and secondary (adjunct device) confirmation methods.

The Cricoid Pressure Maneuver

Why? During tracheal intubation *in adults* a second rescuer should apply cricoid pressure to protect against regurgitation of gastric contents and help ensure tube placement in the tracheal orifice. Maintain cricoid pressure until the cuff of the tracheal tube is inflated and proper tube position is confirmed.

Cricoid Pressure Technique

- Find the prominent thyroid cartilage (Adam's apple).
- Find the soft depression below the thyroid cartilage (cricothyroid membrane).
- Find the hard prominence just below that (cricoid cartilage).
- Apply firm pressure while pinching with the thumb and index finger toward the victim's back and somewhat toward the head. This blocks the esophagus with the firm, cartilaginous back wall of the trachea. Cricoid pressure pushes the tracheal orifice backward and more into the visual field of the person performing the intubation.
- Release pressure *only* when proper tube placement is confirmed and the tube cuff is inflated.

7. Provide primary and secondary confirmation of tracheal tube placement

Correct Placement of Tracheal Tube I: Primary Confirmation by Physical Examination

Confirm tube placement immediately, assessing the first breath delivered by the bag-mask unit. As the bag is squeezed, listen over the epigastrium and observe the chest wall for movement. If you hear stomach gurgling and see no chest wall expansion, you have intubated the esophagus. Stop ventilations. Remove the tracheal tube at once. Then:

- Reattempt intubation after reoxygenating the victim (15 to 30 seconds of bag ventilations using 100% oxygen).
- If the chest wall rises appropriately and stomach gurgling is not heard, listen to the lung fields with *5-point auscultation:* left and right anterior, left and right midaxillary, and over the stomach. Document the location of the patient's breath sounds in his or her medical records. If you have any doubt, stop ventilations through the tube.
- If there is continued doubt about correct tube placement, use the laryngoscope to see whether the tube is passing through the vocal cords.
- If the tube seems to be in place, reconfirm the tube mark at the front teeth (previously noted after inserting the tube 1 to 2 cm past the vocal cords).
- Secure the tube with a commercial device designed for this purpose (preferred).
- Once the tube is secured, insert an oropharyngeal airway or add a bite block or both to prevent the patient from biting down and occluding the airway.
- Look for moisture condensation on the inside of the tracheal tube with exhalation (not 100% accurate: false-positive condensation can be observed with esophageal intubations).

Correct Placement of Tracheal Tube II: Secondary Confirmation

A variety of electronic and mechanical devices are available for use both in-hospital and outside the hospital. These devices range from simple and inexpensive to complex and costly and include several models of end-tidal CO_2 detectors (qualitative, quantitative, and continuous) and several types of esophageal detector devices.

The AHA International Guidelines 2000 Conference addressed this topic in detail to determine whether evidence now supports secondary confirmation devices as a *required* adjunct. No device or adjunct can substitute for proper visualization of the tracheal tube passing through the vocal cords. Careful surveys of consecutive tracheal intubation attempts invariably reach the conclusion that healthcare providers as well as anesthesiologists in operating rooms can still unknowingly

FIGURE 13. Qualitative end-tidal CO_2 detector. The tube should be held in place and secured once correct position is verified.

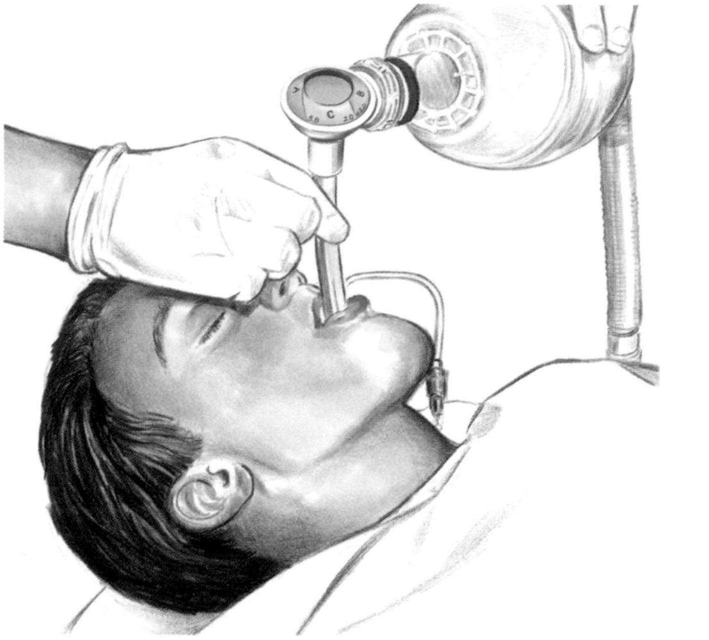

place the tracheal tube in the esophagus and leave it there. Detailed assessment of out-of-hospital intubation attempts have concluded that tracheal tubes are (1) much more difficult to place properly in that setting and (2) highly susceptible to dislodgment. Proper training, supervision, and frequent clinical performance are the keys to achieving successful intubation for every patient.

End-Tidal CO_2 Detectors

Qualitative (Figure 13)

A number of commercial devices can react, usually with a color change, to CO_2 exhaled from the lungs. The qualitative detection device indicating exhaled CO_2 indicates proper tracheal tube placement. The absence of a CO_2 response from the detector generally means that the tube is in the esophagus, particularly in patients with spontaneous circulation.

False-negative readings (the tube is in the trachea, but a false-negative reading leads to unnecessary removal of the tube). False-negative readings most commonly occur because end-tidal CO_2 production is minimal in cardiac arrest. Cardiac arrest patients have only low blood flow to the lungs produced by the chest compressions of CPR; therefore, little if any CO_2 is exhaled. This is also true of patients with a large amount of dead space (eg, significant pulmonary embolus). Inadequate or contaminated readings have been reported in patients who had ingested carbonated liquids before the arrest (tube in the esophagus yet CO_2 detected, leading to prolonged esophageal intubation).

Quantitative

The quantitative end-tidal CO_2 monitor is widely accepted as the best, albeit most expensive, secondary confirmation device. A hand-held *capnometer* provides a single quantitative readout of the concentration of CO_2 at a single point in time. The *capnograph* provides a continuous display of the level of CO_2 as it varies throughout the ventilation cycle.

These monitors can confirm successful tracheal tube placement within seconds of an intubation attempt. Patient deterioration associated with declining clinical status or subsequent tracheal tube dislodgment can also be detected with these devices. Dislodgment is an adverse event that is alarmingly common during out-of-hospital transportation of a patient.

Esophageal Detector Devices

Esophageal detector devices (Figure 14) create a suction force at the tracheal end of the tracheal tube when the operator either pulls back the plunger on a large syringe (60 to 100 mL) or completely compresses a flexible aspiration bulb. Once compressed, the bulb is firmly attached to the end of the tube coming

FIGURE 14. Esophageal detector device: the aspiration bulb technique. The tube should be held in place and secured once correct position is verified.

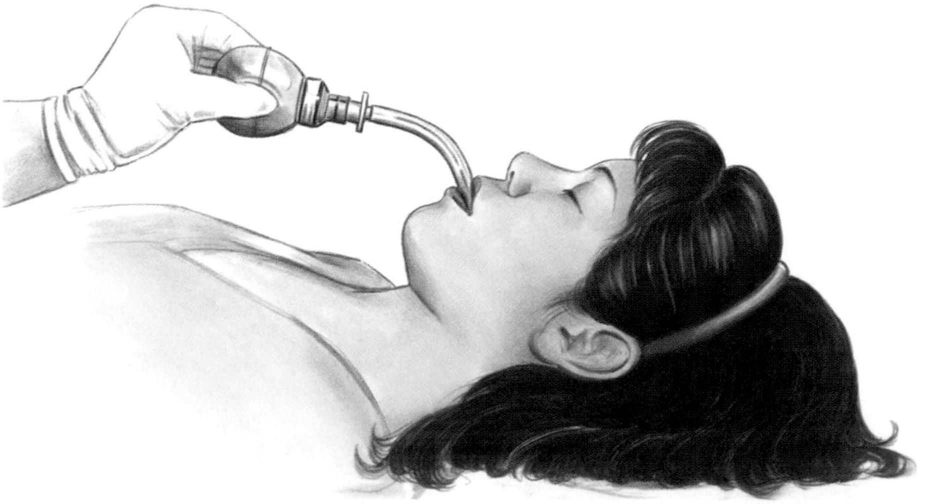

TABLE 1. Causes of False-Positive and False-Negative Results With **(A)** End-Tidal CO_2 Detector and **(B)** Esophageal Detector Devices

A

End-Tidal CO_2 Detector Device Reading	Actual Location of Tracheal Tube: Trachea	Actual Location of Tracheal Tube: Esophagus (or Hypopharynx)
Positive Yellow (positive = CO_2 present)	***True-positive:*** OK. Presence of CO_2 = tube in trachea. Proceed with ventilations.	***False-positive:*** Rescuer thinks tube is in trachea. **Causes:** Distended stomach, recent ingestion of carbonated beverage, nonpulmonary sources of CO_2. **Consequences:** Unrecognized esophageal intubation; can lead to iatrogenic death.
Negative Blue (negative = CO_2 absent)	***False-negative:*** Rescuer thinks tube is in esophagus. **Causes:** Low or no blood flow state, eg, cardiac arrest; any cardiac arrest with no, prolonged, or poor CPR. **Consequences:** Leads to unnecessary removal of properly placed tracheal tube. Reintubation attempts increase chances of more adverse consequences.	***True-negative:*** Rescuer thinks tube is in the esophagus. **Causes:** Rescuer has inserted tracheal tube in esophagus/hypopharynx. A life-threatening adverse event has occurred. **Consequences:** Rescuer recognizes tube is not in trachea; properly and rapidly identified; tracheal tube is removed at once; patient is reintubated.

B

Esophageal Detector Device Reading	Actual Location of Tracheal Tube: Esophagus	Actual Location of Tracheal Tube: Trachea
Positive Suction maintained (bulb does not refill for more than 10 seconds × 2); indicates tracheal tube is in esophagus	***True-positive:*** Rescuer thinks tube is in esophagus. **Causes:** Rescuer has inserted tracheal tube in esophagus/hypopharynx. A life-threatening adverse event has occurred. **Consequences:** Rescuer correctly recognizes tube is in esophagus; tracheal tube is removed at once; patient is reintubated.	***False-positive:*** Rescuer thinks tube is in esophagus. **Causes:** Secretions in trachea (mucus, gastric contents, acute pulmonary edema); right mainstem bronchus insertion; or pliable trachea (morbid obesity, late-term pregnancy). **Consequences:** Leads to unnecessary removal of properly placed tracheal tube. Reintubation attempts increase chances of other adverse consequences.
Negative Suction not sustained (bulb fills immediately); indicates tracheal tube in trachea	***False-negative:*** Rescuer thinks tube is in trachea. **Causes:** ■ Conditions that cause increased lung expansion (eg, COPD, status asthmaticus) ■ Conditions that fill stomach with air (eg, recent bag-mask ventilation, mouth-to-mask/mouth rescue breathing) ■ Conditions that cause poor tone in esophageal sphincter or increased gastric pressure (late pregnancy) **Consequences:** An unrecognized esophageal intubation can lead to **death.**	***True-negative:*** Rescuer thinks tube is in trachea. EDD indicates tube is in trachea. Proceed with ventilations.

Columns indicate true location of tracheal tube; rows indicate expected results from using either calorimetric end-tidal CO_2 detector (A) or bulb-type esophageal detector device (B). Both A and B assume that the operator made a conscientious intubation effort and thinks the tracheal tube is in the trachea.

out of the mouth and then released. If the tube is in the esophagus, the suction will pull the esophageal mucosa against the distal end of the detector, preventing movement of the plunger or re-expansion of the suction bulb. There will be no or very slow re-expansion.

Unlike the end-tidal CO_2 detector, the esophageal detector device does not depend on blood flow. Therefore, the esophageal detector device is preferred for secondary confirmation of tube placement in patients who have been in cardiac arrest, especially prolonged cardiac arrest (more than 3 to 5 minutes). There are several ways, however, in which the esophageal detector device can indicate "tube in trachea" (suction not maintained on bulb) when in fact the tube is in the esophagus. This is the dreaded *type II* or *false-negative* error so feared in clinical medicine. A false-negative error occurs when a patient is pronounced "well" or "OK" ("negative" for disease) when in fact a possible fatal condition or error exists.

TABLE 2. Correct Placement of Tube Confirmed (Tracheal Cuff Inflated): Next Actions

- *Ventilate with a tidal volume of 10 to 15 mL/kg.*
- *Ventilate at a rate of 1 breath every 5 seconds.*
- *Ventilate* 2 seconds for each bag ventilation.
- *Ventilate* with 100% oxygen.
- Insert an oropharyngeal airway.
- Insert a bite protector.
- Secure the tracheal tube to prevent dislodgment, but use a commercial tracheal tube holder rather than an informal tie-and-tape technique.
- Note the depth marking on the tube at front teeth.

Consider use of a cervical spine collar, backboard, and cervical spine collar to backboard if faced with potentially complex patient transfers, eg, bed to floor to stretcher to downstairs across the lawn into back of ambulance.

Prior CPR or prior ventilations on the ventilation bag can fill the stomach or esophagus with air, causing the esophageal detector device to be unable to maintain suction against the esophageal mucosa. The esophageal detector device indicates that the tracheal tube should be in the trachea by rapid reexpansion of the suction bulb. The unwary rescuer, thinking the tube is in the trachea, may therefore leave the tube in the esophagus, a potentially fatal error that could lead to the patient's death.

Table 1 compares the qualitative performance of the esophageal detector and end-tidal CO_2 device in terms of correct responses plus the most common causes of false-positive (type I) and false-negative (type II) errors.

Case 1: Respiratory Emergencies presents a new algorithm, prepared for the ACLS Provider Course, that provides more detailed information on the use of primary and secondary confirmation techniques for tracheal intubation.

How to Ventilate With a Properly Placed Tracheal Tube

The *ECC Guidelines 2000* state specific weight-based ventilation volumes:

- During *cardiac or respiratory arrest* rescuers should provide the following:
  - — **Volume** = 10 to 15 mL/kg
    - ◆ A simpler and easier to follow clinical guide is to attempt to produce several centimeters of visible chest expansion. The volume should make the chest begin to rise and "then some," as one expert advised. Try to spend extra time in skills practice—get a sense of what such a volume feels like when squeezing the bag.
    - ◆ If oxygen is unavailable, increase the volume until the chest has a conspicuous rise of 4 to 6 cm. If using supplemental oxygen, decrease the volume slightly. The chest, however, should still rise visibly.
    - ◆ Provide slightly more volume for very obese patients and slightly less volume for patients with fragile intrathoracic airways or diminished lung volumes.
  - — **Rate** = 10 to 12 breaths per minute, 1 breath every 5 to 6 seconds, each breath lasting 2 seconds
  - — **Compression-ventilation cycles:** Provide chest compressions at a sustained rate of at least 100 per minute without reference to ventilations. Remember: with an unprotected airway, 2 ventilations are delivered in relation to the sets of 15 chest compressions. With a protected airway, the recommended ventilation rate changes to 1 ventilation delivered in relation to the clock; ie, every 5 seconds deliver 1 breath over 1 to 2 seconds.
  - — **Summary:**
    - ◆ Unprotected airway: sets of 15 compressions at 100 per minute, 2 ventilations at 2 seconds per ventilation
    - ◆ Protected airway: continuous compressions at 100 per minute, asynchronous with 1 ventilation at 2 seconds per ventilation every 5 seconds.
    - ◆ When spontaneous circulation has been restored:
  - — Continue to provide a tidal volume of 10 to 15 mL/kg (ie, a volume that causes an obvious chest rise of several centimeters).
  - — Increase the ventilation rate to 12 to 15 breaths per minute (1 breath every 4 to 5 seconds).
  - — Aim for mild-to-moderate hyperventilation (achieved at a rate of 12 ventilations per minute and a volume of 15 mL/kg).

— When continuous oxygen saturation measurements are available, watch for a fall in the O_2 saturation percentage. Respond by adjusting any of several ventilation parameters: ventilations per minute, seconds per ventilation, or flow of supplemental oxygen.

- Obtain a chest x-ray as soon as possible to determine the position of the tracheal tube within the trachea. Look for placement in a single mainstem bronchus. *Never* use a chest x-ray to detect inadvertent esophageal insertion—that is a clinical determination that must be performed immediately after any intubation attempt. Confirm proper tracheal insertion by physical examination and the secondary confirmation techniques discussed above. Review the x-rays of tubes placed too high or too low in the trachea and inserted into a single bronchus.

- Take care not to induce air trapping in patients with conditions associated with increased resistance to exhalation, such as hypovolemia, severe obstructive lung disease, and asthma. Air trapping could result in a positive end-expiratory pressure (PEEP) effect that may significantly lower blood pressure. In these patients use slower ventilation rates to allow more complete exhalation. In cases of hypovolemia, restore intravascular volume.

Complications

Insertion of Tube Into Esophagus

- Accidental insertion of the tracheal tube into the esophagus will result in the patient's receiving no ventilation or oxygenation (unless the patient is still breathing spontaneously). If you or your resuscitation team fail to recognize esophageal intubation, the patient could suffer permanent brain damage or even death.

- Care is required to successfully remove and replace a tube that has been incorrectly placed. A patient in cardiac arrest who is receiving CPR should be reintubated as soon as possible. The tracheal tube will reduce the risk of gastric inflation.

- If a laryngoscope and tube are not readily available or if the intubation attempt is not successful within 20 to 30 seconds, return to the inflatable resuscitator bag and face mask. Provide 100% oxygen until the next attempt is made, 20 to 30 seconds later.

Tube Trauma and Adverse Effects

Tracheal intubation can cause significant trauma to the patient, such as

- Lacerated lips or tongue from forceful pressure between the laryngoscope blade and the tongue or cheek
- Chipped teeth
- Lacerated pharynx or trachea from the end of the stylet or tracheal tube
- Injury to the vocal cords
- Pharyngeal-esophageal perforation
- Vomiting and aspiration of gastric contents into the lower airway
- Release of high levels of epinephrine and norepinephrine stimulated by tracheal intubation, which can cause elevated blood pressures, tachycardia, or arrhythmias

Insertion of Tracheal Tube Into 1 Lung

Insertion of the tracheal tube into either the right (more common) or left main bronchus is a frequent complication. Unrecognized and uncorrected intubation of a bronchus can result in hypoxemia due to underinflation of the other lung.

Listen to the chest for bilateral breath sounds. Look for equal expansion of both sides during ventilation. If you suspect misintubation into either the left or right main bronchus, deflate the tube cuff, slide the tube back 1 to 2 cm, and recheck the patient's clinical signs. Order portable chest x-rays to check placement. Healthcare providers must understand, however, that recognition of this complication is a clinical, not a radiographic responsibility.

Airway Control in Trauma Patients

Excessive movement of the head and neck in patients with an unstable cervical spinal column can cause a disastrous injury to the spinal cord or make a minor cord injury much worse. Avoid unnecessary movement of the spine in trauma patients. Assume that any patient with multiple trauma, head injury, or facial trauma has a cervical spine injury. Maintain a high index of suspicion for spinal column or spinal cord injury. Your suspicion should be based on the mechanism of the accident alone, eg, high-speed motor vehicle crashes, falls from a height, diving into unknown waters, and submersion or near-drowning.

Steps to Follow in Known or Suspected Cervical Spine Trauma

- With a suspected neck injury, perform the chin lift or jaw thrust *without head tilt.*
- Direct a trained rescuer to stabilize the head in a neutral position during all airway manipulation.
- In a patient with facial fractures and fractures at the base of the skull, attempt direct orotracheal intubation while a second rescuer provides spinal immobilization.
- Suction the upper airway as needed.
- If tracheal intubation cannot be performed, consider cricothyrotomy or tracheotomy.
- Blind nasal intubation is generally used in breathing patients, but this is an advanced skill that is not covered in ACLS training. Immobilize the spine continuously during intubation attempts because the stimulus may result in spontaneous neck movement. As an advanced technique, blind nasal intubation should be performed only by someone with experience in this technique.

- Avoid manipulating the patient's head and neck during intubation.
- Use paralytic drugs in patients who cannot be intubated with the techniques described above. These techniques should be used only by persons experienced in these procedures. The use of profound sedation and paralysis to achieve tracheal intubation is outside the scope of skills taught in ACLS provider courses.
- The *ECC Handbook* provides detailed listings of the sequence of actions and medications needed for rapid-sequence intubation.

Additional Techniques for Invasive Airway Control and Ventilation

Several invasive airway devices were developed, evaluated, and marketed during the 1990s. Experts reviewed scientific reports for the *ECC Guidelines 2000* and concluded that there was sufficient evidence to support the following recommendations.

Class IIb recommendation: Two devices were approved for use as advanced airway devices:

- Laryngeal mask airway
- Esophageal-tracheal Combitube™

The Laryngeal Mask Airway

The LMA (Figure 15) provides an airway adjunct with a cuffed (inflatable), masklike projection at the distal end that is introduced into the pharynx and advanced until resistance is felt. The resistance indicates that the distal end of the tube has reached the hypopharynx. When the cuff is inflated, the mask is pushed up against the tracheal opening, providing an effective seal and a clear airway into the trachea.

The LMA has several distinguishing features that account for its enthusiastic acceptance as part of the ACLS airway armamentarium:

FIGURE 15. Laryngeal mask airway. The tube should be held in place and secured once correct position is verified.

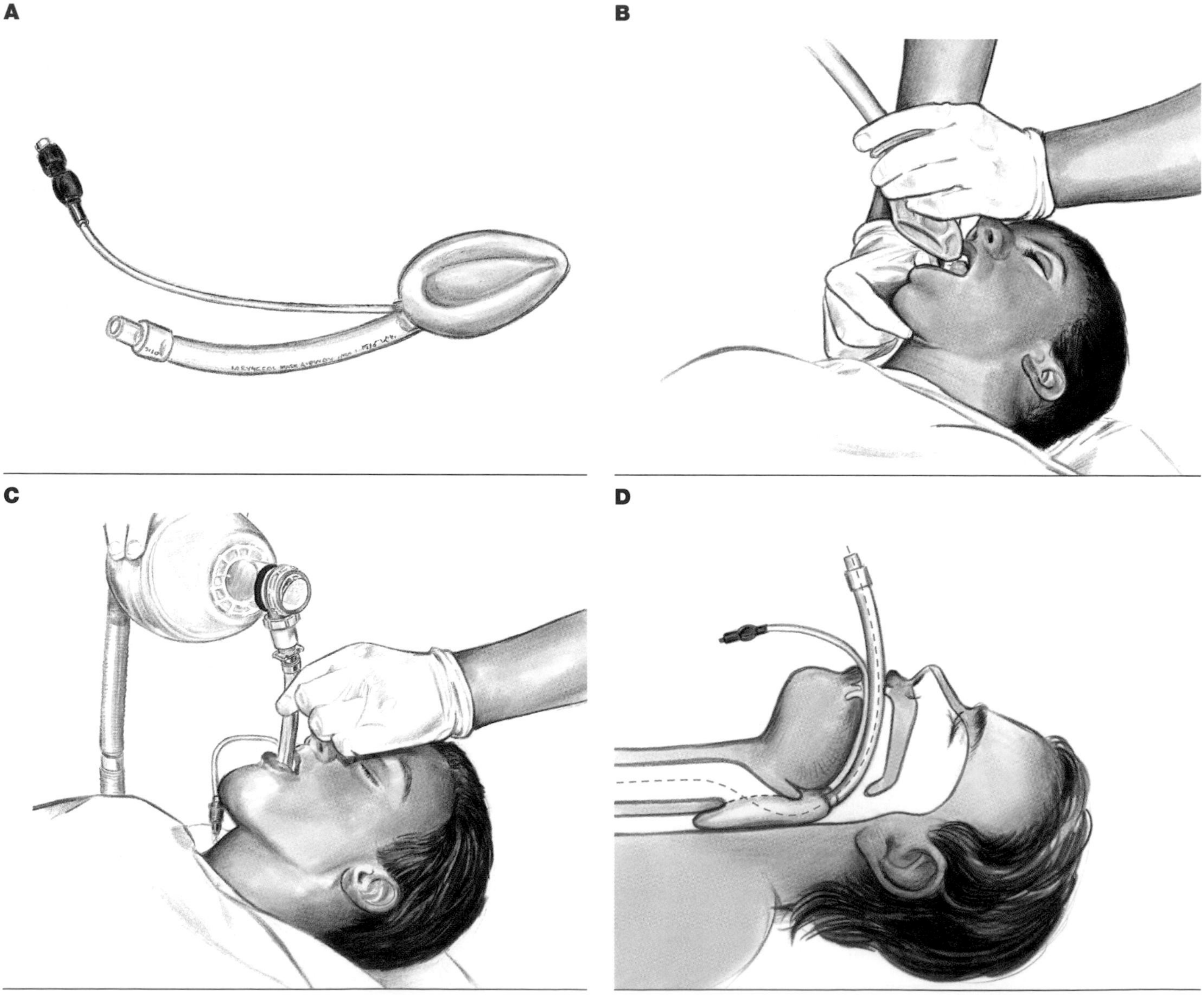

- Blind insertion means that the operator does not have to learn to use a laryngoscope or learn to visualize the tracheal opening.
- The need for proper positioning and alignment of the pharyngeal, oral, and tracheal axes is eliminated because the vocal cords are not visualized. The LMA has significant advantages over the tracheal tube in the following circumstances: when a patient has possible unstable neck injuries, access to the patient is limited, or appropriate positioning of the patient for tracheal intubation is difficult or impossible.
- The possibility of fatal errors with the LMA is much lower than that associated with tracheal tubes. The LMA does not invade the trachea, and consequently there is less risk for the fatal error of ventilating only into the esophagus with the blocked trachea.

The LMA provides slightly less airway protection from regurgitation than the tracheal tube. The device shows great promise for use by healthcare providers who cannot be trained to perform tracheal intubation and for in-hospital and out-of-hospital sites without early responses from advanced-level personnel. The LMA may also prove superior to the tracheal tube for the difficult airway.

Esophageal-Tracheal Combitube™

The combitube is another invasive advanced airway adjunct with many of the advantages of the LMA. The combitube is a tracheal tube bonded side by side with an esophageal obturator (Figure 16). Ventilation can be given through either lumen, depending on where the end inserted in the patient rests. More than 80% of the time the combitube ends up in the esophagus after blind insertion. After the 2 inflatable sealant cuffs are inflated, ventilation should proceed through the esophageal obturator. Ventilations enter the trachea through the side vents on the obturator. Observe carefully for proper chest rise and verification of effective pulmonary ventilation.

If initial ventilations through the esophageal obturator do not produce chest rise, then the combitube is probably in the trachea. Switch the ventilation bag to the other tube (the tracheal tube) and provide several inflations. Chest expansion should be noticeable. Perform secondary confirmation of proper placement with an end tidal CO_2 or esophageal detector device.

Studies of the clinical use of the combitube confirm superior ventilation and oxygenation compared with the face mask and equivalent performance compared with the tracheal tube. Note that the combitube is also a blind insertion device; thus, it eliminates the need for training in laryngoscopy and visualization of the vocal cords and the epiglottic opening. The combitube is included in the difficult airway protocols of the American Society of Anesthesiology and is generally thought to be superior to the tracheal tube when visualization of the tracheal opening is obscured by blood or secretions in the upper airway.

Background

Developers continue to search for devices that can maintain and protect the airway while also providing high oxygenation and effective ventilation. These devices should be equivalent to tracheal intubation but without the need for as much training, practice, and experience. Evidence is lacking that these devices are superior to tracheal intubation. In some EMS systems, however, ACLS providers with effective intubation skills are simply not available. The search therefore has been for devices that are equivalent to the tracheal tube but do not require high-level, sophisticated training, practice, and skills maintenance.

By the year 2000 there was sufficient evidence to support the concept of equivalence—or superiority—among the following:

- The LMA and tracheal tube in the hands of nonparamedics
- The combitube and tracheal tube in the hands of nonparamedics
- The bag mask and tracheal tube in the hands of nonparamedics

At this time the critical question of equivalence between these devices when used by advanced personnel such as paramedics or physicians cannot be answered because the question has not been studied. The new evidence reviewed in the *ECC Guidelines 2000* requires consideration of a new factor: tracheal tubes are dangerous and can cause a fatal outcome. Therefore, the question becomes much more complicated

FIGURE 16. The combitube with labels.

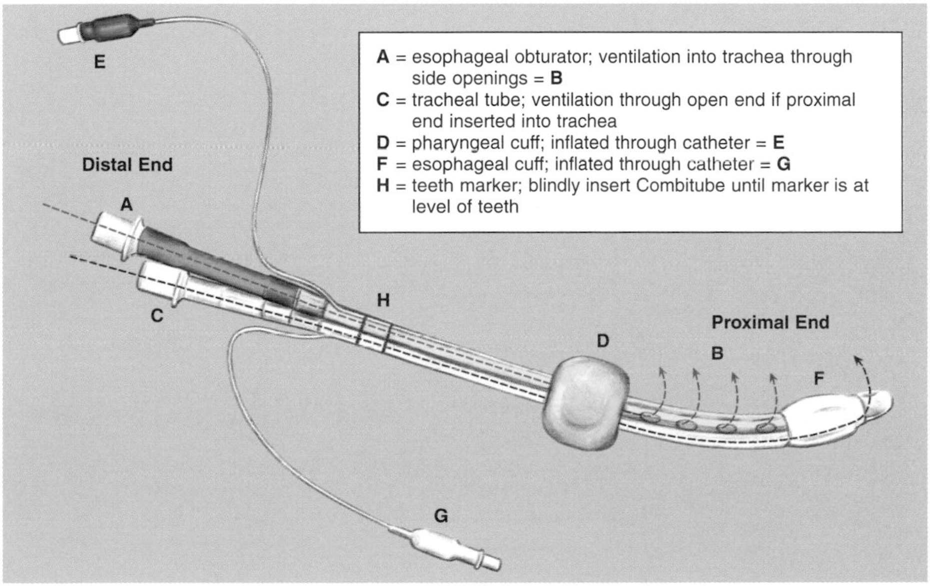

A = esophageal obturator; ventilation into trachea through side openings = B
C = tracheal tube; ventilation through open end if proximal end inserted into trachea
D = pharyngeal cuff; inflated through catheter = E
F = esophageal cuff; inflated through catheter = G
H = teeth marker; blindly insert Combitube until marker is at level of teeth
E
Distal End
A
C
H
D
Proximal End
B
F
G

than the clinical superiority of one device over another. Although most experts consider tracheal intubation to be the gold standard of airway management, that status must be tempered by the awareness that tracheal intubation can lead to death. The other 2 devices, the LMA and the combitube, lack this element of danger. The scientific consensus is that these new alternative invasive techniques—the LMA and the combitube—have a role in complex situations and are acceptable.

Class indeterminate recommendation: the evidence is lacking for inclusion of these devices in the guidelines:

- Esophageal obturator airway
- Esophageal pharyngeal airway
- Pharyngotracheal lumen airway
- Tracheal-esophageal airway
- Berman intubating-pharyngeal airway (BIPA)

Cricothyrotomy

Cricothyrotomy (Figure 17) allows rapid entrance into the airway for temporary ventilation and oxygenation of patients for whom airway control is not possible by other methods. In this technique the cricothyroid membrane is opened with a scalpel and a tube inserted. Percutaneous dilational cricothyrotomy is an emergency variation in which a small vertical incision is made and a cricothyrotomy tube is advanced over a guidewire and dilator. ACLS providers should be aware of a number of techniques that are available but beyond the scope of practice of ACLS providers.

FIGURE 17. Neck with cricoid membrane displayed with an incision indicating location of a cricothyrotomy.

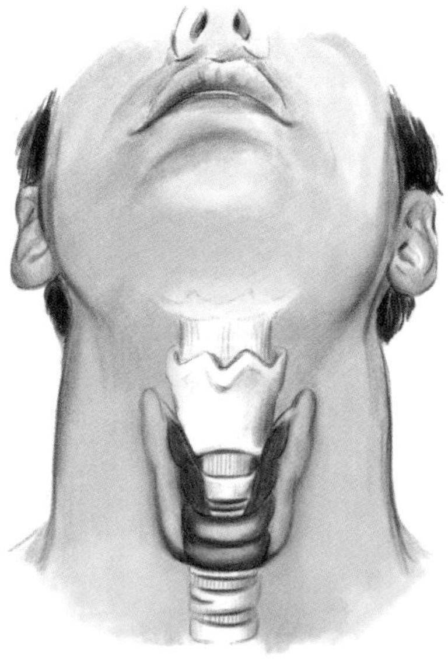

Tracheostomy

Surgical opening of the trachea and insertion of a tracheostomy tube should be performed under controlled conditions in the operating room by a skilled person. Tracheostomies should be performed *after* the airway has first been secured by a tracheal tube, a translaryngeal catheter, or cricothyrotomy. Tracheostomies are not an appropriate procedure for urgent situations such as airway obstruction or cardiac arrest.

Suction Devices

Two types of suction devices are used by ACLS providers:

1. A rigid pharyngeal device (Yankauer) is used to clear secretions, blood clots, and other foreign material from the mouth and pharynx. Pharyngeal suction requires high suction pressure.
2. A tracheobronchial suction catheter is used to clear secretions from deep within the nasopharynx and trachea. The tracheobronchial suction catheter should
   - Produce minimal trauma to the mucosa with molded ends and side holes
   - Be long enough to pass through the tip of the tracheal tube
   - Have minimal frictional resistance during insertion through the tracheal tube
   - Be sterile and disposable

ACLS Skill 2: Recognize the Rhythm

Recognition of Cardiac Arrest Rhythms

The 4 cardiac arrest rhythms are discussed in detail in the cases that focus on those rhythms: ventricular fibrillation (Cases 2 and 3), pulseless ventricular tachycardia (Case 3), pulseless electrical activity (Case 4), and asystole (Case 5).

Recognition of Non-VF/VT Rhythms

Approach to Rhythm Interpretation

For the ACLS provider rhythm interpretation should be simple, practical, and easy to remember. The most important question is not *What is this rhythm?* but rather *How is this rhythm affecting the patient clinically?* The simplest approach is to lump all rhythms into 2 classifications:

1. Cardiac arrest (lethal) rhythms

   or

2. Noncardiac arrest (nonlethal) rhythms

This classification is easy to remember because, broadly speaking, there are only 2 cardiac arrest rhythms:

1. Shockable rhythms (VF and pulseless VT)

   or

2. Nonshockable rhythms (asystole and pulseless electrical activity)

Pulseless electrical activity (PEA) includes rhythms that produce some electrical activity on the monitor but fail to produce a detectable pulse. Terms used for the electrical activity seen in pulseless victims include electromechanical dissociation (EMD), bradyasystolic rhythms, and pulseless idioventricular rhythms.

Noncardiac Arrest Rhythms

ACLS providers must be able to recognize noncardiac arrest rhythms that are, in effect, precollapse or pre-cardiac arrest rhythms. In the context of emergency cardiovascular care, there are only 2 noncardiac arrest rhythms to consider:

1. Rhythm *too* slow (less than 60 beats per minute)
2. Rhythm *too* fast (more than 120 beats per minute)

The Concept of a Rhythm That Is Too Fast or Too Slow

The word *too* is used intentionally because it focuses attention on the critical questions *How fast is "too fast"?* and *How slow is "too slow"?* To answer the questions, determine whether the speed of the rhythm is associated with clinical signs or symptoms such as

- Low blood pressure
- Poor mentation
- Shortness of breath
- Chest pain or angina
- Signs of shock

Do not make decisions or take actions on the basis of the monitor display alone: *treat the patient, not the monitor!* Always concentrate on what is happening with the patient, using the ABCD surveys to review critical clinical parameters.

Intermediate Rhythm Interpretation

The learning objectives for ACLS providers who complete the ACLS Provider Course are to recognize the *shockable* cardiac arrest rhythms of VF and pulseless VT and the *nonshockable*, noncardiac arrest rhythms of too fast or too slow. For the ACLS provider who wants to learn more about rhythm interpretation, see Appendix 3 for a detailed presentation of how to classify more rhythms, including the following:

- *Bradycardias,* including sinus bradycardia, atrioventricular nodal blocks (first-, second-, and third-degree, with wide or narrow complexes)
- *Atrial tachycardias,* including atrial tachycardia with block, atrial flutter with various degrees of block, and premature ventricular complexes
- *Tachycardias,* including sinus tachycardia, atrial fibrillation, atrial flutter, narrow-complex supraventricular tachycardias (junctional tachycardias, ectopic or multifocal, or PSVT), wide-complex tachycardias of unknown type, and stable VT (monomorphic and polymorphic).

Using Automated External Defibrillators

All automated external defibrillators (AEDs) operate using the following basic steps	Details of Operation
1. POWER ON Turn power on.	**1. POWER ON** Turn power on.
2. Attachment Attach to the patient.	**2. Attachment** ■ Open adhesive defibrillator pads. ■ Attach defibrillator cables to pads. ■ Expose adhesive surface. ■ Attach pads to the patient (upper right sternal border and cardiac apex).
3. Analysis Place in ANALYZE mode.	**3. Analysis** ■ Announce to the team members, *"Analyzing rhythm—stand clear!"* (Verify that there is no patient movement and that no one is in contact with the patient.) ■ Press the ANALYZE control (some AEDs omit this control).
4. Shock Press the SHOCK button.	**4. Shock** If VF/VT is present, the device will charge to 150 to 360 J and signal that a shock is indicated. Some AEDs use biphasic waveforms with a constant (nonescalating) energy setting. ■ Announce, *"Shock is indicated—stand clear!"* ■ Verify that no one is touching the patient. ■ Press the SHOCK button when signaled to do so. Repeat these steps until VF/VT is no longer present. The device will signal *"no shock indicated."* In general, shock in sets of 3 without interposed CPR or pulse checks. After a set of 3 shocks, provide 1 minute of CPR.

ACLS Skill 3: Defibrillate

Learning Objectives

At the end of the ACLS course the successful ACLS provider should be able to operate an AED and a conventional monitor/defibrillator to safely and effectively deliver shocks to VF.

Using Conventional (Manual) Defibrillators (Monophasic or Biphasic)

1. Turn on defibrillator.
2. Select energy level at 200 J for monophasic defibrillators (or clinically equivalent biphasic energy level).
3. Set "lead select" switch on "paddles" (or lead I, II, or III if monitor leads are used).
4. Apply gel to paddles, or position conductor pads on patient's chest.
5. Position paddles or remote defibrillation pads on patient (sternum-apex).
6. Visually check the monitor display and assess the rhythm. (Subsequent steps assume VF/VT is present.)
7. Announce to the team members, *"Charging defibrillator—stand clear!"*
8. Press "charge" button on apex paddle (right hand) or defibrillator controls.
9. When the defibrillator is fully charged, state firmly in a forceful voice the following chant (or some suitable equivalent) before each shock:
   - *"I am going to shock on three. One, I'm clear."* (Check to make sure you are clear of contact with the patient, the stretcher, and the equipment.)
   - *"Two, you're clear."* (Make a visual check to ensure that no one continues to touch the patient or stretcher. Do not forget about the person providing ventilations. That person's hands should not be touching the ventilatory adjuncts, including the tracheal tube! Turn oxygen off or direct flow away from patient's chest.)
   - *"Three, everybody's clear."* (Check yourself one more time before pressing the "shock" buttons.)
10. Apply 25 lb of pressure on both paddles.
11. Press the 2 paddle "discharge" buttons simultaneously.
12. Check the monitor. If VF/VT remains, recharge the defibrillator at once. Check a pulse if there is any question about the rhythm display (eg, a lead has been dislodged or the paddles are not displaying the correct signal).
13. Shock at 200 to 300 J, then at 360 J for monophasic defibrillators (or clinically equivalent biphasic energy level), repeating the same verbal statements noted in step 9.

The AHA has developed training material for the use of AEDs and conventional defibrillators. Advances in AED technology have made possible the widespread application of early defibrillation, and defibrillation should be known and understood by all ECC providers as core information (see the *Heartsaver AED* provider manual and the instructor's toolkit). Techniques for using AEDs are presented in Appendix 2 and Case 2. Use of conventional defibrillators is presented in Case 3.

ACLS Skill 4: Cardiovert

Learning Objectives

At the end of the ACLS course the successful ACLS provider should be able to safely and effectively perform synchronized electrical cardioversion for unstable VT with a conventional monitor/defibrillator (see Figure 18).

The most critical action in the management of patients with unstable tachycardia is timely recognition of the patient's condition as unstable and when the instability is due to the tachycardia. In such a situation electrical cardioversion can be lifesaving.

ACLS Skill 5: Provide Transcutaneous Pacing

Learning Objectives

At the end of the ACLS course the successful ACLS provider should be able to safely and effectively use stand-alone transcutaneous pacemakers and the pacing mode in conventional defibrillators.

A transcutaneous pacing system delivers pacing impulses to the heart through the skin via adhesive cutaneous electrodes, causing electrical depolarization and subsequent cardiac contraction. By 2000 most defibrillator manufacturers had added a pacing module to conventional defibrillators. Because transcutaneous pacing is now as close as the nearest defibrillator, ACLS providers need to know the indications for and techniques and hazards of transcutaneous pacing.

Recommendations for Use of Transcutaneous Pacing

The use of transcutaneous pacing for asystole or pulseless electrical activity (PEA) has been disappointing. Several studies have examined whether transcutaneous pacing has any benefit for PEA by speeding up the rate of electrical activity or any benefit for postshock asystole that is only seconds old. These indications have been largely abandoned because of the apparent ineffectiveness of transcutaneous pacing for these conditions. There is, however, an extensive list of indications for patients not in cardiac arrest. These are presented in Table 3. Details on the rationale for and technique of transcutaneous pacing are presented in Case 7: Symptomatic Bradycardia in this manual.

ACLS Skill 6: Gain IV Access to the Circulation

Learning Objectives

At the end of the ACLS course the successful ACLS provider should be able to describe the major advantages and disadvantages of the peripheral and central IV

FIGURE 18. Electrical Cardioversion Algorithm, which displays the major learning points for electrical cardioversion.

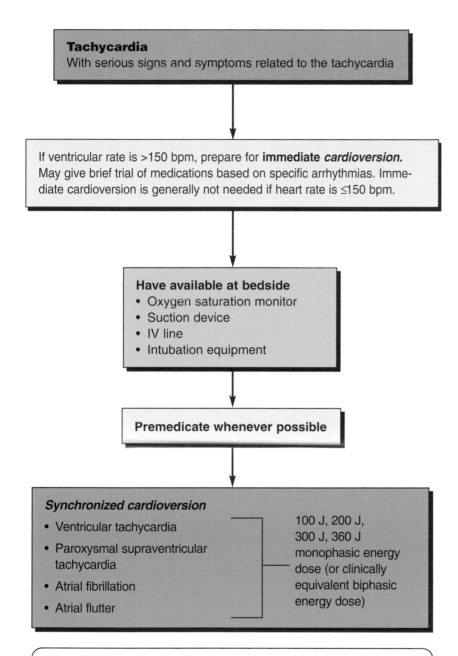

Tachycardia
With serious signs and symptoms related to the tachycardia

↓

If ventricular rate is >150 bpm, prepare for **immediate *cardioversion.*** May give brief trial of medications based on specific arrhythmias. Immediate cardioversion is generally not needed if heart rate is ≤150 bpm.

↓

Have available at bedside
- Oxygen saturation monitor
- Suction device
- IV line
- Intubation equipment

↓

Premedicate whenever possible

↓

Synchronized cardioversion
- Ventricular tachycardia
- Paroxysmal supraventricular tachycardia
- Atrial fibrillation
- Atrial flutter

→ 100 J, 200 J, 300 J, 360 J monophasic energy dose (or clinically equivalent biphasic energy dose)

Notes

1. Effective regimens have included a sedative (eg, ***diazepam, midazolam, barbiturates, etomidate, ketamine, methohexital)*** with or without an analgesic agent (eg, ***fentanyl, morphine, meperidine).*** Many experts recommend anesthesia if service is readily available.
2. Both monophasic and biphasic waveforms are acceptable if documented as clinically equivalent to reports of monophasic shock success.
3. Note possible need to resynchronize after each cardioversion.
4. If delays in synchronization occur and clinical condition is critical, go immediately to unsynchronized shocks.
5. Treat polymorphic ventricular tachycardia (irregular form and rate) like ventricular fibrillation: see Ventricular Fibrillation/Pulseless Ventricular Tachycardia Algorithm.
6. Paroxysmal supraventricular tachycardia and atrial flutter often respond to lower energy levels (start with 50 J).

Steps for Synchronized Cardioversion

1. Consider sedation.
2. Turn on defibrillator (monophasic or biphasic).
3. Attach monitor leads to the patient ("white to right, red to ribs, what's left over to the left shoulder") and ensure proper display of the patient's rhythm.
4. Engage the synchronization mode by pressing the "sync" control button.
5. Look for markers on R waves indicating sync mode.
6. If necessary, adjust monitor gain until sync markers occur with each R wave.
7. Select appropriate energy level.
8. Position conductor pads on patient (or apply gel to paddles).
9. Position paddle on patient (sternum-apex).
10. Announce to teammembers: *"Charging defibrillator—stand clear!"*
11. Press "charge" button on apex paddle (right hand).
12. When the defibrillator is charged, begin the final clearing chant. State firmly in a forceful voice the following chant before each shock:
    - *"I am going to shock on three. One, I'm clear."* (Check to make sure you are clear of contact with the patient, the stretcher, and the equipment.)
    - *"Two, you are clear."* (Make a visual check to ensure that no one continues to touch the patient or stretcher. In particular, do not forget about the person providing ventilations. That person's hands should not be touching the ventilatory adjuncts, including the tracheal tube! Turn oxygen off or direct flow away from patient's chest.)
    - *"Three, everybody's clear."* (Check yourself one more time before pressing the "shock" buttons.)
13. Apply 25 lb pressure on both paddles.
14. Press the "discharge" buttons simultaneously.
15. Check the monitor. If tachycardia persists, increase the joules according to the electrical cardioversion algorithm.
16. **Reset the sync mode after each synchronized cardioversion because most defibrillators default back to unsynchronized mode.** This default allows an immediate shock if the cardioversion produces VF.

TABLE 3. Indications for Transcutaneous Pacing

Immediate Emergent Pacing

Class I

Hemodynamically symptomatic, compromising bradycardias that are too slow and unresponsive to atropine.* Symptoms can include blood pressure less than 80 mm Hg systolic, change in mental status, angina, pulmonary edema.

Class IIa

- Bradycardia with escape rhythms unresponsive to pharmacologic therapy
- Pacing for patients in cardiac arrest with profound bradycardia or PEA due to drug overdose, acidosis, or electrolyte abnormalities
- Standby pacing: prepare for pacing for specific AMI-associated rhythms:
  - — Symptomatic sinus node dysfunction
  - — Mobitz type II second-degree heart block
  - — Third-degree heart block†
  - — New left, right, or alternating BBB or bifascicular block

Class IIb

- Overdrive pacing of either supraventricular or ventricular tachycardia that is refractory to pharmacologic therapy or electrical cardioversion
- Bradyasystolic cardiac arrest

PEA indicates pulseless electrical activity; AMI, acute myocardial infarction; and BBB, bundle branch block.

*Includes complete heart block, symptomatic second-degree heart block, symptomatic sick sinus syndrome, drug-induced bradycardias (ie, amiodarone, digoxin, β-blockers, calcium channel blockers, procainamide), permanent pacemaker failure, idioventricular bradycardias, symptomatic atrial fibrillation with slow ventricular response, refractory bradycardia during resuscitation of hypovolemic shock, and bradyarrhythmias with malignant ventricular escape mechanisms.

†Relatively asymptomatic second- or third-degree heart block can occur in patients with an inferior myocardial infarction. In such patients pacing should be based on symptoms of deteriorating bradycardia.

approaches. The ACLS provider should also recognize the differences in drug administration imposed by cardiac arrest when blood flow is not present and available to deliver administered agents to the tissues.

Purpose of IV Cannulation

IV cannulation provides direct peripheral or central access to the venous circulation. This allows the rescuer to

- Administer drugs and fluids
- Obtain venous blood for laboratory determinations
- Insert catheters into the central circulation, including the right side of the heart and pulmonary artery, for physiological monitoring and electrical pacing

All ACLS providers should be proficient at gaining direct IV access. They should take appropriate universal precautions, use protective barriers, and take care in hand washing. Dispose of all needles and sharp instruments.

The following percutaneous IV techniques and sites are commonly used:

- Peripheral venipuncture
  - — Arm vein (antecubital or hand)
  - — External jugular vein
- Central venipuncture
  - — Internal jugular vein
  - — Subclavian vein
  - — Common femoral vein

ACLS providers should know the general guidelines for choice of access route; the available needles, cannulas, and catheters; the general principles of IV therapy; and the specific anatomy, indications, performance criteria, and complications for each of these techniques. These topics, however, are not discussed in detail during an actual ACLS Provider Course. The *ACLS Reference Textbook* provides a well-illustrated, step-by-step guide to vascular access.

Vascular Access: Choice of Approach

Peripheral Line

Advantages

Peripheral venous access is the procedure of choice, even during CPR. Cannulate the large, easily accessible peripheral veins, such as the cephalic, femoral, or external jugular. Peripheral sites are compressible, which is particularly important for patients who may require thrombolytic therapy.

Disadvantages

Peripheral venous lines may collapse during low-flow states, making access difficult and time-consuming. During a cardiac arrest the time required for a medication given through a peripheral vein to appear in the central circulation is excessive. Therefore, in cardiac arrest use upper-extremity veins, keep the access site elevated, and follow drug administration with a flush of IV fluid.

Central Line

Advantages

Cannulate central veins when peripheral sites are unavailable or access to the central circulation is required. The predictable anatomic location of central vessels permits rapid access in emergencies, avoiding time lost searching for a peripheral site. The large size of the central vessels allows the use of large-bore catheters when rapid volume replacement is needed. Greater flow through the central vessels permits infusion of concentrated solutions that would irritate peripheral vessels.

Disadvantages

Subclavian and internal jugular veins lie close to the carotid and subclavian arteries, the apical pleura of the lungs, the trachea, and various nerves. These structures are frequently damaged when inexperienced operators perform the procedures. Central vein cannulation carries the risks of *air embolus, catheter embolus,* and *hemorrhage* from noncompressible sites. The last may be a particular problem for patients receiving fibrinolytic therapy.

Complication rates decline with increased operator experience, so it is important to choose the technique with which the operator is most familiar. The supraclavicular subclavian and central internal jugular approaches are both relatively easy to perform, with a low incidence of pneumothorax. The supraclavicular subclavian approach has advantages during cardiac arrest because it does not require long interruptions of chest compression (unlike the infraclavicular approach). This approach permits the operator to stand at the side of the patient's head during the procedure. This position involves less interference with airway management than that associated with internal jugular cannulation.

General Principles of IV Therapy

In an emergency, speed is essential (especially outside the hospital), and strict aseptic technique may be impossible. After the patient is stabilized, the cannula should be removed and replaced under sterile conditions. If the patient is awake, anesthetize the overlying skin with 1% lidocaine without epinephrine. Then insert a large-bore cannula. During cardiac arrest follow all administered drugs by bolus administration of at least 20 mL of IV saline to flush the drug into the central circulation.

ACLS Skill 7: Provide Appropriate Resuscitation Medications

Learning Objectives

In ACLS treatment, medications and pharmacologic agents are used to meet the following major objectives:

- To correct **hypoxemia**
- To restore spontaneous **circulation** at an adequate **blood pressure**
- To promote optimal **cardiac function**
- To prevent or suppress significant **arrhythmias**
- To relieve **pain**
- To correct **electrolyte abnormalities,** adjust **acidosis,** and counteract the effects of excessive amounts of **prescribed medications** or **illegitimate agents**
- To treat **congestive heart failure**

Rote Memorization Versus Full Understanding

Cardiac emergencies require many agents with complex actions and overlapping indications. Frequently ACLS personnel must make decisions in a few seconds. In these situations quick mental associations between *"rhythm-drug-and-dose"* are helpful and at times lifesaving. An excellent example is the *characteristic rhythm of severe hyperkalemia:*

Tall-peaked T-waves with bizarre QRS complexes →

Calcium chloride →

500 to 1000 mg IV push

Each order for a medication, however, should be supported by a thorough understanding of the *mechanism of action, indications* and *contraindications, dosages,* and *precautions.*

The Handbook of Emergency Cardiovascular Care for Healthcare Providers

The ECC pocket handbook will be your most valuable and up-to-date resource for ACLS pharmacology. The *ECC Handbook* reproduces the ACLS clinical algorithms, indicating the drug and often the doses. In addition, the *ECC Handbook* contains a detailed alphabetical list of every drug recommended in the ACLS guidelines. This section summarizes the *Why?* (drug actions), *When?* (drug indications), *How?* (drug dosing), and *Watch out!* (precautions) for every agent.

In keeping with the ACLS model of adult professional education, all ACLS provider candidates are encouraged to consult the ECC handbook at any time during the course. This includes during the skills- and case-based small group sessions, evaluation stations, and even during the written examination. As adult professionals, ACLS providers are better served by knowing what is in the handbook and where to look for critical information than by straining to remember—often incorrectly—specific agents and doses.

Summary

This chapter provides a review of the 7 advanced ACLS skills:

1. **Airway** management
2. **Rhythm** recognition
3. **Defibrillation** with conventional monitor/defibrillators
4. **Cardioversion**
5. Transcutaneous **pacing**
6. Direct circulation access through **intravenous catheters**
7. Administration of appropriate resuscitation **medications**

This review isolates these skills and describes the baseline information every ACLS provider needs. The Primary and Secondary ABCD Surveys begin to give the ACLS provider a sense of the sequential integration of these advanced ACLS skills when used in actual resuscitation attempts. The role of the basic ACLS skills is also conveyed in the Primary ABCD Survey. The ACLS algorithms add considerably more details to the ACLS provider's information base.

These facts, descriptions, and recommendations, however, have meaning only when applied to actual patients with specific problems and conditions. Part 2 of this manual presents the 10 core ACLS cases. It is only through actual case management that ACLS providers learn to integrate all basic and advanced ACLS skills.

Chapter 4

The Human Dimension of CPR and ACLS: Human, Ethical, and Legal Issues

How Often Will CPR, Defibrillation, and ACLS Succeed?

Since 1973 more than 40 million people in the United States have learned CPR. Many public health experts consider CPR training to be the most successful public health initiative of modern times. Millions of people have been willing to prepare themselves to take action to save the life of a fellow human being. Despite our best efforts, however, we know that more than half of resuscitation attempts do not succeed. CPR at home or in public helps to restart the heart and restore breathing only about 50% of the time, even in the most "successful" communities.

Tragically even when their hearts restart, only about half of the VF cardiac arrest victims admitted to the Emergency Department and the hospital survive and go home. This means that 3 of 4 CPR attempts will be unsuccessful. We must consider and plan for the emotional reactions from rescuers and witnesses to any resuscitation attempt. This is particularly true when their efforts appear to have made no difference.

Learning Objectives

By the end of this chapter you should be able to

1. Explain how CPR and defibrillation seldom restore normal heartbeat and breathing out of hospital
2. Give 2 different definitions of "rescuer success" in resuscitation for cardiac arrest
3. State the importance of debriefing after a resuscitation attempt
4. Discuss the possibility of lawsuits and legal actions in relation to the performance of out-of-hospital CPR or defibrillation by EMS professionals and by lay rescuers
5. Explain the purpose of Good Samaritan laws
6. List 3 conditions under which BLS rescuers can stop CPR efforts and 3 different conditions under which ACLS rescuers can stop CPR efforts
7. List 3 conditions under which BLS rescuers do not have to start CPR efforts and 3 different conditions under which ACLS rescuers do not have to start CPR efforts
8. Explain the differences between living wills and advance directives

Take Pride in Your Skills as an ACLS Provider

You should be proud of the fact that you are learning to become an ACLS provider. Now you can be confident that you will be better prepared to do the right thing when your professional skills are needed.

Of course these emergencies can have negative outcomes. You and the other emergency personnel who arrive to help in the resuscitation may not succeed in restoring life. Some people have a cardiac arrest simply because they have reached the end of their life. Your success will not be measured by whether a cardiac arrest victim lives or dies but rather by the fact that you tried. Simply by taking action, making an effort, just trying to help, you will be judged a success.

Stress Reactions of Rescuers and Witnesses After Resuscitation Attempts

A cardiac arrest is a dramatic and emotional event, especially if the victim is a friend or loved one. The emergency may involve disagreeable physical details, such as bleeding, vomiting, or poor hygiene. Any emergency can be an emotional burden, especially if the rescuer is closely involved with the victim. The emergency can produce strong emotional reactions in physicians, nurses, bystanders, lay rescuers, and EMS professionals. Failed attempts at resuscitation can impose even more stress on rescuers. This stress can result in a variety of emotional reactions and physical symptoms that may last long after the original emergency.

It is common for a person to experience emotional aftershocks when he or she has gone through an unpleasant event. Usually such stress reactions occur immediately or within the first few hours after the event. Sometimes the emotional response may occur later. These reactions are frequent and quite normal. There is nothing wrong with the rescuer or other witnesses.

Psychologists working with professional emergency personnel have learned that rescuers may experience grief, anxiety, anger, and sometimes guilt. Typical physical reactions include difficulty sleeping, fatigue, irritability, changes in eating habits, and confusion. Many people say that they are unable to stop thinking about the event. Remember that these reactions are *common* and *normal*. They do not mean that you are "disturbed" or "weak." Strong reactions simply indicate that this particular event had a powerful impact on you. With the understanding and support of friends and loved ones, the stress reactions usually pass quickly.

Techniques to Prevent and Reduce Stress in Rescuers, Families, and Witnesses

Psychologists have learned that the most successful way to reduce stress after rescue efforts is very simple: *Talk about it.* Sit down with other people who witnessed the event and talk it over. EMS personnel responding to calls from public access defibrillation sites are encouraged to offer emotional support to lay rescuers and bystanders. More formal discussions should include not only the lay rescuers but also the professional responders.

In these discussions you will be encouraged to describe what happened. Do not be frightened about "reliving" the event. It is natural and healthful to do this. Describe what went through your mind during the rescue effort. Describe how it made you feel at the time. Describe how you feel now. Be patient with yourself. Understand that most reactions will diminish within a few days. Sharing your thoughts and feelings with your companions at work, fellow rescuers, EMS personnel, friends, or clergy will either prevent stress reactions or help with your recovery.

Critical Incident Stress Debriefings

In some locations—for example, busy Emergency Departments or EMS systems, the homes of high-risk patients, or commercial worksites—program leaders may plan more formal discussions some days after attempted resuscitations. Such sessions have been called *critical incident stress debriefings,* or CISDs.

Teams of specially trained persons organize and conduct these debriefings. Such persons are usually associated with EMS services, employee assistance programs, community mental health centers, or public school systems. Other sources of psychological and emotional support can be local clergy, police chaplains, fire service chaplains, or hospital and Emergency Department social workers. Your course instructor may be able to tell you what plans are established for critical event debriefings in your professional setting.

A critical event debriefing is a confidential group process. The facilitator leads persons involved in a stressful situation to express their thoughts and feelings about the event. You do not have to talk during the briefing, but if you do, what you say may help and reassure others. Rescuers and witnesses to an event can express and discuss shared feelings they experienced during and after a resuscitation attempt. These may be feelings of guilt, anxiety, or failure, especially if the resuscitation attempt had a negative outcome. Rescuers most involved in the resuscitation should be present for the debriefing. For example, in some public access defibrillation programs EMS personnel are encouraged to visit the lay rescuers who were involved in the resuscitative effort.

In some ACLS and CPR courses instructors overlook this human dimension of resuscitation, often because of time limitations and a full teaching agenda. The AHA encourages medical directors and course instructors to introduce the possible emotional impact that may follow resuscitation attempts.

Psychological Barriers to Action

Performance Anxiety

The ACLS Provider Course helps prepare you to respond appropriately to a future emergency. Here are common concerns ACLS providers express about responding to sudden cardiac emergencies: Will I be able to take action? Will I remember the steps of the ACLS Approach? the skills of CPR, defibrillation, and intubation? the details of drug doses and algorithm branches? *Will I really have what it takes to respond to a true emergency?* Any emergency involving a patient you have grown close to, a friend, a family member, or a loved one will produce strong emotional reactions.

Disagreeable Aspects of CPR

What about the unpleasant and disagreeable aspects of doing CPR either in hospital or out of hospital? Would you really be able to do mouth-to-mouth rescue breathing on a stranger? What if the victim is bleeding from facial injuries that occurred when the victim collapsed? Would this not pose a risk of disease for a rescuer without a CPR barrier device? CPR and defibrillation outside the hospital or in the Emergency Department require the rescuer to remove clothing from the victim's chest. You cannot attach defibrillation electrodes unless the pads are placed directly on the skin of the chest. The rescuer must open the shirt or blouse of the cardiac arrest victim and remove her undergarments. Common courtesy and modesty inhibit many people from removing the clothing of strangers, especially in front of many other people in a public location.

Everyone is familiar with defibrillation shocks from television and movies. Everyone knows to expect the "jump" and muscle contractions whenever a character yells "clear." These shocks appear painful. Can you overcome your natural tendency not to hurt others, even in an emergency when your actions could be lifesaving? Often friends and relatives will be at the scene of an emergency. If you respond and take action, these people will look to you to perform precisely and confidently. Yet confidence will be hard to come by at such a rare and challenging event.

These psychological barriers can hinder a quick emergency response, especially in medical settings or community settings where such events are rare. There are no easy solutions to help overcome these psychological barriers. Your instructor will encourage you to anticipate many of the scenes described above. The case scenarios will include role-playing and rehearsals. Think through how you would respond when confronted with such a circumstance. Mental practice, even without hands-on practice, is a good technique for improving future performance.

Summary of the Human Dimensions of CPR

CPR programs train hundreds of thousands of people every year in CPR. Rapid changes in technology have led to AEDs that are simple to operate, safe to use, and effective. Flexible course requirements have allowed thousands of public safety and healthcare providers to be trained in ACLS. Now AEDs and innovative emergency medical leaders are opening the door for lay rescuers to perform not only CPR but also early defibrillation.

Be proud of your initiative to take an ACLS Provider Course. Be proud of your new skills in using the ACLS Approach.

Despite the promise of AEDs and public access defibrillation, there are limitations to what you can do. Your efforts will not always succeed. What is important is to take action and to try to help another human being. Some people must overcome barriers to action if asked to respond to a dramatic emergency such as cardiac arrest. Many of these barriers will be reduced by taking an ACLS Provider Course or by taking a Heartsaver AED Course. Feel free to express your concerns openly during the course and the small group sessions.

Leaders of all courses that follow the AHA guidelines are aware of the mental and emotional challenge of rescue efforts. You will have support if you ever participate in a resuscitation attempt. You may not know for several days whether the victim lives or dies. If the person you try to resuscitate does not live, take comfort from knowing that in taking action you did your best.

Legal and Ethical Issues

The AHA has supported community CPR training for more than 3 decades. Citizen CPR responders have helped save thousands of lives. The AHA believes that the addition of training in the use of AEDs will dramatically increase the number of survivors of cardiac arrest.

Anyone can perform emergency CPR without fear of legal action.

Chest compressions and rescue breathing require direct physical contact between rescuer and victim. Often these 2 people are strangers. Too often the arrest victim dies. In the United States people may take legal action when they perceive damage or think that a person has harmed another, even unintentionally. Despite this legal environment, CPR remains widely used and remarkably free of legal issues and lawsuits. Although attorneys have included rescuers who performed CPR in lawsuits, no "Good Samaritan" has ever been found guilty of doing harm while performing CPR.

All 50 states have Good Samaritan laws that grant immunity to anyone who attempts CPR in an honest, "good-faith" effort to save a life. A person is considered a Good Samaritan if

- The person is genuinely trying to help
- The help is reasonable (you cannot engage in gross misconduct, such as doing chest compressions on someone's neck)
- The rescue effort is voluntary and not part of the person's job requirements

Under most Good Samaritan laws, laypeople are protected if they perform CPR even if they have had no formal training. This is to encourage broader awareness of resuscitative techniques and to remove a small barrier to involving more people. Unless you are expected to perform CPR as part of your job responsibilities, you are under no *legal* obligation to attempt CPR on a victim of cardiac arrest. Failure to attempt CPR when there is no danger to the rescuer and the rescuer has the ability is considered an *ethical* violation by some.

When to Stop CPR

Many rescuers are troubled by the thought of performing CPR on someone who may never respond. How long do you keep on doing CPR in such a situation? Stories are told, for example, about passengers in overseas commercial aircraft having a cardiac arrest when the nearest airport is hours away. How long should you perform CPR for such a person? The AHA recommends using common sense and reasonable judgment in unusual circumstances. Widely accepted guidelines for stopping CPR include the following:

- The victim responds, regains an adequate pulse, and begins to breathe.

- A trained professional responder arrives, takes over, and assumes responsibility.
- The rescuers are too exhausted to continue or continued CPR poses a danger to rescuers. For example, if CPR is being performed for an in-flight cardiac arrest, do not hesitate to stop CPR during landings. Stop CPR, occupy the nearest seat, and fasten your seatbelt. Resume CPR as soon as possible after touching the ground.
- A medical professional tells you to stop.
- Obvious signs of death are apparent.

When Not to Start CPR

Professional responders follow several widely accepted criteria as reasons not to start CPR. These include

- A valid order not to attempt resuscitation in the event of an apparent cardiac arrest. These are called "Do Not Attempt Resuscitation" (DNAR) orders.
- Obvious signs of death. The most reliable are
  - — Dependent livido; blotchy, black and blue, or reddish discoloration of the skin; this begins in the parts of the body closest to the floor within minutes of death and progresses over the rest of the body.
  - — Rigor mortis, a postmortem contraction of the muscles without relaxation; this causes a rigidity found first in the neck and jaw.
  - — Algo mortis, the steady lowering of body temperature after death.
  - — Injuries that are incompatible with life.
- Other reasons not to attempt to resuscitate are threats to rescuers' safety, family objections, and written DNAR orders or a "living will" that appears unofficial or informal.

"Do Not Attempt Resuscitation" (DNAR)

You may encounter a victim of cardiac arrest who has expressed a wish to forego resuscitation attempts if cardiac arrest occurs. Friends or relatives of the victim may supply this information. Medic Alert® bracelets or wallet cards are often used as a way of communicating the victim's prearrest wishes. Many states have "Do Not Attempt Resuscitation" (DNAR) programs. Clear expressions of the victim's wishes must be respected by emergency medical personnel. They are legally obligated to do so.

Living Wills and Advance Directives

The Patient Self-Determination Act of 1991 recognizes the right of an individual to make decisions about his or her medical care, including care at the end of life.

Living Wills

A person may express preferences about care at the end of life by preparing a "living will." The living will documents the *person's* wishes, providing instructions for family members, physicians, and other healthcare providers. Everyone, particularly persons entering their senior years, should prepare a living will.

Advance Directives

Advance directives differ from living wills. Advance directives are prepared by the attending physician or other care provider rather than by the individual patient. In general a responsible physician writes the advance directive, guided by the patient's living will. More often, however, physicians write advance directives for patients who have been hospitalized with a terminal condition. Frequently patients are too ill to participate in the decision making. Physicians and families should talk with patients about their preferences regarding CPR in various clinical settings.

EMS No-CPR Programs

A number of states have adopted no-CPR programs. These programs allow patients and family members to call 911 for emergency care, support, and treatment for end-of-life distress (for example, shortness of breath, bleeding, or uncontrolled pain). At the same time patients do not have to fear unwanted resuscitative efforts.

In a no-CPR program the patient, who usually has a terminal illness, signs a document requesting "no heroics" if there is a loss of pulse or if breathing stops. In some states this document directs the patient to wear a no-CPR identification bracelet. In an emergency the bracelet or other documentation signals rescuers that CPR efforts, including use of an AED, are prohibited.

If an ACLS provider arrives at the side of a person in apparent cardiac arrest (unresponsive, no pulse, not breathing) and sees that the person is wearing a no-CPR bracelet (or has some other indication of no-CPR status), the provider should respect the person's wishes. Report the problem as a "collapsed, unresponsive person who is wearing a no-CPR bracelet." Report that you think CPR should not be performed.

Legal Aspects of AED Use

Defibrillators, including AEDs, are restricted medical devices. Most states have health practice acts that require a physician to authorize the use of any restricted medical device. Public access defibrillation programs that make AEDs available to lay rescuers and in some cases EMS providers are required to have a *medical authority* who oversees the purchase of AEDs, treatment protocols, training, and EMS providers. In one sense the medical authority *prescribes* the AED for use by the lay responder and therefore makes the use of the AED consistent with the medical regulations.

In the United States malpractice accusations and product liability lawsuits increase every year. Innovative programs to bring early CPR and early defibrillation into every community have fallen under the shadow of fear of malpractice suits. Physicians, trainers, program directors, corporation heads, and legal counsel for many groups have often refused to support early defibrillation programs for fear of being involved in a lawsuit. Without medical authority lay rescuers cannot use an AED. Yet physicians are extremely reluctant to support programs that place defibrillators in homes, worksites, and public places if that support exposes them to legal risk. Likewise, lay rescuers, even with physician authorization, fear being sued if they try to help someone by using an AED and "something goes wrong."

To solve this problem, all states have changed existing laws and regulations. Many states have amended Good Samaritan laws to include the use of AEDs by lay rescuers. This means that the legal system will consider lay rescuers to be Good Samaritans when they attempt CPR and defibrillation on someone in cardiac arrest. As a Good Samaritan you cannot be sued for any harm or damage that occurs during the rescue effort (except in cases of gross negligence). As of 2000, plaintiffs and attorneys have filed lawsuits against facilities for failure to train and equip employees to perform CPR and use an AED. The converse is legal action against a layperson or commercial entity for making a defibrillator available and using it in an attempt to save someone's life. Legal actions against *use* of an AED, however, have not occurred or have not been reported.

In some public access defibrillation legislation the state grants immunity from lawsuits only when specific recommendations are fulfilled. These recommendations state that the rescuer must

- Have formal training in CPR and use of an AED (for example, the AHA Heartsaver AED Course or equivalent)
- Use treatment protocols, such as the CPR-AED algorithm, that are approved by a recognized medical authority
- Perform routine checks and maintenance on the AED as specified by the manufacturer
- Notify local EMS authorities of the placement of the AED so that EMS personnel, particularly the emergency medical dispatcher system, are aware when emergency calls are made from a setting in which an AED is available

Summary of Ethical and Legal Aspects of Resuscitation

Our legal system has never found a lay rescuer guilty of doing harm in attempting CPR on a victim of cardiac arrest. Our legal system has never found a professional responder guilty of doing harm by using an AED on a cardiac arrest victim. Good Samaritan laws exist in every state to give immunity to rescuers who try to help a person who is experiencing a medical emergency. The lay rescuer must act voluntarily in a *good-faith* effort to help another person. (*Good faith* means that the rescuer does not have a professional duty to respond.) The rescuer's efforts must be based on common sense and must be reasonable. For example, a rescuer cannot attempt to help in a manner that exceeds his or her skills or violates training.

The right of patients to self-determination over health care means that a patient can choose not to receive CPR or resuscitative efforts. All rescuers should respect this right. To ensure this right, some people use a living will to document their wish to forego resuscitation attempts in a cardiac arrest. A number of states have established "Do Not Attempt Resuscitation," or DNAR, programs. Patients may wear notifying bracelets or carry wallet cards as a means of communicating their wishes in case of a cardiac arrest.

Final Comments

Resuscitation is a complex area. Issues of living or dying are immensely personal and dramatic. There are no right or wrong answers in most cases. This is especially true when the issues involve people who simply may be at the end of their life due to advanced age or the effects of disease. Letting go is difficult for both family members and rescuers.

In many ways the phrase "do not resuscitate" does ACLS a disservice because it implies that we could resuscitate a patient if we exercised that choice. In reality we only *attempt* to resuscitate people. Whether the patient regains a pulse and is restored to a normal life is something rescuers cannot determine. For some patients, however, a cardiac arrest is not the natural end of life but only a reversible response to treatable events. Identifying and treating those people is the mission of ACLS.

Chapter 5

Final, Take-Home ACLS Concepts

This chapter reviews some important concepts and principles not stated explicitly in the earlier chapters. These principles provide the foundation for what we do in emergency cardiovascular care.

Learning Objectives

By the end of this chapter you should try to restate in your own words the principle behind each of the following concepts:

1. Resuscitate the heart, restore the brain
2. Treat the patient, not the arrhythmia
3. The value of an unbroken Chain of Survival: BLS–defibrillation–ACLS
4. Time is critical
5. Seek and treat the cause, not just the condition
6. Postresuscitation care: restart the heart and *keep* it restarted
7. Advance planning: know the phases of resuscitation
8. Expect deaths and futile resuscitations: there is a right time to die
9. The Chain of Survival can be applied in the community *and* in the hospital
10. Strengthen the Chain of Survival in *your* community—both home and hospital

1. Resuscitate the Heart, Restore the Brain

Cerebral resuscitation is the most important goal of ACLS.

ECC personnel take the first step toward that goal when they restart the heart. Cerebral resuscitation—returning the patient to the level of neurological functioning he or she had before the arrest—stands as the ultimate purpose of all resuscitative efforts. Peter Safar proposed the term *cardio-pulmonary-cerebral resuscitation* (CPCR) to convey our objective, which is to restart the heart to restore the brain. Unless spontaneous ventilation and circulation are restarted quickly, successful cerebral resuscitation cannot occur.

2. Treat the Patient, Not the Arrhythmia

Never forget the patient.

Resuscitations challenge emergency care providers to make decisions quickly, under pressure, and in dramatic settings. Human nature pushes providers to focus on specific resuscitation challenges: get the IV started, insert the tracheal tube, identify the arrhythmia, remember the "right" medication to use. These actions are the means to the end. Emergency care providers must constantly aim for an overall view of every resuscitative effort. Maintain constant clinical vigilance:

- Is the airway clear and open?
- Are ventilations effective?
- What could have caused this arrest?
- What else could be wrong?
- What am I missing?

Constant clinical alertness will help you achieve the ultimate goal—resuscitating the heart and brain.

The ACLS Approach uses the Primary and Secondary ABCD Surveys in combination with the algorithms. This will keep you centered on the most important acts of resuscitation: airway maintenance, ventilation, basic CPR, defibrillation, and all medications indicated for a specific patient under specific conditions.

3. Value of the Unbroken Chain of Survival: BLS–Defibrillation–ACLS

Resuscitation is a tight continuum starting with basic life support and ending with advanced cardiovascular life support.

BLS occupies one end of this continuum. The steps in BLS give the victim of cardiopulmonary arrest the benefits of an early call to 911, an open airway, adequate ventilation, and (through chest compressions) mechanical circulation to the heart, brain, and vital organs.

ACLS occupies the other end of this continuum. ACLS attempts to restore spontaneous respiration and circulation by ACLS-only interventions: defibrillation, synchronized cardioversion, transcutaneous pacing, and IV medications.

The middle of this continuum has been blurred by the introduction of AEDs, invasive airway devices that extend into the mouth but not into the trachea, and sublingual and subcutaneous medications. Some of the traditional "advanced" skills are now included in the training of a variety of in-hospital personnel, such as nurses and respiratory therapists, and an even greater variety of out-of-hospital personnel, such as first responders, EMTs, and paramedics. Many observers now use the term *intermediate* life support for these crossover treatments.

As an ACLS provider you must know BLS. ACLS rescuers cannot discount BLS skills. They must maintain an acceptable level of competency. The day will come when you will be the first person at the scene of a cardiac arrest, and CPR will be *your* responsibility. In addition, you often must supervise and monitor the performance of others. Proper ACLS leadership requires constant and careful monitoring of the BLS objectives: an open airway, adequate breathing, adequate circulation, and a spontaneous heartbeat after defibrillation of VF.

As an ACLS rescuer you must be able to work with different team members who have different skills. The scene can be in the hospital or outside the hospital. The response team might include 2 responders trained in BLS plus defibrillation. The team might have 3 responders with advanced training. Be flexible, be embracing, and accept and celebrate the skills—and limitations—of your fellow rescuers. You are all there, at the patient's side, on the same mission.

4. Time Is Critical

A short time interval from *collapse to care* decides all patient outcomes.

The probability of patient survival decreases rapidly with every passing minute of poor blood flow and poor oxygenation. Some interventions—the "pump-'n-blow" of CPR is the best example—slow the rate of decline in the probability of survival. Other interventions, such as opening an obstructed airway or defibrillating VF, can restore a beating heart within seconds; this changes the probability of survival dramatically. Never forget the clock: the longer it takes to restore the heartbeat, the lower the chances of successful resuscitation.

5. Seek and Treat the Cause, Not Just the Condition

Emergency personnel must quickly identify medical conditions that led to the cardiac arrest.

People who experience arrest in VF need a *defibrillator;* people who experience arrest in asystole or pulseless electrical activity need a *diagnosis.* Once rescuers identify a diagnosis, they must start appropriate therapy quickly. VF is a unique condition in sudden cardiac arrest: a single intervention can completely reverse an otherwise lethal arrhythmia. Fortunately VF is observed frequently in sudden cardiac arrest.

For the non-VF rhythms, however, there is often no specific therapy. To reverse asystole and pulseless electrical activity, reverse the immediate cause of the collapse. These causes include electrolyte abnormalities, toxicological problems, hypovolemia, anaphylaxis, cardiac tamponade, pulmonary embolism, and pneumothorax.

This manual lists recommendations for the prearrest period, conditions to look for, and what interventions to provide. Acute myocardial infarction is the most dramatic example of a condition that leads to cardiac arrest if left untreated. Effective therapy is now widely available. Time is the critical element. The effectiveness of fibrinolytic therapy declines dramatically with the length of time it takes medical personnel to diagnose the acute myocardial infarction and start therapy.

6. Postresuscitation Care: Restart the Heart and Keep It Restarted

Rescuers must continue to provide appropriate assessment and treatment when spontaneous cardiac activity returns: this is the postresuscitation period.

Emergency care personnel are often the only rescuers present immediately after resuscitation. These personnel are responsible for the care of the patient while awaiting transport of the patient to an Emergency Department or a critical care area of the hospital. Rescuers must stay alert to changes in the patient's condition. Patients are particularly vulnerable to cardiac or respiratory compromise immediately after the heartbeat and breathing are restored. Rescuers must remain vigilant once they have helped to resuscitate a victim.

The ACLS Provider Course concentrates on resuscitation *during* a cardiac arrest, especially the first 10 minutes of a VF arrest. ACLS providers, however, must not neglect the critical actions to take in 2 other periods: (1) the vulnerable period *after* the cardiac arrest when the pulse is restored but not stabilized and (2) the prearrest period for ill patients at high risk for cardiac deterioration.

7. Advance Planning: Know the Phases of Resuscitation

Every resuscitation attempt has a structure that evolves over time through intermediate phases.

Anticipate each phase and plan for it in advance. The phases of resuscitation from the perspective of an Emergency Department, an EMS mobile response unit, or an in-hospital response team include

- *Anticipation* of patient arrival at the Emergency Department or the team's arrival at the patient's side
- *Transfer* to/*reception* of the patient by the receiving resuscitation team
- *Resuscitative* efforts by the primary response team
- *Maintenance* of the patient with return of circulation
- *Notification of the patient's family* of the final outcome or frequent updates of the patient's status. The family or loved ones may be present during the resuscitation attempt. The AHA endorses the concept of the patient's family being present in the resuscitation area (see the *ECC Guidelines 2000).*
- *Transfer* of the patient to a higher or equal level of care
- *Critical incident stress debriefing* about the resuscitative effort, with special attention to emotional reactions that professional personnel, rescuers, bystanders, and lay rescuers are experiencing but often are not expressing

Advance planning for each of these resuscitation phases can help organize resuscitative efforts in a rural community, an Emergency Department, a sophisticated urban EMS system, or the intensive care unit of a tertiary care medical center. Resuscitative efforts have a greater chance of success if we recognize this structure, plan for it, and follow the appropriate steps.

8. Expect Deaths and Futile Resuscitations: There Is a Right Time to Die

For many people the last beat of their heart *should* be the last beat of their heart.

These people simply have reached the end of their life. A disease process reaches the end of its clinical course, and a human life stops. In these circumstances resuscitation is unwanted, unneeded, and impossible. If started, resuscitative efforts for these people are inappropriate, futile, undignified, and demeaning to both the patient and rescuers. Good ACLS requires *careful thought* about *when to stop* resuscitative efforts and—even more important—*when not to start.*

9. The Chain of Survival Can Be Applied in the Community and the Hospital

Successful outcomes depend on how well a community or a hospital links together all emergency efforts in the *Chain of Survival:*

- *Early access:* someone must recognize a cardiac emergency and a rescuer must respond.
- *Early CPR:* someone must make an effort to open the airway, provide ventilation, and restore blood circulation as soon as possible.
- *Early defibrillation:* rapid identification and treatment of VF is the single most important intervention.
- *Early ACLS:* advanced airway control and rhythm-appropriate IV medications must be administered quickly.

ECC providers must never forget that the principles and recommendations for ECC, whether BLS or ACLS, apply in all settings. This is true whether the cardiac arrest is outside the hospital, in the hospital, or in the Emergency Department. The continuum taught in courses in BLS, BLS with an AED (the Heartsaver AED Course), and ACLS applies equally in the intensive care unit, the patient's home, and the local shopping mall. As an example of this continuum, all levels of ECC courses now include training in the use of an AED and the integration of CPR and use of an AED.

10. Strengthen the Chain of Survival in Your Community—Both Home and Hospital

Successful resuscitation depends on how strongly the *Chain of Survival* is linked in your community, including the community of your hospital.

ACLS cannot exist in a vacuum. The ultimate effect of advanced care such as intubation, defibrillation, identification of rhythms, and proper medications depends on the performance of others. The people who respond before the ACLS team reaches the patient are particularly critical to the success of the resuscitative effort. The concept of a linked chain applies to cardiac arrests in-hospital as well as to arrests in the prehospital arena. We must closely examine the links in both settings. Failure to examine and strengthen all of the links condemns emergency personnel and the patient to an inferior outcome.

Respiratory Compromise: From Shortness of Breath to Respiratory Arrest (With a Pulse)

Description

Case 1 requires that you assess an unconscious/unresponsive patient with a pulse. Respirations may be present, absent, or compromised. Case 1 uses the Primary and Secondary ABCD Surveys even though the patient is not in full cardiac arrest. You must determine the appropriate management:

- Should you compress the chest?
- Should you open the airway?
- Should you place the patient in the recovery position?
- Should you insert an advanced airway device?

In Case 1 you will learn the priorities to follow when you assess and manage an unconscious/unresponsive patient who may or may not be in cardiac arrest. This case covers how to

- Assess the patient
- Position the patient to open the airway
- Give supplemental oxygen
- Give positive-pressure ventilation
- Manage the airway with simple, noninvasive airway adjuncts and advanced invasive devices

Case 1 covers respiratory arrest or near-respiratory arrest. The case does not discuss evaluation of arterial blood gases, the presence or absence of respiratory failure, or the use of ventilators.

What's New in the Guidelines...

Ventilation, Oxygen, and Airway Management

1. To provide effective oxygenation and ventilation and reduce the risk of gastric inflation with regurgitation and aspiration of stomach contents
   - Provide supplemental oxygen to nearly every patient
   - Use continuous oxygen saturation measurements to adjust oxygen delivery
   - Provide 15 compressions with 2 breaths during 2-rescuer CPR
   - Take 2 seconds for each of the 2 breaths given during CPR
2. If supplemental oxygen is given
   - Reduce the volume of each ventilation (*old:* 800 to 1200 mL; *new:* 400 to 600 mL)
   - Increase the duration of each breath (*old:* up to 2 seconds; *new:* 2 seconds)
3. In nonintubated patients these changes in ventilation volume, rate, and duration are applicable only when supplemental oxygen can be given.
4. Bag-mask ventilation is emphasized as the *method of choice* for initial ventilatory support.
5. This upgrade in the use of bag-mask ventilation is particularly applicable for out-of-hospital caregivers, who have limited opportunities for regular field experiences in intubation, short transport intervals, or both (Class IIa recommendation; see the *ECC Guidelines 2000,* pp 267-268).
6. Once the gold standard of airway management, tracheal intubation has become the advanced airway of choice *only* when intubation skills are supported by intense programs of performance monitoring, skills maintenance, and quality improvement.
   - Without such programs, the probability of lethal complications from tracheal intubation becomes unacceptably high.

(Continued on next page)

Settings and Scenarios

In Case 1 instructors will present patients similar to those in the following scenarios.

Setting: Prehospital, Unmonitored Patient

EMTs have just walked into the home of a 69-year-old man who is a 4-pack-per-day smoker. His wife says that he has been short of breath the last few days and quit breathing 1 minute ago. He has been on a ventilator in the past.

Setting: Emergency Dept, Unmonitored Patient

A 69-year-old 4-pack-per-day smoker with severe chronic obstructive pulmonary disease (COPD) enters the Emergency Department (ED) complaining of increasing shortness of breath and lethargy. While his vital signs are being assessed, he becomes unresponsive.

Setting: In-Hospital, Unmonitored Patient

A 69-year-old 4-pack-per-day smoker with severe COPD was transferred to the ward from the critical care unit 2 days ago. About 2 hours ago the patient was evaluated for increased dyspnea, and his medications were adjusted. His daughter runs to the nursing station and says he is not breathing.

Setting: Critical Care Unit, Monitored Patient

A 69-year-old heavy smoker has been mechanically ventilated for 3 days and was successfully extubated 5 hours ago. His blood gas values reveal hypercarbia (elevated P_{CO_2}), but the values have all been stable. The nurse notes that his heart rate has fallen from 95 to 45 beats per minute during the past minute.

- This guideline applies equally to all healthcare providers in all settings, including out-of-hospital, Emergency Departments, critical care units, or general medical care.

7. To achieve a goal of "zero risk" for lethal errors with tracheal tubes, the guidelines provide important new recommendations for verification of tracheal tube placement. Healthcare providers should always confirm proper tracheal tube placement by performing a sequence of confirmation techniques: (1) primary confirmation with physical examination criteria; (2) secondary confirmation with the following criteria, which are not a part of the physical exam:

- End-tidal CO_2 detection (qualitative or quantitative), the preferred approach in patients with a pulse
- Esophageal detection (either the bulb- or syringe-aspiration approach), the preferred technique for patients in full cardiac arrest who are unable to produce expired CO_2. These approaches are described in more detail later.

8. To prevent tracheal tube dislodgment after proper insertion, the guidelines recommend

- The use of commercial tracheal tube holders rather than tape-and-tie techniques
- Consideration of immobilization of the patient's head and cervical spine in relation to the thoracic and lumbar spine. This recommendation is particularly important for transport of the intubated patient, which occurs most commonly outside the hospital as well as in-hospital for procedures and diagnostic testing. Cervical spine collars and spinal backboards are required.

9. To detect tracheal tube dislodgment, the guidelines recommend either continuous (capnography) or intermittent (capnometry) measurements of end-tidal CO_2.

10. The effectiveness of some alternative advanced airway methods approaches that of tracheal intubation but without requiring the same high level of skill. Two new airway devices are recommended:

- The laryngeal mask airway (LMA), which is inserted blindly through the mouth and hypopharynx into the tracheal opening. The LMA is designed for use by emergency providers whose work setting lacks the clinical volume necessary to easily maintain tracheal intubation skills.
- The esophageal-tracheal Combitube® is a more complex, double-lumen tube that can be inserted in the trachea by direct visualization (functioning as a tracheal tube) but is more commonly inserted blindly. After blind insertion the tip can rest in either the esophagus or the trachea. Insertion of the Combitube requires more skill than insertion of the LMA because the Combitube has 2 cuffs and 2 lumens.
  - The 2 cuffs of the Combitube are the proximal large pharyngeal cuff and the distal smaller cuff. The 2 lumens are actually 2 tubes fused together.

(Continued on next page)

- The proximal or pharyngeal tube is blue, and it ends blindly above the level of the distal cuff. Just before the blind end are 8 side holes that open into the pharynx between the pharyngeal and distal cuffs.
- The second tube is open from the white or clear adapter to the distal tip of the tube beyond the distal cuff.
- The healthcare provider may deliver ventilations through either lumen, but he or she must select the correct lumen for ventilation based on placement of the Combitube.
  - The blue lumen, or the primary or proximal lumen (also called tube 1), is open only to the pharyngeal side holes. It is not open to the end of the Combitube. You provide ventilations through the proximal lumen if the tip of the tube lies in the patient's esophagus.
  - The white/clear lumen, or the secondary or distal lumen (tube 2), is open to the distal tip of the tube, beyond the distal cuff. You provide ventilations through the distal lumen only if the tip of the tube lies in the patient's trachea.
  - If the Combitube is inserted so that the tip of the tube rests in the trachea, you must provide ventilations through the white/clear (secondary or distal) lumen directly into the trachea.
  - If the tip of the tube rests in the esophagus, you must provide ventilations through the blue lumen into the pharynx. The 2 cuffs will then ensure that ventilations through the pharyngeal side holes can enter only the trachea. The pharyngeal cuff prevents gas from escaping, and the distal cuff, located in the esophagus, blocks ventilation into the esophagus.
  - The American Society of Anesthesiology (ASA) prefers the use of the Combitube, which is recommended in the ASA Difficult Airway Protocol. The Combitube is most useful when direct visualization of the vocal cords is obscured by edema, blood, tissue damage, or anatomic distortion.
  - For more details about insertion of the Combitube, see Chapter 3 of this manual and the box Blind Insertion of the Esophageal Tracheal Combitube in this case.

11. To increase the range of patients and variety of problems for which advanced airway control can be achieved, the *ECC Guidelines 2000* noted the need for emergency use of paralytic agents to aid intubation in patients with cardiac arrest. The guidelines also commented on the usefulness of the rapid-sequence intubation technique ("the use of deep sedation and paralysis to facilitate endotracheal intubation," page 302, quoted from *Annals of Emergency Medicine)*. These more advanced topics are not included in the ACLS Provider Course curriculum; however, the ACLS and PALS Subcommittees are preparing specialized, advanced modules on specific topics. Modules on advanced airway management, covering the use of paralytic agents and rapid-sequence intubation, are also planned. The interested reader is referred to the *ECC Handbook* or the *ACLS Reference Textbook*.

Learning and Skills Objectives

At the end of Case 1 you should be able to answer the following questions, describe or demonstrate the requested skills, and manage a patient with respiratory compromise.

1. Describe the ACLS Approach (Primary and Secondary ABCD Surveys) in suspected cardiopulmonary emergencies:

- Describe the 3 indications for starting CPR
- State the indications for placing a patient in the recovery position
- Describe the primary A and B steps for a patient with respiratory compromise who has a pulse and other signs of circulation
- Demonstrate the Heimlich maneuver for a conscious choking victim versus the Heimlich maneuver for an unconscious victim with presumed airway obstruction. How does the procedure followed by the healthcare provider differ from that followed by the lay rescuer?

Type I and Type II Errors

Tracheal intubation provides an excellent example of the common clinical problem of type I and type II errors:

- A type I error occurs when the clinician mistakenly thinks the tracheal tube is in the esophagus when it is actually in the trachea. This leads to a minor error, the unnecessary removal of a tracheal tube that was correctly placed.
- A type II error occurs when the clinician thinks the tracheal tube is in the trachea when it is actually in the esophagus. This causes the clinician to leave the tube in the esophagus, a potentially lethal error with devastating consequences.

2. Describe the clinical situations in which each of the following airway adjuncts are the preferred and most appropriate devices to help clear and open an obstructed airway and maintain patency (see Chapter 3 for illustrations of these devices):
   - Oropharyngeal airways
   - Nasopharyngeal airways
   - LMA
   - Combitube
   - Tracheal tube
   - Suctioning
3. Demonstrate how to provide positive-pressure ventilation with the following techniques (see illustrations in Chapter 3):
   - Mouth-to-mask ventilation with a pocket face mask
   - Bag-mask ventilation (face mask attached to a self-inflating ventilation bag)
4. Demonstrate how to give supplemental oxygen using
   - Nasal cannula
   - Pocket face mask with oxygen port
   - Venturi mask with oxygen attachments
   - Face mask with oxygen reservoir bags
5. Describe *and* demonstrate the proper performance of tracheal intubation.
6. Describe (you need not demonstrate) the use of an LMA or the Combitube (see illustrations in Chapter 3). See box below.

Blind Insertion of the Esophageal Tracheal Combitube

1. Equipment preparation: Check the integrity of both cuffs according to the manufacturer's instructions and lubricate the tube.
2. Preparation of patient: Provide oxygenation and ventilation, sedate as indicated, and position the patient. Rule out the following contraindications to insertion of the Combitube (according to the instructions posted on the manufacturer's website):
   - Age younger than 16 years or height less than 60 inches
   - Active gag reflex
   - Known or suspected esophageal disease
   - Ingestion of a caustic substance
3. Insertion technique:
   a. Hold the device with cuffs deflated so that the curvature of the tube matches the curvature of the pharynx.
   b. Lift the jaw and insert the tube gently until the black lines on the tube are positioned between the patient's teeth (do not force and do not continue the attempt for more than 30 seconds).
   c. Inflate the pharyngeal/proximal (blue) cuff with 100 mL of air and then inflate the distal (white/clear) cuff with 12 mL of air.
4. Verify the tube location and select the lumen for ventilation: to select the appropriate lumen to use for ventilation, the rescuer must determine where the tube tip is located. The tip of the tube can rest in either the esophagus or the trachea.
   a. *Esophageal placement:* Breath sounds should be present bilaterally with no epigastric sounds. Provide ventilation through the blue (proximal/pharyngeal) lumen. This delivers ventilation through the pharyngeal side holes between the 2 cuffs, and the gas will enter the trachea. Because the tip of the tube rests in the esophagus, do not use the distal (white/clear) tube for ventilation. The distal cuff will also lie within the esophagus; inflation of this cuff prevents the ventilations that you deliver through the pharyngeal tube from entering the esophagus. Detection of exhaled CO_2 (through the ventilation or blue tube) can be used for secondary confirmation, particularly if the patient has a perfusing rhythm.
   b. *Tracheal placement:* Breath sounds are absent and epigastric sounds are present when you attempt to provide ventilation through the blue lumen. Immediately stop providing ventilation through the blue lumen and provide ventilation through the secondary (white/clear) lumen that opens at the tip of the tube in the trachea. With tracheal placement of the tube, the distal cuff performs the same function as a cuff on a tracheal tube. Detection of exhaled CO_2 (through the ventilating white or clear lumen) can be used for secondary confirmation, particularly if the patient has a perfusing rhythm.
   c. *Unknown placement:* Breath sounds and epigastric sounds are absent. Deflate both cuffs and withdraw the tube slightly, reinflate the blue cuff, and then reinflate the white (clear) cuff. See steps a and b, above. If breath sounds and epigastric sounds are still absent, remove the tube.
5. Insert an oropharyngeal and nasopharyngeal airway, provide ventilation, and continue to monitor the patient's condition and the position of the tube.

7. Describe and demonstrate where you should listen when performing 5-point auscultation to verify proper tube placement.

8. Describe how to confirm tracheal intubation with the following secondary verification systems. Be prepared to discuss some situations in which these systems may yield misleading results:
   - An end-tidal CO_2 qualitative detector
   - An esophageal detection device

9. Describe how to secure the tracheal tube at the patient's mouth to prevent dislodgment—in your work setting.

10. Describe at least 1 technique to prevent dislodgment of the tracheal tube during transportation.

11. Demonstrate how to provide ventilation with the tracheal tube or other advanced airway device and a ventilation bag.

12. Describe how to obtain IV access through the appropriate peripheral veins.

Note: Course directors may include a skills teaching station on peripheral and central venous access, depending on the participants' needs and skills level.

Major Learning Points

- Basic airway management without devices
- Basic airway management with devices, including tracheal intubation
- Rescue breathing
- Giving supplemental oxygen
- Establishing peripheral IV access

New Rhythms to Learn

- No new cardiac rhythms to learn
- Bradycardia is the rhythm most commonly associated with respiratory compromise. Case 7 teaches about bradycardias and the bradycardia algorithm.

New Drugs to Learn

- No specific medications
- The exceptions are locations where paralysis and/or rapid-sequence intubation is allowed.
- Review oxygen administration through airway adjuncts in terms of flow rate and percentage of oxygen.

See the *ECC Handbook.*

Airway Issues in the ACLS Algorithms

In the 3 ACLS cardiac arrest algorithms (*ECC Handbook*, Figures 3 through 5), the Primary and Secondary ABCD Surveys contain references to the airway. The boxes and box notes that display the surveys are nearly identical (only minor wording differences) in the 3 algorithms:

Primary ABCD Survey

***Focus:** basic CPR and defibrillation*

- **Check** responsiveness
- **Activate** emergency response system
- **Get** AED

A **Airway:** open the airway
B **Breathing:** provide positive-pressure ventilations
C **Circulation:** give chest compressions
D **Defibrillation:** assess for and shock VF/pulseless VT up to 3 times (200 J, 200 to 300 J, 360 J; or equivalent *biphasic*) if necessary

Secondary ABCD Survey

***Focus:** more advanced assessments and treatments*

A **Airway:** place advanced airway device as soon as possible
B **Breathing:** confirm advanced airway device placement by physical exam and confirmation device ***(Note 1)***
B **Breathing:** secure advanced airway device; use of purpose-made tube holders preferred ***(Note 2A)***
B **Breathing:** confirm effective oxygenation and ventilation ***(Note 2B)***
C **Circulation:** establish IV access
C **Circulation:** identify rhythm → monitor
C **Circulation:** administer drugs appropriate for rhythm and condition
D **Differential Diagnosis:** search for and treat identified reversible causes

Notes

1. *Confirm* tube placement with
   - Primary physical exam criteria *plus*
   - Secondary confirmation device (end-tidal CO_2; EDD) *(Class IIa)*

2A. *Secure* the advanced airway device (tracheal tube, LMA, Combitube):
   - To prevent dislodgment, especially in patients at risk for movement, use purpose-made tracheal tube holders, which are superior to tie-and-tape methods *(Class IIb)*
   - Consider cervical collar and backboard for transport *(Class Indeterminate)*
   - Consider *capnography:* continuous, quantitative end-tidal CO_2 monitor display *(Class IIa)*

2B. Confirm oxygenation and ventilation with
   - End-tidal CO_2 monitor and oxygen saturation monitor

Critical Actions: Assessment and Management

- The checklist below contains the critical actions needed to manage severe respiratory compromise in a patient with a pulse. These actions combine the knowledge and skills you bring from previous training in medical procedures, the ACLS course, and your experience.
- You should master each of these critical actions because they are needed for initial assessment and management of all cardiorespiratory emergencies.
- The course instructors will evaluate your knowledge and how you perform the skills in treating a case of severe respiratory compromise in a patient with a pulse. The instructors use a critical action checklist similar to that below.
- The checklist is keyed to each of the assess-then-manage steps in the ACLS Approach using the Primary and Secondary ABCD Surveys. Review the checklist until you understand the order and rationale for all the assess-then-manage steps. You will learn the details and practice the procedures during the case discussions.

Critical Actions Checklist: ACLS Case 1 Respiratory Arrest With a Pulse		
Scene Survey Steps	**Assess: Do or Monitor**	**Manage: Do or Delegate**
Recognize an emergency; respond. (Follow the initial steps of basic CPR.)	***Rescuer and patient safety?*** ☐ Check for rescuer and patient safety ***Responsive?*** ☐ Stimulate for responsiveness (touch and talk; shake and shout)	***Unresponsive*** ☐ In-hospital: shout for help/activate a code plan and bring resuscitation cart ☐ Out-of-hospital: phone 911, activate EMS, get the AED (if lone rescuer) ☐ Put on protective gloves ☐ Position the victim ☐ Position yourself as rescuer
Primary ABCD Survey		
Airway	***Airway open? Chin up? Head tilted? Correct position for ventilation?*** ☐ Look at head, neck, chin position ☐ Look in mouth if foreign body suspected	***Head, neck, or chin out of position or FBAO:*** ☐ Head tilt–chin lift; jaw thrust (refer to Chapter 3, Figures 2 and 3) ***Foreign body in airway:*** ☐ Attempt, reattempt ventilation; perform tongue-jaw lift, finger sweep, abdominal thrusts
Breathing	***Breathing? Air movement?*** ☐ Look for chest rise ☐ Listen for air movement ☐ Feel breath against your skin	***Not breathing—breathless:*** ☐ Use mouth-to-mouth breathing *or* ☐ Apply noninvasive airway device (pocket face mask preferred) with/without oxygen *or* ☐ Use a face shield ☐ Use a bag-mask device with/without oxygen ☐ Give 2 rescue breaths ☐ Observe for bilateral chest rise ☐ Use obstructed airway protocols if FBAO is a possibility

Primary ABCD Survey (continued)		
Scene Survey Steps	**Assess: Do or Monitor**	**Manage: Do or Delegate**
Circulation	***Pulse?*** ☐ Check for pulse at carotid or femoral artery	***Pulse present***
Defibrillation	***Hunt for VF?*** ☐ When available, attach AED or other monitor source and determine whether VF/VT is present	***AED indicates VF is present:*** ☐ If yes, treat appropriately
Secondary ABCD Survey		
Airway	***Breathing? Air movement?*** ***Check again:*** ☐ Look for chest rise ☐ Listen for air movement ☐ Feel breath against your skin ***Endotracheal/tracheal intubation indicated?*** ☐ Responsive patient unable to ventilate adequately? ☐ Unresponsive patient unable to protect airway (coma, no gag reflex)? ☐ Rescuer unable to ventilate with other methods?	***Gurgling, noisy breathing:*** ☐ Suction airway ☐ If inadequate spontaneous breathing: use abdominal thrusts to remove obstruction according to obstructed airway protocols ***Yes, endotracheal/tracheal intubation indicated:*** ☐ Prepare for intubation ☐ Get second rescuer to apply cricoid pressure ☐ Perform endotracheal/tracheal intubation in the standard manner (see the *ACLS Reference Textbook*) ☐ Inflate cuff on tube ☐ Attach ventilation bag ☐ Prepare to confirm correct placement (use stethoscope to listen for 5-point auscultation)
Breathing	***Confirm tracheal tube in correct position:*** ***a. With physical signs?*** ☐ Look at bilateral chest movement with first ventilation? Moisture collects in tube with each breath? ☐ Listen by performing 5-point auscultation (over stomach with first bag-valve ventilation; left and right axilla; left and right anterior chest)? ☐ Feel ventilation-bag resistance?	***No, suspect tube not in trachea past vocal cords:*** ☐ Remove tube immediately if any doubt about proper tube placement ☐ Resume positive-pressure bag ventilations with 100% oxygen at 8 to 10 L/min ☐ Reattempt intubation; do not exceed 30 seconds on each attempt ***Correct placement of tube confirmed:*** ☐ Ventilate with tidal volume: 10 to 15 mL/kg ☐ Ventilate with rate: 10 to 15 breaths/min ☐ Ventilate with duration: 2 seconds/breath ☐ Ventilate with 100% oxygen ☐ 5-point auscultation, monitor for chest expansion

Secondary ABCD Survey (continued)		
Scene Survey Steps	**Assess: Do or Monitor**	**Manage: Do or Delegate**
Breathing (continued)	***b. With second verification techniques?*** ☐ Qualitative end-tidal CO_2 detector? ☐ Esophageal detector device? ☐ Portable chest radiograph? ***Continue to assess breathing while intubated*** ***Recognize signs of misplaced/displaced tube*** ***Recognize causes of acute deterioration in intubated patient (mnemonic):*** ☐ Displaced tube ☐ Obstructed tube ☐ Pneumothorax ☐ Equipment failure	***Secondary confirmation:*** ☐ End-tidal CO_2 monitor ☐ Esophageal detector device ☐ Chest radiograph ☐ Appropriate pulse oximetry, blood gases ☐ Insert oropharyngeal airway ☐ Insert bite protector ☐ Secure tube in place (using tape or commercial devices), noting depth marking on tube at front teeth ☐ Consider cervical spine collar and backboard if transportation is required ☐ Recognize signs of tube misplacement/displacement and complications of positive-pressure ventilation (eg, tension pneumothorax)
Circulation	***Status of circulation?*** ☐ Determine blood pressure and rate ☐ Attach ECG monitor leads ☐ Identify rhythm ☐ Check for signs of hypoperfusion and shock	***Gain IV access to circulation:*** ☐ Establish peripheral IV ☐ Provide medications and fluids as indicated by rate, blood pressure, rhythm, and clinical signs
Differential Diagnosis	***Consider possible reversible causes?*** ☐ Consider 5 H's and 5 T's mnemonic* (see Cases 4 and 5) ☐ Gather relevant patient history ☐ Order indicated lab tests	☐ Manage and treat identified reversible causes of respiratory compromise ☐ Move to indicated algorithm according to suspected cause

*Note: Advanced providers may use 6 H's by adding hypo-/hyperglycemia and 6 T's by adding trauma.

Unacceptable Actions: Perils and Pitfalls

Avoid all of the "unacceptable actions" noted below. Your instructors will watch carefully for these common errors and pitfalls and correct any unacceptable actions at once. Learners who are unfamiliar with the correct and incorrect actions may be asked to return later in the course for further instruction and practice (or remediation).

During case assessment and management, avoid these unacceptable actions. It is considered unacceptable if the ACLS learner

- Fails to adequately assess and manage a patient with the steps of the Primary and Secondary ABCD Surveys
- Fails to assess and manage a patient throughout the entire case
- Initiates treatment before assessment establishes the need for treatment (eg, starting chest compressions in a patient with a pulse or attempting to defibrillate a patient before assessment shows a shockable rhythm)
- Omits ventilations for more than 30 seconds during intubation or reassessment
- Fails to give the proper amount of supplemental oxygen through the proper airway adjunct
- Uses an inappropriate airway adjunct (eg, inserts an oropharyngeal airway in a patient with a gag reflex)
- Fails to recognize a "difficult airway" and to use alternative airway management approaches
- Fails to confirm successful tracheal tube placement using multiple clinical reference points; fails to use secondary verification methods when available
- Fails to recognize signs of a misplaced tube or displaced tube and correct immediately
- Fails to oxygenate and ventilate the patient between intubation attempts

Hazards of Aggressive Hyperventilation

Many years ago hyperventilation was routinely performed following intubation for cardiac arrest in the belief that it would help correct existing metabolic acidosis. More recent resuscitation guidelines, including the *ECC Guidelines 2000,* recommend effective ventilation and avoidance of hyperventilation. It is now clear that hyperventilation can cause complications, including relative or absolute hypocarbia and decreased cerebral blood flow. In addition, hyperventilation can result in "auto-PEEP."

Auto-PEEP is a positive pressure generated in the lung that can cause hypotension. Auto-PEEP results from air trapping and "breath stacking" (inhaled air enters the lung and is unable to escape). This sometimes, but not always, occurs during mechanical ventilation. Patients with severe asthma or exacerbations of COPD experience some obstruction to inflation and marked obstruction of exhalation.

To prevent auto-PEEP, the person responsible for ventilating the patient after intubation should be instructed before intubation to ventilate at only 6 to 8 breaths per minute to avoid auto-PEEP and its consequence, severe hypotension. Overzealous hyperventilation and auto-PEEP can cause a sudden extreme drop in blood pressure. Prevention of this problem is preferable to treatment.

Hyperventilation immediately following intubation can also cause complications other than auto-PEEP. For example, a 71-year-old man taking diuretics presents with exacerbated asthma/COPD. Blood gas measurement on 100% oxygen by mask reveals the following:

- pH 7.29
- P_{CO_2} 100 mm Hg
- P_{O_2} 164 mm Hg
- HCO_3 47 mEq/L

Clinically the patient requires tracheal intubation. After immediate tracheal intubation this patient is hyperventilated because his P_{CO_2} was so high in an effort to return this value to the normal range. The patient suddenly develops a seizure, slow pulseless electrical activity (PEA), then asystole on ECG.

This patient presented with an exacerbation of emphysema. He is also receiving long-term diuretic therapy for mild-to-moderate heart failure due to emphysema. At baseline he is chronically hypercarbic, but renal compensation restores his pH to near-normal, and long-term diuretic therapy produces a hypochloremic or hypokalemic metabolic alkalosis. Therefore, his baseline arterial blood gas measurement probably resembles the following:

- pH of 7.50
- P_{CO_2} 62 mm Hg
- P_{O_2} of 52 mm Hg
- HCO_3 of 47 mEq/L

This patient has a compensated chronic respiratory acidosis from emphysema and a superimposed mild metabolic alkalosis from the diuretics. If an arterial blood gas measurement had been obtained immediately after intubation and initial hyperventilation, the following arterial blood gas measurement would have been obtained on F_{IO_2} of 100%:

- pH 7.82
- P_{CO_2} 30 mm Hg
- P_{O_2} 224 mm Hg
- HCO_3 of 47 mEq/L

The P_{CO_2} responds promptly to hyperventilation, leaving an unopposed metabolic alkalosis caused by the high HCO_3.

This example illustrates the severe consequences that can ensue when a patient with chronic respiratory acidosis is intubated and hyperventilated: P_{CO_2} drops into the alkalotic range and in combination with the alkalotic effects of the high HCO_3, a severe respiratory and metabolic alkalosis ensues.

When patients with chronic (compensated) respiratory failure are mechanically ventilated, they should be ventilated to correct pH, *not* Pa_{CO_2}.

Workbook Review

1. If there is continued doubt about correct placement of a tube after tracheal intubation and 5-point auscultation of breath sounds, the rescuer should visually check to see that the tube passes through the ______ ______________________________.

Read more about it in the ECC Guidelines 2000, *pages 101-102: "How to Confirm Accurate Placement of Tracheal Tube: Primary Confirmation" and "How to Confirm Accurate Placement of Tracheal Tube: Secondary Confirmation"*

2. To confirm proper placement of tracheal tube or advanced airway device through 5-point auscultation, which of the following observations are appropriate? (Check all that apply.)

___ check breath sounds in the left and right lateral chest and lung bases

___ auscultate breath sounds in the left and right anterior sides of the chest

___ listen for gastric bubbling noises from the epigastrium

___ ensure equal and adequate chest expansion bilaterally

Read more about it in the ECC Guidelines 2000, *page 101: "How to Confirm Accurate Placement of Tracheal Tube: Primary Confirmation"*

3. Which of the following is true about an oropharyngeal airway?

a. it eliminates the need to position the head of the unconscious patient

b. it eliminates the possibility of an upper airway obstruction

c. it is of no value once a tracheal tube is inserted

d. it may stimulate vomiting or laryngospasm if inserted in the semiconscious patient

Read more about it in the ECC Guidelines 2000, *page 98: "Airway Adjuncts"*

4. You have just attempted tracheal intubation. You hear stomach gurgling over the epigastrium, you see no chest expansion, and you are unable to hear breath sounds on either side of the chest during hand ventilation with a bag. Pulse oximetry indicates that the hemoglobin saturation has failed to rise. Which of the following is the most likely explanation of this finding?

a. intubation of the esophagus

b. intubation of the left main bronchus

c. intubation of the right main bronchus

d. unilateral tension pneumothorax

Read more about it in the ECC Guidelines 2000, *pages 101-102: "How to Confirm Accurate Placement of Tracheal Tube: Primary Confirmation" and "How to Confirm Accurate Placement of Tracheal Tube: Secondary Confirmation"*

5. Which of the following is an indication for tracheal intubation?

a. difficulty encountered by qualified rescuers in ventilating an apneic patient with a bag-mask device

b. a respiratory rate of less than 20 breaths per minute in a patient with severe chest pain

c. the presence of premature ventricular contractions

d. to provide airway protection in a responsive patient with an adequate gag reflex

Read more about it in the ECC Guidelines 2000, *page 100: "Tracheal Intubation," right column*

6. You are treating a victim of trauma who is in shock and a deep coma. Which of the following is the airway of choice for this patient?

a. a tracheal tube

b. the patient's own airway

c. a nasopharyngeal airway

d. an oropharyngeal airway

Read more about it in the ECC Guidelines 2000, *pages 100-101: "Tracheal Intubation"; and page 245: "ACLS for Cardiac Arrest Associated with Trauma: Airway"*

7. Once a tracheal tube is inserted and the position verified (with both primary and secondary confirmation) during CPR, which of the following best describes the ventilations that should be provided?

a. an average of 12 to 15 ventilations per minute without pauses for chest compressions

b. ventilations should provide prompt hyperventilation to correct acidosis, with a pause after every fifth compression

c. ventilations should be delivered with an estimated tidal volume of 3 to 5 mL/kg

d. ventilations should be delivered with room air to avoid hyperoxygenation

Read more about it in the ECC Guidelines 2000, *page 102, top left column*

8. You are providing hand ventilations with a bag mask for a patient with no spontaneous ventilation. You are explaining the use of bag-mask ventilation to a group of new nurses and residents who are observing your technique. Which of the following statements would most accurately describe the use of bag-mask ventilation during resuscitation?

a. bag-mask ventilation can be performed effectively with minimal training and little practice

b. bag-mask ventilation will deliver nearly 100% oxygen if a reservoir with a high oxygen flow rate is used

c. bag-mask ventilation cannot be performed effectively by one person during resuscitation

d. bag-mask ventilation should not be used if the patient makes any spontaneous respiratory effort

Read more about it in the ECC Guidelines 2000, *page 95: "Bag-Valve Devices" and page 97: Figure 2, legend*

9. Which of the following is the *most important* step to restore oxygenation and ventilation for the unresponsive, breathless submersion (near-drowning) victim?

a. attempt to drain water from breathing passages by performing the Heimlich maneuver

b. begin chest compressions

c. provide cervical spine stabilization because a diving accident may have occurred

d. open the airway and begin rescue breathing as soon as possible, even in the water

Read more about it in the ECC Guidelines 2000, *pages 234-235: "Modifications to Guidelines for BLS for Resuscitation From Submersion"*

10. You have completed a tracheal intubation attempt for a patient in cardiac arrest. The tracheal tube appears to be in place after primary confirmation: you hear no stomach gurgling over the epigastrium, and breath sounds and chest expansion are equal and adequate bilaterally over the chest. You check the end-tidal CO_2 and do not detect exhaled CO_2. Which of the following actions would be appropriate at this time?

a. immediately remove the tracheal tube because the absence of exhaled CO_2 always indicates esophageal placement of the tube

b. use an esophageal detector device because low pulmonary blood flow during cardiac arrest can result in low exhaled CO_2 despite correct tracheal placement of the tube

c. check pulse oximetry and remove the tube unless the hemoglobin saturation rises above 95%

d. leave the tube in place and do not attempt further verification of tube placement because no confirmatory device is accurate for the patient in cardiac arrest

Read more about it in the ECC Guidelines 2000, *pages 101-102: "How to Confirm Accurate Placement of Tracheal Tube: Primary Confirmation" and "How to Confirm Accurate Placement of Tracheal Tube: Secondary Confirmation"*

VF Treated With CPR and Automated External Defibrillation

Description

Case 2 was developed to help the ACLS provider prepare to respond as a lone rescuer to an out-of-hospital emergency, equipped with only CPR skills and an AED.

The case scenario presents a victim who collapses from either VF or pulseless ventricular tachycardia (VT) in front of a single—or *lone*—rescuer. The only equipment available to this ACLS-trained rescuer is an AED stocked with a pocket face mask and a pair of gloves. Additional rescuers may not be available, so the ACLS provider must know how to care for the victim without assistance.

The ACLS interventions advanced airway control and intravenous medications are not options in this scenario. In the first 10 minutes of a witnessed VF arrest, the ACLS provider's initial response must be to care for the victim using only the AED and the provider's hands and lungs.

Settings and Scenarios

The ACLS Provider Course instructor will present a VF case similar to one or more of the following.

Setting: Prehospital, Unmonitored Patient

While flying on a commercial aircraft to Hawaii you hear an overhead announcement: "If you are a healthcare provider,

What's New in the Guidelines...

VF Treated With CPR and Automated External Defibrillation

To better prepare the ACLS provider for responding to a victim who has collapsed in this era of automated external defibrillators (AEDs) and public access defibrillation, Case 2 concentrates on witnessed ventricular fibrillation (VF) arrest treated by a lone rescuer using CPR and an AED.

- The *ECC Guidelines 2000* continue to strongly emphasize early defibrillation generally and the growing acceptance of AEDs specifically. The guidelines also continue to advocate the concepts of the Chain of Survival and public access defibrillation.
- Increasingly there is a strong possibility that the ACLS provider will someday face the challenge of responding as a lone rescuer in a nonmedical setting with little or no equipment.
- Important observations have come from the Las Vegas Casino Study, Chicago-O'Hare International Airport's public access defibrillation program, and American Airlines' in-flight medical emergency response plan for commercial aircraft. The results from these and other studies dramatically confirm the validity of the concepts "the earlier the better" and "CPR makes defibrillation work better."
- The *ECC Guidelines 2000* strongly support wider use of AEDs in medical centers, outpatient clinics, and individual physician's offices. The evidence reviewed for the guidelines confirms that for witnessed VF arrest, immediate bystander CPR and early use of an AED can achieve outcomes equivalent to those achieved with the full ACLS armamentarium.
- Responsible ACLS providers recognize these trends and want to be prepared to respond appropriately. The proper response requires skills in CPR and use of an AED.

please notify a flight attendant." You enter the galley and see 2 flight attendants doing chest compressions and pocket-mask ventilation on a 55-year-old man. Nearby is an unopened AED. What would you do next?

Setting: Emergency Dept, Unmonitored Patient

As an emergency medical technician (EMT), you transport a 55-year-old man with intermittent chest pain to the Emergency Department (ED) of a small community hospital. With the man lying on a stretcher, you stop at the registration desk. Suddenly the man's chest pains become severe. Just as the triage nurse arrives seeking more information, the man falls back unconscious on the stretcher. A portable AED without a monitor screen is stored beneath the stretcher. The nurse states that the ED physician has just answered a "show of force" alarm in radiology. Clearly you are expected to "do something! Don't just stand there!" What would you do next?

Setting: In-Hospital, Unmonitored Patient

You are a general floor nurse in the rehabilitation unit, which recently added an AED at each nursing station. A 55-year-old man is visiting his mother, who is a patient in the unit. Without warning, the man suddenly grabs his chest, says he is in severe pain, and crumples slowly to the floor. What would you do next?

Setting: Out-of-Hospital, Medical Office

You are a nurse working in an oral surgeon's office. A 55-year-old man has been receiving IV sedation and analgesia for a wisdom tooth extraction. He is slow to recover and resting in a postprocedure recovery area. His wife, who is sitting with him, suddenly shouts "Someone, come look at my husband! He doesn't look right!" Begin management of this case now.

Learning and Skills Objectives

At the end of Case 2 you should be able to successfully manage a patient who collapses in VF arrest using only an AED, a pair of protective gloves, and a pocket face mask. You should be able to describe

1. The initial steps to take, starting with seeing the victim collapse
2. The 1-rescuer CPR sequence, including the appropriate time to phone 911 and when to get the AED
3. The steps the lone rescuer takes in the AED sequence, beginning with the arrival of the AED at the victim's side until the device advises *"no shock indicated"*
4. How to include a second rescuer in the resuscitation attempt should one arrive on the scene
5. "Special situations" that might arise with the use of an AED and how to manage them

Specific Skills to Master

The ACLS provider must be able to demonstrate the following skills:

1. Defibrillation with an AED
2. Basic CPR skills
3. Noninvasive airway techniques, including pocket face mask, bag-mask device, oropharyngeal airway, barrier methods, and oxygen delivery systems (if not covered in Case 1)

New Rhythms to Learn

With an AED there are no rhythms for the ACLS provider to learn. The ACLS provider must answer only 2 rhythm-related questions:

1. Does the victim have a pulse?
2. Is the rhythm "shockable," ie, VF or VT?

New Drugs to Learn

There are no medications to learn in Case 2.

Major Learning Points

The ACLS provider should use the ACLS Approach. Start with the **Primary ABCD Survey.** Note that defibrillation is part of the Primary ABCD Survey. Although ACLS providers must often perform the Secondary ABCD Survey as well, this case does not cover those topics.

1. The Primary ABCD Survey: Use It in All Cases of Cardiac Arrest

The first steps in treatment of any emergency are to quickly assess responsiveness, activate the EMS system, assess the ABCs, and if indicated, start CPR. The **Primary ABCD Survey** of the ACLS Approach is the most effective way to remember these steps. Some people in apparent cardiac arrest will respond to the initial actions:

A: open the airway

B: provide ventilations

C: perform chest compressions

These first steps also identify victims with an obstructed airway, which must be cleared.

The Primary ABCD Survey keeps you from treating the patient before you have established that the patient needs treatment. For example, the ABCD Survey keeps you from attaching and operating an AED before you determine that the victim has no pulse.

For patients without a pulse, the Primary ABCD Survey makes no mention of IV access. This is intentional. Although medications provide a clinical benefit in cardiac resuscitation, they remain a distant second in the Primary ABCD Survey.

2. Noninvasive Airway Techniques, Including Mouth-to-Mouth Ventilations and Chest Compression–Only CPR

In most scenarios involving 1 rescuer with an AED, you will arrive without advanced airway support. The pocket face mask is the airway device of choice. You have your CPR skills, a pocket face mask, and the AED. In the absence of a second rescuer to perform CPR, how do you choose between the urgent need to provide airway support and the high priority of phoning 911 and getting the AED? Evidence presented at the Guidelines 2000 Conference suggested the following:

- If the AED arrives early (in less than 1 to 3 minutes*), place the highest priority on attaching the AED and delivering the first 1 to 3 shocks.
- In the absence of bystander CPR, if the AED arrives 3 or more minutes later, it may be beneficial and not harmful to provide 1 minute or more of initial CPR before stopping to attach and operate the AED.
- Otherwise, never delay defibrillation! Airway and ventilation are secondary to prompt defibrillation if defibrillation can be performed in the first minutes after arrest.
- If VF is secondary to respiratory arrest or coincides with respiratory

*ACLS has many variables (time events, time intervals, blood pressure, heart rate, rales, wheezes), many of which are "fuzzy." When making clinical decisions it is wise not to be absolute, dogmatic, or inflexible. The "less than 1 to 3 minutes" time interval for arrival of the AED is a "fuzzy" variable. Understand the point being made; do not memorize the exact amount of time.

Mouth-to-Mouth Ventilation by ACLS Providers Responding Without a Barrier or Shield Device

In the more than 40 years since the inception and teaching of CPR there have been only 15 reports of disease transmission related to CPR. No cases of transmission of HIV, hepatitis B virus, hepatitis C virus, or cytomegalovirus have been reported in the literature. Performance of mouth-to-mouth ventilation or invasive procedures, however, can result in the exchange of blood between the victim and rescuer. For this reason rescuers with a duty to provide CPR should follow precautions and guidelines such as those established by the Centers for Disease Control and Prevention and the Occupational Safety and Health Administration. These guidelines recommend the use of barriers, such as latex gloves, and manual ventilation equipment, such as a bag mask and other resuscitation masks with a valve designed to divert the victim's expired air away from the rescuer. In every other case in the ACLS Provider Course, healthcare providers are expected to provide ventilation *with* a barrier device (face shield or pocket face mask).

The training scenarios in Case 2, however, feature the "off-duty" ACLS provider. These scenarios mimic real situations. The ACLS provider may be asked to respond to a cardiopulmonary emergency in-flight, at the airport, or in the community, the neighborhood, or even the home. Healthcare providers do not always carry a pocket face mask or face shield with them. Under these conditions the provider will have to decide whether to provide mouth-to-mouth ventilation without a barrier device or to forgo ventilation and provide chest compressions only.

Mouth-to-mouth rescue breathing is a safe and effective technique that has saved many lives. Despite decades of experience indicating its safety for victims and rescuers alike, some published surveys have documented reluctance by professional and lay rescuers to perform mouth-to-mouth ventilation for unknown victims of cardiac arrest. This reluctance is related to fear of transmission of infectious disease. **If a rescuer is unwilling or unable to perform mouth-to-mouth ventilation for an adult victim, he or she should still attempt resuscitation by providing chest compressions.**

Current evidence indicates that in adult cardiac arrest the outcome of chest compressions without mouth-to-mouth ventilation is significantly better than *no resuscitation attempt*. Some evidence in animals and limited adult clinical trials suggests that positive-pressure ventilation is not essential during the initial minutes of resuscitation after adult sudden cardiac arrest. Several mechanisms may account for the effectiveness of chest compressions alone. Studies have shown that spontaneous gasping can maintain near-normal minute ventilation and arterial oxygen and carbon dioxide tensions during chest compression without ventilations. In addition, because the cardiac output generated during chest compression is only 25% of normal, there is also a reduced requirement for ventilation to maintain optimal ventilation-perfusion relationships.

The ACLS provider must make an individual decision about providing mouth-to-mouth ventilation during attempted resuscitation when a barrier device is not available. However, to avoid the need to make a choice, whenever possible the ACLS provider should carry a barrier device. In addition, pocket masks should be stored in the AED carrying case.

compromise (as is commonly the case in pediatric VF), then A and B have the highest priority. In these cases defibrillation will work only when the rescuer ensures that the airway is adequate and provides effective ventilations.

- After 3 defibrillation attempts or in cases in which respiratory arrest or compromise induces VF, manage the airway and support ventilations by
  - Using barrier devices for CPR: mouth-to-mask or bag-mask devices
  - Inserting an oropharygeal airway
  - Providing supplemental oxygen
  - Providing mouth-to-mouth ventilation (see sidebar on mouth-to-mouth ventilation)

3. The Purpose of Defibrillation

Defibrillation does not "jump start" the heart. When effective, a defibrillatory shock completely "stuns" or depolarizes the myocardium. A brief period of asystole typically follows this complete depolarization. Then cardiac automaticity can resume if sufficient stores of high-energy phosphates remain in the myocardium. This automaticity may represent resumption of normal activity by pacemaker centers of the heart. The stores of high-energy phosphates are a key variable in the response to a defibrillation attempt. A fibrillating myocardium consumes the high-energy stores at a rate faster than normal cardiac rhythms. Thus, it is critical to provide early defibrillation—before fibrillation consumes all these energy stores.

4. Know Your Defibrillator

You must know your defibrillator and be ready to use it at any time. Study the quick troubleshooting checklist supplied by most AED manufacturers. Learn to perform the daily maintenance checks (see checklist, next page), which serve as an effective review of the steps of operation as well as a means of verifying that the AED is ready for use.

Studies of alleged defibrillator "failures" reveal that operator error rather than defibrillator defect is the cause of most problems reported with defibrillators. Operators may not be experienced in using the AED, may not understand how to give proper care, or may fail to properly maintain the device with service checks and upgrades.

Whenever you attempt to use a defibrillator clinically, review the steps of operation *before* you arrive at the victim's side. If something appears to go wrong at the scene, troubleshoot the steps of operation quickly. Review each step:

1. POWER ON the AED
2. Attach electrode pads to the patient
3. Clear the patient and analyze the rhythm
4. Charge; clear the patient and deliver a shock if indicated

If the defibrillator does not immediately analyze the rhythm, give voice commands, or charge appropriately, review your actions and ensure that all connections between the AED and the victim are intact. Check the device you have before you get another AED. It will take much longer for you to locate and attach another AED than it will to troubleshoot the one you are already using.

User-Critical Steps in AED Defibrillation

In defibrillation a "user-critical step" is any step that *must* be performed by the operator for the device to function successfully. All AEDs require that the operator use the following user-critical steps:

1. Attach the electrode pads when a patient is unresponsive, breathless, and pulseless.
2. Attach the pads to the AED cables (if not already attached by the manufacturer).
3. Attach the AED cables to the AED (if not already attached by the manufacturer).
4. POWER ON the AED.
5. Clear the patient and analyze the signal for VF/VT.
6. Charge the AED if VF/VT is present (some devices charge automatically).
7. Press the SHOCK button to defibrillate.

Each of these steps is critical: if a single step is omitted or done incorrectly, a shock will not be delivered to the patient in VF. Any error at this point would mean losing the chance to save a life. Some AEDs perform some of the steps listed above. The more user-critical steps an AED performs, the fewer the chances for error. For example, some AED models power up automatically when the AED lid is opened. In some models the cables are already attached to the AED and the adhesive defibrillator pads. Some AEDs perform constant background analysis and will automatically "precharge" if VF is detected. One model has reduced the number of actions required of the operator to just 3: open the lid, attach the pads to the patient, and press the SHOCK button.

A Quick Review of AED Operation

Here is a quick review of AED operation. These steps are covered in greater detail in Appendix 1.

1. **POWER ON the AED.**
2. **Attach the AED to the patient (pads to patient, pads to cable, cable to AED).**
3. **Clear the patient and analyze the patient's rhythm with the AED.** Depending on the model, AEDs require approximately 5 to 15 seconds to analyze the rhythm. There must be no movement of the patient during analysis. To avoid the small possibility of electromagnetic field interference, do not use radios during analysis. In many devices, pressing the ANALYZE button will also charge the AED if the rhythm is VF.

CHECKLIST.

Readiness-for-Use Checklist: Automated External Defibrillators for Healthcare Providers: Daily/Weekly Checklist

Date ____________ **Covering Period** ______________ **to** ______________

Organization Name/Identifier ________________ **Mfr/Model No.** ______________________ **Serial/ID No.** ______________

At the beginning of each shift or at the scheduled time, inspect the device using the checklist below. Note any inconsistencies, deficiencies, and corrective actions taken. If the device is not ready for use or is out of service, write OOS on the "day of month" line and note deficiencies in the corrective action log.

1. Defibrillator unit
- a. Clean, no spills, unobstructed
- b. Casing intact

2. Defibrillation cables and connectors
- a. Inspect for cracks, broken wires, or damage
- b. Connectors engage securely

3. Supplies available
- a. Two sets of unexpired hands-free defibrillator pads in sealed packages
- b. PPE—gloves, barrier device, or equivalent
- c. Razor and scissors
- d. Hand towel
- e. *Spare event documentation device
- f. *ECG paper
- g. *ECG monitoring electrodes
- h. *ALS module/key/equivalent

4. Power supply
- a. Verify fully charged battery(ies) in place
- b. *Spare charged battery available
- c. *Rotate batteries per manufacturer's specifications
- d. *AC power plugged into live outlet

5. Indicators and screen display
- a. *POWER ON display and self-test OK
- b. *ECG monitor display functional
- c. *No error or service required indicator/message
- d. Correct time displayed/set; synchronized with dispatch center

6. ECG paper and event documentation device
- a. *Event documentation device in place and functional
- b. *Adequate ECG paper
- c. *ECG recorder functional

7. Charge/display cycle for defibrillation
- a. Test per manufacturer's recommended test procedure
- b. *Identifies shockable rhythm
- c. *Charges to appropriate energy level
- d. *Acceptable discharge detected

8. AED returned to patient ready status

**Applicable only if the device has this capability/feature or if required by medical authorization.*

Corrective Action Log

____

Day of Month/Signature/Unit No.

1. ____________
2. ____________
3. ____________
4. ____________
5. ____________
6. ____________
7. ____________
8. ____________
9. ____________
10. ____________
11. ____________
12. ____________
13. ____________
14. ____________
15. ____________
16. ____________
17. ____________
18. ____________
19. ____________
20. ____________
21. ____________
22. ____________
23. ____________
24. ____________
25. ____________
26. ____________
27. ____________
28. ____________
29. ____________
30. ____________
31. ____________

Example: *5. John Jones (signature)/Aid 2 checked Aid 2's device on the 5th day of this month and found it ready for use.*

4. **Clear the patient and deliver a shock if indicated: deliver *stacked shocks* if indicated.** For VF or pulseless VT, deliver up to 3 shocks in succession as close together as the analysis and charging cycles allow. The term *stacked shocks* refers to shocks delivered consecutively (one immediately after another) without performing CPR between shocks. Several AED models are programmed to deliver shocks of increasing strength (200 J, 200 to 300 J, up to 360 J). These 3 shocks are delivered in a stacked shocks sequence.

   Several AED models now available use defibrillation waveforms that differ from traditional monophasic waveforms. In most patients biphasic waveform shocks have proved to be as effective at lower current levels as monophasic waveforms. In general, AEDs that use biphasic waveforms are acceptable and appear to be equivalent despite numerous claims to the contrary by manufacturers. It is ***early*** defibrillation that increases the patient's chance of survival, regardless of whether it is *monophasic truncated exponential (TE), monophasic damped sinusoidal (DS), biphasic plain, biphasic deluxe,* or *biphasic extra special.*

5. **Always use a "clearing" chant for safety.** Operator and bystander safety is *critical* in defibrillation. The person who presses the SHOCK button is responsible for ensuring that no one is touching the victim when a defibrillatory shock is provided. See the sidebar "A Clearing Chant for Defibrillation Safety."

A Clearing Chant for Defibrillation Safety

To ensure the safety of conventional or automated defibrillation, the defibrillator operator must always announce when he or she is about to deliver a defibrillatory shock. The person who is operating the defibrillator should state a "warning chant" firmly and in a forceful voice before each shock. For example,

- "I am going to shock on three. One, I am clear." (The operator checks and makes sure he or she has no contact with the patient, the stretcher, or other equipment.)
- *"Two, you are clear."* (The operator checks to see that no one is touching the patient, including providers who are doing chest compressions, starting IVs, inserting catheters, or performing ventilation and airway maintenance.)

  The operator should make sure that all personnel step away from the patient, remove their hands from the patient, and end contact with any device or object touching the patient. This clearing should also include any personnel in indirect contact with the patient, such as the therapist holding a ventilation bag attached to a tracheal tube. The person responsible for airway support and ventilation should ensure that oxygen is not openly flowing around the electrode pads or paddles.
- *"Three, everybody is clear."* (The operator makes a visual check to ensure that no one else has contact with the patient or stretcher.)

The person operating the defibrillator need not use these exact words but must warn others that he or she is about to deliver defibrillation shocks and that everyone needs to stand clear.

A Walk Through the AED Treatment Algorithm

This case does not take a step-by-step walk through the AED Treatment Algorithm. These steps are already presented in detail in Appendix 1. Take several minutes to review the algorithm and details in the Appendix. Then review the critical action checklist that follows. Educators have established that repetitive mental "review" or "rehearsal" is a powerful learning technique, even for tasks that require psychomotor skills.

Critical Actions: Assessment and Management

The critical actions checklist presents the critical actions that the lone rescuer with an AED must take to treat a person in VF or pulseless VT. The checklist is keyed to the standard BLS sequence and the Primary ABCD Survey. Review the checklist until you understand the order and rationale for all the steps.

Critical Concepts: Special Situations in AED Use

ACLS instructors may refer to a variety of special situations that can be encountered during AED use. New information presented in the *ECC Guidelines 2000* provides more clarity on how to respond to these scenarios.

1. **Children under 8 years of age:** AED technology has changed rapidly since *ECC Guidelines 2000* was published. Several manufacturers now have been cleared by the FDA to market AEDs that accommodate both adult electrode pads and pediatric cable-pad systems that attenuate the delivered energy to a dose more appropriate for children under the age of 8 years.

   After evaluation of the evidence, the AHA and the International Liaison Committee on Resuscitation (ILCOR) revised the *ECC Guidelines 2000* recommendations for use of AEDs in children under the age of 8 years as follows:

   - AEDs may be used for children 1 to 8 years of age with no signs of circulation (Class IIb). Ideally the device should deliver a child dose and should demonstrate high specificity for pediatric shockable rhythms (using **child** pads).
   - Currently there is insufficient evidence to recommend for or against the use of AEDs in infants <1 year of age.
   - For a single rescuer responding to a child without signs of circulation, 1 minute of CPR is recommended before any other action, such as activating EMS or attaching an AED.
   - Defibrillation is recommended for documented VF/pulseless VT (Class I).
   - Rescuers should *not* use child pads for any victim 8 years of age or older.

   Refer to the AHA website for the full text (**www.americanheart.org/cpr**).

2. **Victim lying in water:** Before publication of the *ECC Guidelines 2000,* EMS personnel were advised to *"avoid shocking a victim who is lying in water or on a wet surface, as it may cause burns or shocks to the rescuers."* Realistically the chances of a rescuer receiving a significant shock are negligible, even if the victim is lying on a wet surface and the rescuer is standing on the same wet surface. If the surface of the chest is extremely wet, the current may arc from one electrode pad to the other, reducing the effectiveness of shock delivery to the heart. If the victim is immersed in water or water is on the victim's chest, do not attempt defibrillation until first removing the victim from the water and then drying the chest quickly.

   Recommmendations

   - Remove the victim from water before defibrillation. Drag the victim gently by the arms or legs or on a blanket or towel.
   - Dry the victim's chest quickly before attaching the AED.

3. **Implanted pacemakers or defibrillators:** These devices create a hard lump beneath the skin of the upper chest or abdomen (usually on the victim's left side). The lump or scar is often clearly visible or can be felt. An implanted pacemaker is about half the size of a deck of cards. Placing an AED electrode pad directly over an implanted medical device may reduce the effectiveness of defibrillation.

   Recommendation:

   - Do not place an AED electrode pad directly over an implanted device.
   - Place an AED electrode pad at least 1 inch to the side of an implanted device.

4. **Transdermal medication patches*:** Placing an AED electrode pad on top of a transdermal medication patch may decrease the energy delivered by a shock, making it less effective.

   Recommendation:

   Remove the patch and wipe the area clean before attaching the AED or monitor electrodes.

5. **Victim lying on or in contact with metal surfaces:** Before publication of the *ECC Guidelines 2000,* EMS personnel were advised to *"avoid shocking a victim who is lying on a metal surface."* Even though metal conducts electric current, the risk of injury to a rescuer by this mechanism is so insignificant that operator shock is more a theory than a reality. This issue has been removed from the list of special resuscitation situations in the ECC guidelines and educational materials.

   Recommendation:

   Proceed with the AED treatment protocols. It is unnecessary to move the victim from a metal surface.

---

*Apocryphal stories abound about nitroglycerin ointment applied to the skin and then covered with a paper, plastic, or metal (legend-only) backing. Will a gap between defibrillator pads/paddles and the nitroglycerin-covered skin produce a spark during defibrillatory shocks that will cause the nitroglycerin to explode? Only in legends!

AED Treatment Algorithm for Emergency Cardiovascular Care Pending Arrival of Emergency Medical Personnel.

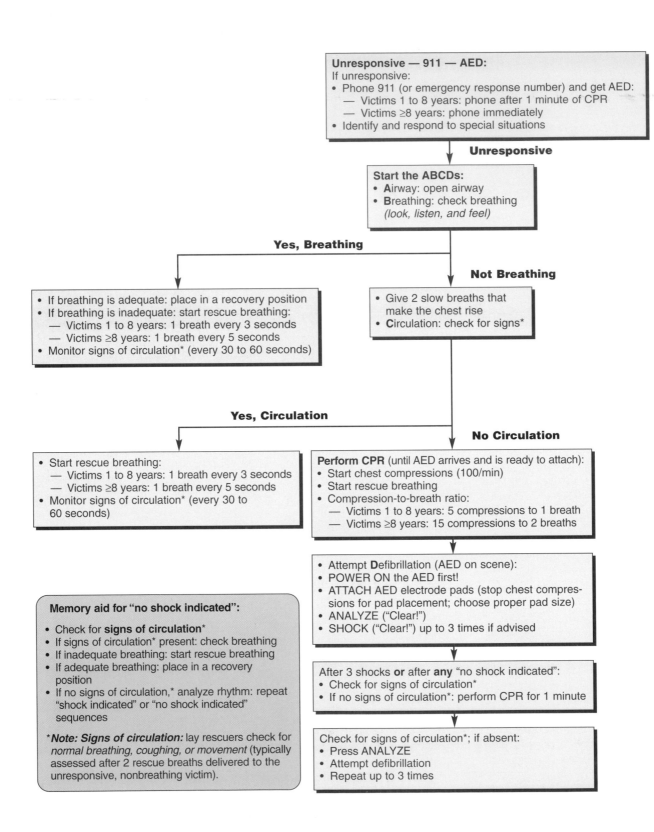

Unresponsive — 911 — AED:
If unresponsive:
- Phone 911 (or emergency response number) and get AED:
  - — Victims 1 to 8 years: phone after 1 minute of CPR
  - — Victims ≥8 years: phone immediately
- Identify and respond to special situations

Unresponsive

Start the ABCDs:
- **A**irway: open airway
- **B**reathing: check breathing *(look, listen, and feel)*

Yes, Breathing

- If breathing is adequate: place in a recovery position
- If breathing is inadequate: start rescue breathing:
  - — Victims 1 to 8 years: 1 breath every 3 seconds
  - — Victims ≥8 years: 1 breath every 5 seconds
- Monitor signs of circulation* (every 30 to 60 seconds)

Not Breathing

- Give 2 slow breaths that make the chest rise
- **C**irculation: check for signs*

Yes, Circulation

- Start rescue breathing:
  - — Victims 1 to 8 years: 1 breath every 3 seconds
  - — Victims ≥8 years: 1 breath every 5 seconds
- Monitor signs of circulation* (every 30 to 60 seconds)

No Circulation

Perform CPR (until AED arrives and is ready to attach):
- Start chest compressions (100/min)
- Start rescue breathing
- Compression-to-breath ratio:
  - — Victims 1 to 8 years: 5 compressions to 1 breath
  - — Victims ≥8 years: 15 compressions to 2 breaths

- Attempt **D**efibrillation (AED on scene):
- POWER ON the AED first!
- ATTACH AED electrode pads (stop chest compressions for pad placement; choose proper pad size)
- ANALYZE ("Clear!")
- SHOCK ("Clear!") up to 3 times if advised

After 3 shocks **or** after **any** "no shock indicated":
- Check for signs of circulation*
- If no signs of circulation*: perform CPR for 1 minute

Check for signs of circulation*; if absent:
- Press ANALYZE
- Attempt defibrillation
- Repeat up to 3 times

Memory aid for "no shock indicated":

- Check for **signs of circulation***
- If signs of circulation* present: check breathing
- If inadequate breathing: start rescue breathing
- If adequate breathing: place in a recovery position
- If no signs of circulation,* analyze rhythm: repeat "shock indicated" or "no shock indicated" sequences

**Note: Signs of circulation:* lay rescuers check for *normal breathing, coughing, or movement* (typically assessed after 2 rescue breaths delivered to the unresponsive, nonbreathing victim).

Critical Actions Checklist: ACLS Case 2
VF Treated With CPR and AED

Scene Survey Steps	Assess: Do or Monitor	Manage: Do or Delegate
Recognize the emergency and respond. *Note: Specific details on assessment and management vary, based on the setting (in-hospital or out of hospital) and number (1 or 2) of rescuers present.*	***Responsive?*** ☐ Check for danger to rescuers ☐ Check for risk of spinal trauma ☐ Shake and shout; touch and talk	***Unresponsive?*** ☐ Shout for help ☐ If alone, phone 911; activate EMS ☐ Get AED ☐ Position victim, AED appropriately ☐ Position self (rescuer)
Start the Primary ABCD Survey/Follow the AED Algorithm		
Airway	***Mouth and upper airway clear and in position for ventilation?*** ☐ Look in mouth	***Contents in mouth; airway appears blocked?*** ☐ Put on protective gloves ☐ Perform a finger sweep ☐ Perform a head tilt–chin lift or jaw thrust
Breathing	***Check for breathing:*** ☐ Look ☐ Listen ☐ Feel	***No spontaneous air movement:*** ☐ Apply barrier device/face shield ☐ Apply appropriate noninvasive airway device
Circulation	***Pulse?*** ☐ Check for a pulse	***No pulse:*** ☐ Start basic CPR if an AED is unavailable ☐ When an AED is available, attach electrodes
Defibrillation	***Rhythm?*** ☐ Assess using "analyze" mode	***VF or pulseless VT:*** ☐ Analyze: "hunt for VF" ☐ Deliver shock (if VF) <90 seconds after AED becomes available ☐ Use all safety precautions for defibrillation ☐ Follow "analyze-shock" sequence and shock as indicated by AED ☐ Perform 1 minute of CPR after every 3 shocks ***"No shock indicated" signal:*** ☐ Check breathing, check pulse ☐ As indicated, either resume CPR, place in recovery position, or provide rescue breaths ☐ Reanalyze every 3 to 5 minutes or when indicated by AED

Unacceptable Actions: Perils and Pitfalls

The following actions contribute to complications or poor patient outcome. The instructor should immediately identify and correct these actions. Unacceptable actions include

1. Inability to satisfactorily complete the Heartsaver AED skills checklist
2. *Errors in defibrillator maintenance:* arriving on the scene with a nonfunctioning AED due to battery failure, inadequate maintenance, or failure to use the AHA-FDA–recommended daily readiness-for-use checks
3. *Errors in defibrillator operation:* failure to make proper cable and electrode connections, malposition of the adhesive defibrillator pads, pressing the SHOCK button without pressing the ANALYZE button, not pressing SHOCK when indicated, and returning frequently to the ANALYZE-SHOCK sequence
4. *Errors in defibrillation safety:* for example, not "clearing" the patient before pressing the SHOCK button
5. *Sequencing errors:* for example, performing CPR for several minutes before attempting to assess for VF/VT
6. Failing to check for a pulse after a series of 3 defibrillatory shocks

Read More About It

For in-depth information on the topics covered in this case please see the following:

- The *ECC Guidelines 2000:*
  - Part 4: The Automated External Defibrillator: Key Link in the Chain of Survival, pages 60-76
  - Part 6: Section 2: Defibrillation, pages 90-94

Workbook Review

1. Which of the following choices lists *in correct order* the major steps of CPR and AED operation for an unresponsive victim?

a. send someone to phone 911, check for a pulse, attach the AED electrode pads, open the airway, provide 2 breaths if needed, then turn on the AED

b. wait for the AED and barrier device to arrive, then open the airway, provide 2 breaths if needed, check for a pulse, and if no pulse is present, attach the AED and follow the sequence of AED prompts

c. send someone to phone 911 and get the AED, open the airway, provide 2 breaths if needed, check for a pulse, and if no pulse is present, attach the AED and follow the sequence of AED prompts

d. provide 2 breaths, check for a pulse, call for the AED, provide chest compressions until the AED arrives, attach the AED

Read more about it in the ECC Guidelines 2000, *page 67: Figure 4: The AED Treatment Algorithm*

2. In correct order, what are the 4 "universal steps" required to operate an AED?

a. POWER ON the AED, attach the AED to the victim, analyze the rhythm, deliver a shock if indicated

b. attach the AED to the victim, POWER ON the AED, analyze the rhythm, deliver a shock if indicated

c. attach the electrode pads to the victim, attach the electronic cables to the AED, POWER ON the AED, analyze the rhythm, deliver a shock if indicated

d. POWER ON the AED, attach the AED to the victim, deliver the first shock, analyze the rhythm

Read more about it in the ECC Guidelines 2000, *page 65: "The Universal AED: Common Steps to Operate All AEDs"*

3. A 12-year-old child collapses in a crowded museum. A museum employee is first on the scene and has an AED. She finds the victim unresponsive, so she immediately tells a bystander to activate EMS. The victim is not breathing, so the employee delivers 2 rescue breaths, checks for signs of circulation, and finds none. Next she POWERS ON the AED and attaches it correctly to the victim. She "clears" the victim and the AED analyzes the rhythm. The AED advises a shock, and the employee clears the victim and delivers a shock. What should the employee do next?

a. immediately give 2 rescue breaths to provide oxygen to the circulation

b. allow the AED to analyze the rhythm and deliver a shock up to 2 more times

c. provide chest compressions for approximately 1 minute

d. check for signs of circulation; if signs of circulation are present, begin rescue breathing

Read more about it in the ECC Guidelines 2000, *page 66: top left paragraph*

4. You respond with 2 other rescuers to a 50-year-old man who is unresponsive, pulseless, and not breathing. What tasks would you assign the other rescuers while you set up the AED?

a. one rescuer should phone 911 and the other rescuer should begin CPR

b. both rescuers should help set up the AED and provide CPR

c. one rescuer should open the airway and begin rescue breathing, and the second rescuer should begin chest compressions

d. recruit additional first responders to help

Read more about it in the ECC Guidelines 2000, *page 66: "Integration of CPR and AED Use"; and page 67: Figure 4: The AED Treatment Algorithm*

5. You are participating in the attempted resuscitation of a man who collapsed in the airport. You are operating the AED. After 3 successive shocks the victim is still pulseless. What should you do next?

a. resume delivering shocks immediately

b. do not attempt to shock again until EMS personnel arrive

c. perform CPR for 1 minute and reanalyze the victim's rhythm

d. remove the AED and transport the victim to the ED

Read more about it in the ECC Guidelines 2000, *pages 65-66: "Step 4: Clear the victim and press the SHOCK button"*

6. You attach an AED to a 43-year-old victim who is pulseless and not breathing, and the AED advises *"no shock indicated."* What should you do?

a. reanalyze immediately

b. perform CPR for 1 minute and reanalyze

c. perform CPR until EMS personnel arrive

d. remove the AED

Read more about it in the ECC Guidelines 2000, *page 66: "'No Shock Indicated' Message"*

7. An AED hangs on the wall in the radiology suite where you work. Suddenly a code is called. You grab the AED and run to the room where the resuscitation attempt is ongoing. A colleague has begun CPR and confirms that the patient is in pulseless arrest. As you begin to attach the AED to the victim, you see a transdermal medication patch on the victim's upper right chest, precisely where you were going to place an AED electrode pad. What is your most appropriate *next* action?

a. ignore the medication patch and place the electrode pad in the usual position

b. avoid the medication patch and place the second electrode pad on the victim's back

c. remove the medication patch, wipe the area dry, and place the electrode pad in the correct position

d. place the electrode pad on the victim's right abdomen

Read more about it in the ECC Guidelines 2000, *pages 64-65: "Transdermal Medications"*

✵VF/Pulseless VT: Persistent/Refractory/ Recurrent/Shock Resistant

Description

The cases for refractory VF/pulseless VT focus on assessment and management of *witnessed* cardiac arrest due to *VF or pulseless VT* that is *resistant* (unresponsive) to the first set of defibrillation shocks. In the Case 2 scenarios you successfully treated witnessed VF/pulseless VT with CPR and defibrillation shocks from an AED (the patient regained a perfusing rhythm). In the Case 3 scenarios you will use all of the ACLS interventions, including advanced airway techniques and IV medications. Case 3 teaches the ACLS provider to integrate the following interventions:

- CPR
- Rhythm recognition (shockable rhythms versus nonshockable rhythms)
- Conventional defibrillation
- Advanced airway interventions
- IV access
- Resuscitation pharmacology

Settings and Scenarios

In Case 3 the ACLS instructors will present a victim who experiences sudden VF in one or more of the following scenarios:

What's New in the Guidelines...

VF/Pulseless VT: Persistent/ Refractory/Recurrent/Shock Resistant

In the treatment of ventricular fibrillation (VF), the *ECC Guidelines 2000* revise existing perspectives, add new recommendations, and alter old guidelines. The title itself reflects an altered perspective on VF. Patients in VF who fail to respond to the initial 3 shocks fall quickly into several categories requiring advanced airway interventions, multiple IV medications, and thoughtful diagnostic consideration. Their course becomes complicated because VF may persist after the first 3 shocks ("shock-resistant"); VF may be continuous despite *all* interventions ("persistent" or "refractory"); or VF may disappear briefly after shocks or medications and then reappear ("recurrent"). The promise that new antiarrhythmic agents may provide better survival rates when given for one or more of these subtypes has not yet been realized. The hope, if not promise, remains.

- Newly available defibrillators (conventional and automated) that deliver defibrillatory shocks using biphasic waveforms are acceptable.
- Clinical researchers have not demonstrated that any waveform or current-delivery pattern is superior to any others in out-of-hospital transthoracic defibrillation.
- The new airway devices and techniques discussed in Case 1 (secondary confirmation of proper tracheal tube placement, techniques to prevent tube dislodgment, alternative advanced airway devices) apply equally to Case 3, the patient in VF.
- Vasopressin, a vasoactive agent new to these guidelines, appears acceptable and equal in efficaciousness to epinephrine for VF arrest.
- The VF guidelines recommend "consider antiarrhythmics" if a patient remains in VF after 3 attempts at defibrillation. Amiodarone has been added to the list of antiarrhythmics to consider, having received support from a randomized, controlled clinical trial in the out-of-hospital setting.
- Bretylium has been removed from the list of "antiarrhythmics to consider."

(Continued on next page)

Setting: Prehospital, Unmonitored Patient

A 60-year-old woman collapses while cleaning her empty hot tub. A neighbor witnesses the event and phones 911, and her son, a local lifeguard, performs CPR. An EMS unit of 2 paramedics arrives within 4 minutes after the 911 call. How should they manage the patient?

Setting: Emergency Dept, Unmonitored Patient

A 60-year-old electrocardiography technician collapses in the Emergency Department while attaching a 12-lead ECG to a patient. The technician had not complained of discomfort before her collapse. A laboratory technician begins CPR immediately. Describe how you would direct the management of this patient.

Setting: In-Hospital, Unmonitored Patient

A 60-year-old woman who underwent a cholecystectomy 24 hours earlier complains of increased abdominal pain. When the nurse leaves the room to consult a physician, the patient presses her call button again. The doctor enters a few minutes later and finds her lying in bed unconscious and unresponsive. Describe what the doctor should do immediately. How should she direct the other rescuers as they enter the room?

Setting: Critical Care Unit, Monitored Patient

A 60-year-old woman is admitted to the CCU from the ED. She has been complaining of severe chest pain that is unrelieved by nitroglycerin. She notices an increase in her pain, and the ECG monitor alarm sounds. The patient crumples back on the bed unconscious and unresponsive. The bedside ECG monitor shows VF.

- The role of procainamide for recurrent or intermittent VF has been better defined. "Hot" VF patients, those patients who convert from VF to a perfusing rhythm for short periods of time, appear to benefit from "procainamide loading" during their inter-VF periods. Loading may require several minutes.
- Late in 2000 data published the same month as the *ECC Guidelines 2000* indicated that patients with "hot VF," or so-called "electric-storm" victims, do better with administration of β-blockers during the period of intermittent VF than with standard ACLS VF guidelines. The *ECC Guidelines 2000* experts could not address this specific recommendation before publication deadlines. The ECC evidence-based process, now well established, is being applied constantly to such new developments in resuscitation. Any new recommendation will be communicated to the training network.

Learning and Skills Objectives

At the end of Case 3 you should be able to

- Describe the steps of the **ACLS Approach.** Describe the *Primary ABCD Survey* used to assess and guide initial treatment (CPR and initial defibrillation shocks) for an unresponsive, breathless, and pulseless victim.
- Describe how, after unsuccessful attempts at defibrillation, you immediately apply the *Secondary ABCD Survey* and provide advanced management of the airway, effective ventilation, continued chest compressions, and appropriate IV drugs—all integrated with repeated attempts to defibrillate.
- Discuss the merits of antiarrhythmics versus electricity (shocks) for treatment of persistent, refractory VF.
- Describe the best overall approach to take with each of the following postresuscitation problems that patients may demonstrate immediately after a cardiac arrest:
  - — Hypotension
  - — Recurrent VF/pulseless VT in the postresuscitation period
  - — Postresuscitation tachycardia
  - — Postresuscitation bradycardia
  - — Postresuscitation premature ventricular contractions

New Skills to Learn

At the end of Case 3 you should be able to demonstrate

- Correct attachment of ECG monitor leads (this is also discussed in Case 2)
- Defibrillation with a conventional defibrillator
- How to administer medications by tracheal tube
- IV access to deliver fluids and medications
- Providing direction to a resuscitation team with multiple available interventions

New Rhythms to Learn

At the end of Case 3 you should be able to recognize

- VF
- VT
- ECG artifact that looks like VF

New Drugs to Learn

At the end of Case 3 you should be able to describe the general indications, contraindications, and dosages (as presented in the *ECC Guidelines 2000* and the *ECC Handbook*) of the following medications used for persistent VF/pulseless VT:

- Epinephrine
- Vasopressin
- Amiodarone
- Lidocaine
- Magnesium sulfate
- Procainamide
- Sodium bicarbonate

A Walk Through the VF/Pulseless VT Algorithm

Overview

The Ventricular Fibrillation/Pulseless Ventricular Tachycardia Algorithm is the most important algorithm to know for adult resuscitation. Most people who collapse in cardiac arrest are in VF. Rapid treatment according to the VF/pulseless VT algorithm provides the best scientific approach to restore spontaneous circulation.

Pulseless VT is included in the algorithm because it is electrical activity gone awry—just like VF—leading to ineffective circulation of the blood to the brain, heart, and other vital organs. Pulseless VT is also treated with defibrillatory shocks—just like VF.

Box 1: The Primary ABCD Survey

The first steps in this algorithm are the same as those to respond to any potential cardiorespiratory emergency:

- Ensure rescuer and victim safety
- Assess responsiveness
- "Phone fast"
- Position the victim
- Position yourself as the rescuer

Ventricular Fibrillation/Pulseless Ventricular Tachycardia Algorithm.

1

Primary ABCD Survey
Focus: *basic CPR and defibrillation*
- **Check** responsiveness
- **Activate** emergency response system
- **Call** for defibrillator

A **Airway:** open the airway
B **Breathing:** provide positive-pressure ventilations
C **Circulation:** give chest compressions
D **Defibrillation:** assess for and shock VF/pulseless VT, up to 3 times (200 J, 200 to 300 J, 360 J, or equivalent *biphasic*) if necessary

↓

2

Rhythm after first 3 shocks?

↓

3

Persistent or recurrent VF/VT

↓

4

Secondary ABCD Survey
Focus: *more advanced assessments and treatments*

A **Airway:** place airway device as soon as possible
B **Breathing:** confirm airway device placement by exam plus confirmation device
B **Breathing:** secure airway device; purpose-made tube holders preferred
B **Breathing:** confirm effective oxygenation and ventilation
C **Circulation:** establish IV access
C **Circulation:** identify rhythm → monitor
C **Circulation:** administer drugs appropriate for rhythm and condition
D **Differential Diagnosis:** search for and treat identified reversible causes

↓

5

- ***Epinephrine*** 1 mg IV push, repeat every 3 to 5 minutes
or
- ***Vasopressin*** 40 U IV, **single dose**, 1 time only

↓

6

Resume attempts to defibrillate
1 × 360 J (or equivalent *biphasic*) within 30 to 60 seconds

↓

7

Consider antiarrhythmics:
- ***Amiodarone*** (IIb for persistent or recurrent VF/pulseless VT)
- ***Lidocaine*** (Indeterminate for persistent or recurrent VF/pulseless VT)
- ***Magnesium*** (IIb if known hypomagnesemic state)
- ***Procainamide*** (Indeterminate for persistent VF/pulseless VT; IIb for recurrent VF/pulseless VT)

↓

8

Resume attempts to defibrillate

Primary ABCD Survey
Focus: *basic CPR and defibrillation*

- **Check** responsiveness
- **Activate** emergency response system
- **Call** for defibrillator

A **Airway:** open the airway
B **Breathing:** provide positive-pressure ventilations
C **Circulation:** give chest compressions
D **Defibrillation:** assess for and shock VF/pulseless VT, up to 3 times (200 J, 200 to 300 J, 360 J, or equivalent *biphasic*) if necessary

Box 1 contains the all-important **Primary ABCD Survey:**

- Check the ABCs
- Perform CPR until the defibrillator is attached for defibrillation
- Assess the rhythm (look for VF)
- If VF persists deliver—in a close sequence—up to 3 defibrillatory shocks if needed:
  - — Shock 1: 200 J
  - — Shock 2: 200 to 300 J
  - — Shock 3: up to 360 J

Does the Emperor of ACLS Have No Clothes?

The VF/VT algorithm incorporates many important ACLS interventions, including the challenges of advanced airway control and establishing IV access and selecting appropriate medications and doses from an expanding list of options. It should be acknowledged that of the total number of people who survive after treatment for VF cardiac arrest, 85% to 90% have regained spontaneous circulation by this point in the algorithm, needing only CPR and 1 to 3 shocks.

The estimated cumulative percentage response of all survivors to each of the first 3 shocks is as follows: after the first shock, approximately 60%; after the second shock, approximately 80%; and after the third shock, approximately 90%. These facts should not elicit the reaction *"Then why are we learning so much advanced therapy, applied later in the Secondary ABCD Survey?"*[1] Instead the reaction should be a sharper understanding of why the AHA emphasizes the importance of basic CPR and early defibrillation and why the ACLS Provider Course requires demonstration of satisfactory skills in CPR and use of an AED.

[1]Another example of Pareto's 80%/20% rule: *80% of the work yields 20% of the outcome.*

Whatever Happened to the Precordial Thump?

- The precordial thump is an acceptable intervention (Class IIb) for healthcare providers to use for a *witnessed arrest* when the victim has no pulse and no defibrillator is immediately available.
- A forceful precordial thump can convert patients from VF/pulseless VT into a perfusing cardiac rhythm. However, it can also convert patients from coordinated cardiac activity into VF/pulseless VT or asystole.
- The *1986 ECC Guidelines* recommended the precordial thump when a defibrillator/monitor *was available* to use if the thump converted the patient from VF/VT into asystole, which was generally considered a deterioration rather than an improvement. Publications from the 1970s and 1980s suggested that the thump would rarely have any effect, although it looks good in the movies and on television. When a thump was associated with a change in rhythm, the probability of a post-thump perfusing rhythm was balanced by an equal probability of asystole.
- The *1992 ECC Guidelines* recommended the opposite approach: use the precordial thump only when a defibrillator/monitor is *not* available. The rationale was that a thump may help a victim in VF and there is no alternative way to convert the arrhythmia. Post-thump asystole was arguably no worse than VF without a defibrillator available.
- If a defibrillator/monitor *is* available, it makes sense to go directly to rhythm assessment and defibrillation as indicated rather than engage in thumping.
- Experts involved with the *ECC Guidelines 2000* attempted an evidence-based review of the precordial thump only to find a dearth of acceptable evidence, with very little published after the 1980s. Searches of online medical databases do reveal a fascinating potpourri of bizarre case reports. Reports of death due to unplanned "mechanical stimulation to the chest" by a variety of methods appears to be balanced against a number of less macabre reports in which the precordial thump saved someone who suffered unexpected onset of VF/pulseless VT without immediate access to a defibrillator.
- The astute ACLS provider will have noted that the precordial thump is included in the ILCOR Universal/International ACLS Algorithm (Figure 1 in the *ECC Handbook*). Resuscitation experts in Europe and elsewhere around the world consider the precordial thump to be of value on rare occasions, with a more than acceptable risk profile.
- The AHA accepts the use of precordial thumps only by healthcare professionals, not lay rescuers. The thump is not taught by the AHA as part of either the BLS or ACLS course.

Therefore, before moving to the *Secondary ABCD Survey,* this *walk-through-the-VF/pulseless VT algorithm* provides details on the **D (Defibrillation)** of the **Primary ABCD Survey.**

Identifying VF/Pulseless VT With a Conventional Defibrillator/Monitor

When using a conventional defibrillator/monitor in an advanced treatment setting, the first action after the **ABCs** of CPR is to analyze the cardiac rhythm with the defibrillator/monitor. A "quick-look" feature is present in virtually every contemporary conventional defibrillator. With this feature the operator places the defibrillation paddles on the chest to serve as monitor electrodes. This feature provides the quickest way to assess for and shock VF/VT. It is acceptable, however, to forego *through-the-paddles assessment* and first attach the 3-lead monitor cables. The monitor cables have several advantages over quick-look paddle defibrillation, but their use delays the first shock by 20 to 30 seconds. Once you identify VF/pulseless VT, *immediately* start the defibrillation sequence (details provided in Chapter 3 and Appendix 1).

Where to Place the 3 Monitor Leads

The 3 monitor leads are conspicuously colored white, red, green (or brown, the color of earth or ground). Here is a suggested memory aid for where to attach the leads on the patient:

- *WHITE lead goes to RIGHT:* right side of the chest, just beneath the right clavicle
- *RED lead goes to RIBS:* left mid-axillary line, below the expected point of maximum impulse of the heart
- *LEFT-OVER goes to the LEFT SHOULDER:* left side of the torso, just beneath the distal end of the left clavicle
- Say it fast: *"WHITE-to-RIGHT"*
  "RED-to-RIBS"
  "LEFT-OVER to the LEFT SHOULDER"

Identifying VF/Pulseless VT With an AED

The AED is a computerized defibrillator that can analyze cardiac rhythm, charge to the appropriate shock energy level, and provide the rescuer with voice prompts to guide actions.

- AEDs provide excellent visual clues to defibrillation pad placement: the pads themselves are color-coded and imprinted with illustrations for proper placement.
- Follow the visual (flashing or glowing red or yellow lights), auditory (voice chips in the AED), and printed instructions from the AED to analyze the rhythm and then deliver a shock to the patient (see Case 2 and Appendix 1).
- If defibrillation is unsuccessful, move to the **Secondary ABCD Survey** (and the VF/pulseless VT algorithm) if the necessary equipment, drugs, and personnel are available.
- The Secondary ABCD Survey is activated when rescuers and victims arrive at the ED (for EMS responders) or when the code team has reached the hospitalized patient or when an ACLS-trained emergency response team has reached a patient in the out-of-hospital setting.

Sequential/Escalating/Stacked Shocks

As long as VF/VT persists, attempts to defibrillate must continue. Emergency personnel quote an axiom "never call the

Waveforms and Energy Levels: Biphasic vs Monophasic and Fixed Current vs Escalating Current

Some biphasic waveform-based AEDs deliver shocks at a fixed current level, eg, 200 J. Other devices allow the operators to escalate the current, ranging from less than 200 J to more than 360 J.

Biphasic waveform transthoracic defibrillators that do *not* escalate the current between the first and second and between the second and third shocks raise important questions.

Manufacturers and some researchers allege that low-energy, fixed-current, biphasic waveform devices cause less damage to the myocardium than escalating-current, monophasic waveform defibrillators. However, no convincing clinical evidence has confirmed that one waveform or current level is more or less damaging than another.

Escalating-current devices are alleged to produce more "saves" because the higher current defibrillates patients who are not defibrillated with lower-energy shocks. However, for reasons that are not clear, nonescalating biphasic waveform defibrillators have been consistently more successful than monophasic defibrillators in first-shock defibrillation rates and defibrillation with 3 or fewer shocks, both in-hospital and out of hospital.

The AHA strongly supports all efforts to bring early defibrillation to patients in VF. In 2001 it is recognized that all commercially available defibrillators save lives. These devices have an almost miraculous capability of resuscitating people from clinical death. But is one waveform type clinically and significantly superior to another? Does having a range of energy capabilities produce differences in outcomes?

The AHA considers defibrillators using different types of defibrillation waveforms, with or without changing current levels, equally acceptable. All types are definitely effective but probably not equivalently effective. By the year 2000 the medical device industry, in international collaboration with clinical researchers, had not yet published convincing human evidence that any specific combination of waveform plus current levels is superior to another.

Clearing Chant for Defibrillation

This is a short review of the "clearing chant" presented in Case 2. Defibrillator operators must always announce when they are about to deliver a shock to a patient. The person who controls the defibrillator should state firmly and in a forceful voice a "warning chant" before each shock. This gives everyone in contact with the patient time to step back and end contact with the patient, the bed, and any equipment that may be touching the patient. The warning chant should be clear to everyone. The following is an example of a chant that may be used:

- *"I am going to shock on three. One, I am clear."* (The operator checks and makes sure he or she has no contact with the patient, the stretcher, or other equipment.)
- *"Two, you are clear."* (The operator checks personnel doing ventilations and chest compressions, who should remove their hands from the ventilatory adjuncts, including the tracheal tube and other advanced airway devices and ventilation bags. Operator considers turning the oxygen off or directing the flow away from patient's chest.)
- *"Three, everybody is clear."* (The operator makes a visual check to ensure that no one else has con-

Pulse Checks Between Shocks

During a stacked-shock sequence, do not pause to check the pulse if a properly connected monitor clearly displays persistent VF/pulseless VT. Push the charge control button as soon as the first and second shocks are delivered. Look immediately at the monitor screen (while the defibrillator is recharging) to check for persistent VF/pulseless VT. If a rhythm other than VF/pulseless VT appears on the monitor, remove the paddles from the chest (leave adhesive pads in place), disarm the charged defibrillator, and check for a pulse.

code on a patient in VF," meaning that as long as the myocardium has the energy to produce VF, it has the energy to produce a perfusing rhythm. A resuscitation attempt can be terminated after return of spontaneous circulation or persistent asystole but not while VF is present.

The default scenario in the ACLS case-based teaching course is persistent, refractory VF that continues without conversion through many "rounds of shocks and medications." This case assumes that defibrillation (successful conversion of VF to a perfusing rhythm or any other rhythm) does not occur. The first *set* of defibrillatory shocks consists of 1, 2, or 3 shocks of increasing current, delivered *sequentially*. The rescuer pauses between shocks only to check the monitor screen to determine if VF persists as the postshock rhythm.

Three sequential shocks are delivered in a so-called "stacked shocks" sequence, with *escalating* current levels for the second shock (200 to 300 J) and the third shock (360 J). If a second rescuer is available to operate the defibrillator control buttons, the defibrillator operator should leave the paddles pressed to the chest while administering the stacked shocks. Do not lift the paddles from the chest between shocks. Alternatively the operator can defibrillate "remotely" through adhesive defibrillation pads. If working alone the defibrillator operator will need to operate various controls on either the defibrillator control panel or the paddle handles.

Recharge the defibrillator *before* or *during* postshock rhythm assessment. This will minimize the time between shocks should another shock be needed. During a stacked-shock sequence do not resume CPR between shocks while the defibrillator recharges and rhythm is assessed unless there is an unavoidable delay. Research has shown that shocks given close together with escalating current produce better outcomes than shocks interrupted by pauses to administer adjunctive drug therapy or CPR. Delays between shocks may be detrimental.

Defibrillation in Hypothermic Cardiac Arrest?

Hypothermic cardiac arrest is treated differently after this point in the algorithm. (See the *ECC Guidelines 2000,* page 230, and the *ECC Handbook,* Figure 12: Hypothermia Algorithm.) Do not continue to deliver shocks to a patient in hypothermic cardiac arrest (core temperature less than 30°C) if the patient remains in VF/pulseless VT after 3 defibrillation attempts. This person needs rewarming before the fibrillating heart will respond to further bursts of electric current.

Rhythm after first 3 shocks?

Box 2: Rhythm After First 3 Shocks?

After the first stacked-shock sequence the victim without spontaneous circulation will need chest compressions and rescue ventilations. Examine the monitor to identify one of the following possibilities:

- **VF/pulseless VT?** If after 3 shocks you observe *persistent, refractory, recurrent, or shock-resistant VF/pulseless VT,*[2] the victim requires intubation, epinephrine, antiarrhythmics, and more defibrillation attempts. Proceed to Box 3 (Persistent or recurrent VF/VT); and Box 4 (Secondary ABCD Survey).

- **Potentially perfusing rhythm?** (Check pulse to identify return of spontaneous circulation.) If you observe a potentially perfusing rhythm *and* the pulse check indicates return of spontaneous circulation, you have successfully defibrillated the patient. If the victim is not breathing, give *rescue breathing now.* If the victim has spontaneous breathing, place the victim in the *recovery position.*
- **Pulseless electrical activity?** (Case 4: PEA) Asystole? (Case 5) If you observe PEA, treat the patient according to the PEA algorithm (see Case 4).
- If you observe a **"flat line,"** do not immediately assume **asystole.** Check the flat line protocol (discussed in more detail in Case 5: Asystole) to identify or rule out causes of an isoelectric ECG:
  - — Loose leads
  - — Not connected to the patient
  - — Not connected to the defibrillator/ monitor
  - — No power
  - — Signal *gain* (amplitude/signal strength) turned too low
  - — Isoelectric VF/pulseless VT or "occult VF/pulseless VT"[3]
  - — True *asystole* (total absence of cardiac electrical activity)

Persistent or recurrent VF/VT

Box 3: Persistent or Recurrent VF/VT

If the rhythm after the first 3 shocks is *"persistent VF/VT,"* the ACLS provider moves quickly through Box 3 to Box 4: Secondary ABCD Survey. The rhythm after the first 3 shocks may display non-VF complexes that may or may not be associated with a pulse. After a variable period if the heart refibrillates, use the term *recurrent VF.*

Does each of these subsets of VF require individualized treatment? Despite a number of theories, clinical evidence fails to give the nod to any specific approach. Antiarrhythmic agents may be useful for victims of persistent and recurrent VF, but there is little evidence (see below). The ACLS experts for the *ECC Guidelines 2000* recommended a general approach that is the same for all subsets of VF (see Box 4: Secondary ABCD Survey), with some variations acceptable for recurrent VF (eg, procainamide) or severely resistant *"electrical storm"* VF (eg, β-blockers). These topics are presented below under Box 7: Consider Antiarrhythmics.

Box 4: The Secondary ABCD Survey

If VF/pulseless VT persists after 3 shocks, the ACLS provider moves to the Secondary ABCD Survey to manage the **airway,** provide invasive support of **breathing,** and support the **circulation.**

For treatment purposes the Secondary ABCD Survey for the VF/pulseless VT algorithm is the same as that used for all 3 cardiac arrest algorithms: advanced airway management, effective ventilation, access to the bloodstream, and administration of rhythm-appropriate medications.

The effective team leader will have already assigned 4 tasks at the start of the resuscitation attempt:

- A rescuer to perform chest compressions
- A rescuer to manage the airway, including ventilation adjuncts and advanced airway control
- A rescuer to establish IV or IO access for administration of medications
- A rescuer to monitor rhythm and perform defibrillation

The sequential flow of an algorithm visually suggests that a resuscitation team follows an intervention sequence. In clinical reality, however, ACLS providers perform several multistep tasks in parallel if not simultaneously. Rescuers should realize that a flow algorithm serves better to convey priority or importance rather than to present an absolute sequence of actions.

Algorithms are constructed for pedagogic reasons. They address the "worst case" scenario, which is the scenario in which only one rescuer is available to perform the interventions. With this design, algorithms can answer the unspoken question, *"If alone for the early minutes of a rescue attempt, what should I do first, what should I do second?"* and so on. In well-organized resuscitative efforts, however, other personnel (if available) prepare for and perform their assigned tasks simultaneously as much as possible.

Box 5: Epinephrine and Vasopressin: Agents to Optimize Cardiac Output and Blood Pressure

In the 3 cardiac arrest algorithms (VF/VT, PEA, Asystole) only 2 agents are recommended to optimize cardiac output and

Secondary ABCD Survey

Focus: *more advanced assessments and treatments*

A	**Airway:** place airway device as soon as possible
B	**Breathing:** confirm airway device placement by exam plus confirmation device
B	**Breathing:** secure airway device; purpose-made tube holders preferred
B	**Breathing:** confirm effective oxygenation and ventilation
C	**Circulation:** establish IV access
C	**Circulation:** identify rhythm → monitor
C	**Circulation:** administer drugs appropriate for rhythm and condition
D	**Differential Diagnosis:** search for and treat identified reversible causes

[2]These imprecise terms have emerged from common usage and refer to a patient who continues in VF/pulseless VT after the first 3 stacked shocks.

[3]VF/pulseless VT rarely may have a vector of VF that produces "false asystole" in one lead. This rare phenomenon can be detected by checking 2 or more leads or by orienting the axis of the paddles 90 degrees. Data have demonstrated, however, that operator errors in using the equipment are a more common cause of false asystole than an isoelectric vector of VF.

- ***Epinephrine*** 1 mg IV push, repeat every 3 to 5 minutes

or

- ***Vasopressin*** 40 U IV, **single dose**, 1 time only

blood pressure: epinephrine is recommended for all 3; vasopressin is an alternative agent recommended only in the VF/VT algorithm.

Epinephrine

Epinephrine has been the adrenergic agent of choice for cardiac arrest patients in every version of the ECC Guidelines published. No other adrenergic agent has proved superior to epinephrine for increasing blood flow to the heart and brain. Clinicians should place a high priority on early administration of this agent. Epinephrine stimulates adrenergic receptors, producing vasoconstriction, increasing blood pressure and heart rate, and rerouting blood to the brain and heart.

The recommended *first* dose of epinephrine is 1 mg IV push. For the patient with VF/pulseless VT, epinephrine should be administered if VF/VT persists after 3 shocks at 200 J, 200 to 300 J, and 360 J. After administration of 1 mg of epinephrine, administer a second 360-J shock within 30 to 60 seconds. These directions do not indicate use of epinephrine unless VF/VT persists after 3 shocks.

Establishment of vascular access is often the rate-limiting step to epinephrine administration. If the arrest rhythm is asystole or PEA and a vascular catheter is in place, the ACLS provider should administer epinephrine as soon as possible. When the arrest rhythm is VF/VT, however, 3 shocks should be provided first if a defibrillator is immediately available. If there are delays in defibrillation, ACLS providers should administer the first dose of epinephrine. Throughout resuscitation the epinephrine dose should be repeated every 3 to 5 minutes.

Both beneficial and toxic effects of epinephrine administration during CPR have been reported in animal and small clinical trials. In large randomized clinical trials, however, doses of epinephrine greater than 1 mg were not beneficial and did not improve survival. These higher epinephrine doses may contribute to return of spontaneous circulation, but they have also been associated with greater postresuscitation myocardial dysfunction, and they may create what has been called a "toxic hyperadrenergic" state in the postresuscitation period.

In a retrospective analysis, higher *cumulative* doses of epinephrine (such as those achieved with escalating doses) were also associated with a worse neurologic outcome. For these reasons, the conventional dose of epinephrine is recommended for routine use. Doses of epinephrine greater than 1 mg IV for treatment of cardiac arrest *are not recommended for routine use.* If 1-mg doses of epinephrine fail, higher doses of epinephrine (up to 0.2 mg/kg) may be considered (Class IIb), but these higher doses are not recommended and may be harmful.

IV epinephrine should be administered every 3 to 5 minutes during cardiac arrest. Each dose given by peripheral injection should be followed by a 20-mL flush of IV fluid to ensure delivery of the drug into the central compartment.

The optimal dose of epinephrine for tracheal delivery is unknown. Delivery of drugs by the tracheal route is presented later in this chapter.

Vasopressin

Vasopressin, the naturally occurring antidiuretic hormone, becomes a powerful vasoconstrictor when used at much higher doses than those normally observed in the body. Vasopressin produces the same positive effects as epinephrine in terms of vasoconstriction and increasing the blood flow to the brain and heart during CPR. Moreover, vasopressin does not have the negative, adverse effects of epinephrine on the heart, such as increased ischemia and irritability and, paradoxically, the propensity for VF.

The experts who participated in the adrenergic agents panel at the Evidence Evaluation Conference gave vasopressin a Class IIb recommendation (acceptable, not harmful, supported by only fair evidence) for persistent VF arrest. Vasopressin is not recommended for asystole and PEA at this time simply because its value in the treatment of these cardiac arrest rhythms has not yet been documented in human trials. Give vasopressin as a single, 1-time dose (40 U IV), a regimen based on the much longer half-life of vasopressin (10 to 20 minutes) compared with epinephrine (3 to 5 minutes).

After the single dose of vasopressin, if there is no clinical response in 10 to 20 minutes, it is acceptable to return to 1 mg epinephrine every 3 to 5 minutes (Class Indeterminate). The possibility of giving a second dose of vasopressin at the 10- to 20-minute mark seems rational but is not supported by human data (Class Indeterminate).

Box 6: Resume Attempts to Defibrillate

Resume attempts to defibrillate
1 × 360 J (or equivalent *biphasic*)
within 30 to 60 seconds

After giving the first dose of epinephrine, reassess the rhythm as displayed on the monitor screen after 1 minute, and if VF/pulseless VT is present, deliver additional shocks. The algorithm displays a *drug-shock, drug-shock* sequence. This is a common sequence followed in clinical practice, but multiple sets of 3 shocks at 360 J may also be stacked one after another (Class I), especially when medications are delayed. Any additional shocks after intubation and epinephrine may also be stacked one after another. For example, when indicated the entire sequence could be

- ***Shock-shock-shock***
- **Intubate, IV access, epinephrine**
- ***Shock-shock-shock***

Numerous reports confirm the efficacy of stacked shocks. Successful defibrillation has been reported after 6, 9, 12, or more shocks, even in the absence of pharmacologic therapy. The AHA considers the use of stacked shocks a Class I recommendation (acceptable, definitely effective).

A "natural" or "found" experiment provides evidence relevant to the use of different patterns of shocks, CPR, and medications. Before the *ECC Guidelines 2000* the European Resuscitation Council (ERC) guidelines recommended 4 sets of 3 shocks, with 1 mg of epinephrine between each set. This approach resulted in delivery of up to 12 shocks and a total of 3 mg of epinephrine before other antiarrhythmics were used. Subsequent research has observed that *when all factors are equal,* outcomes resulting from the ERC approach are similar to outcomes resulting from the AHA approach. Experts interpret these observations as confirmation of the principle of early defibrillation. This principle holds that the benefits and outcomes of treating VF are determined by shocking VF, shocking it early, and shocking it until VF is gone. Antiarrhythmic agents; standard, intermediate, or escalating doses of epinephrine; buffer therapy; and various defibrillation waveforms, escalating-energy levels, or stacked vs unstacked shocks—appear to have much less effect on the ultimate outcome of VT/VF arrest than early defibrillation.

Antiarrhythmics and Other Therapies to Consider if VF/Pulseless VT Continues or Recurs After Fourth Shock:

- **Amiodarone** 300 mg IV push for cardiac arrest from VF/VT that *persists* after multiple shocks. If VF/pulseless VT *recurs,* consider administration of a second dose of 150 mg IV. Maximum cumulative dose: 2.2 g over 24 hours (Class IIb)
- **Lidocaine** 1.0 to 1.5 mg/kg IV push for cardiac arrest from VF/VT that persists after multiple shocks. Consider repeating in 3 to 5 minutes to a maximum dose of 3 mg/kg. A single dose of 1.5 mg/kg in cardiac arrest is acceptable (Class Indeterminate).
- **Magnesium sulfate** 1 to 2 g IV in torsades de pointes or when it is suspected that the arrhythmia is caused by a hypomagnesemic state (Class IIb for these indications).
- **Procainamide** up to 50 mg/min (maximum total 17 mg/kg) given to VF/VT victims who respond to shocks with intermittent return of a pulse or a non-VF rhythm, but then VF/VT recurs (Class Indeterminate).
- **Consider buffers: sodium bicarbonate** may be harmful (Class III) in hypercarbic acidosis. Sodium bicarbonate 1 mEq/kg IV is indicated for several conditions associated with sudden VF arrest:
  - — Known, preexisting *hyperkalemia* (Class I)
  - — Known, preexisting bicarbonate-responsive acidosis (Class IIa)
  - — Tricyclic antidepressant overdose (Class IIa)
  - — To alkalinize urine in aspirin or other drug overdoses (Class IIa)
  - — For intubated and ventilated patients with a long arrest interval (Class IIb)
  - — Return of circulation after a long arrest interval (Class IIb)

Box 7: Consider Antiarrhythmics

In the *ECC Guidelines 2000,* ACLS providers should consider these antiarrhythmic agents for shock-refractory VF/pulseless VT: ***amiodarone, lidocaine, magnesium,*** and ***procainamide.*** We do not know, however, whether these agents have *any* incremental value in improving survival to hospital discharge for patients with persistent VF/pulseless VT when compared with continued shocks alone.

Consider antiarrhythmics:

- ***Amiodarone*** (IIb for persistent or recurrent VF/pulseless VT)
- ***Lidocaine*** (Indeterminate for persistent or recurrent VF/pulseless VT)
- ***Magnesium*** (IIb if known hypomagnesemic state)
- ***Procainamide*** (Indeterminate for persistent VF/pulseless VT; IIb for recurrent VF/pulseless VT)

Amiodarone

IV amiodarone is a complex agent with multiple effects on sodium, potassium, and calcium channels. Amiodarone possesses both α- and β-adrenergic blocking properties. Amiodarone in a dose of 300 mg IV push is a Class IIb agent for treatment of cardiac arrest due to shock-resistant VF or pulseless VT. One out-of-hospital randomized controlled trial observed that the number needed to treat with amiodarone to get 1 additional person admitted to the hospital when compared with placebo was 10.

To administer, draw up the contents of 2 glass ampules though a large-gauge needle (to reduce foaming) diluted in a volume of 20 to 30 mL of D_5W. If VF/pulseless VT *recurs,* consider administration of a second dose of 150 mg IV.

Lidocaine

Previous recommendations of lidocaine were based on animal research on fibrillation thresholds and levels of current needed for defibrillation. Limited clinical trials in humans, however, have not shown a superiority of lidocaine over placebo, bretylium, or procainamide. A lidocaine vs amiodarone trial was under way as of late 2000.

The initial recommended dosage of lidocaine is 1.0 to 1.5 mg/kg IV push. For refractory VF give additional boluses of 0.5 to 0.75 mg/kg every 5 to 10 minutes as needed with an additional shock provided after each dose. Maximum dose is 3 mg/kg, which may be excessive in the arrested patient. Lack of blood flow profoundly alters pharmacokinetics and distribution volume. Several clinical conditions, such as advanced age and compromised liver function, dictate lower loading doses of lidocaine. Such patients should receive a single loading dose of 1 mg/kg. For patients who remain in VF/pulseless VT despite multiple shocks, epinephrine, and proper oxygenation and ventilation, the more aggressive dosing regimen remains rational and acceptable (1.5 mg/kg, then 1.5 mg/kg in 3 to 5 minutes). Clinicians must watch vigilantly for seizures, respiratory compromise, and other signs of lidocaine toxicity in those patients who do regain spontaneous circulation after higher doses of lidocaine.

Magnesium Sulfate

The routine use of magnesium sulfate in VF/pulseless VT cardiac arrest is considered a Class Indeterminate recommendation because its efficacy has not been shown in randomized controlled clinical trials. Magnesium sulfate, in a dose of 1 to 2 g IV push, is a Class IIa recommendation for patients with known low or suspected low serum magnesium, such as patients with alcoholism or other conditions associated with malnutrition or hypomagnesemic states. Use magnesium at the same dose or higher for patients with a torsades de pointes pattern of VF or VT. The routine prophylactic use of magnesium sulfate for patients with acute myocardial infarction is no longer recommended.

Procainamide

Procainamide can be used for VF/pulseless VT that *recurs* after periods of non-VF rhythms (Class IIb for recurrent VF/pulseless VT). Procainamide has not been studied extensively for cardiac arrest due to VF/pulseless VT, and the need to infuse this agent slowly limits its usefulness in this setting (Class Indeterminate recommendation with little direct evidence to support its use). An infusion of procainamide of up to 50 mg/min (to a total maximum of 17 mg/kg) can be administered to VF/VT victims who respond to shocks with an intermittent return of a pulse or a non-VF rhythm but then experience recurrent VF/pulseless VT.

Under most conditions the recommended rate of administration of procainamide is 30 mg/min up to a total of 17 mg/kg. At this rate a person weighing 70 kg would reach the recommended amount of 17 mg/kg only after 40 minutes. This slow rate of infusion is impractical during treatment of cardiac arrest or life-threatening recurrent VF/pulseless VT. In urgent situations procainamide can be administered at the faster rate of 50 mg/min. This would shorten administration time for a 70-kg patient to 24 minutes. At the time of publication of the guidelines, no published studies had been found that addressed this specific question.

Resume attempts to defibrillate

Box 8: Resume Attempts to Defibrillate: Electricity vs Antiarrhythmics

The spread of early defibrillation programs provided a natural experiment about the relative effectiveness of *early defibrillation alone* versus *delayed defibrillation plus medication.* Human clinical studies have not confirmed an independent positive benefit from either adrenergics or antiarrhythmics in achieving higher hospital discharge rates after cardiac arrest.

Some research suggests that there may be special resuscitation situations in which rescuers should administer medications, particularly adrenergic agents, before defibrillation. In the deterioration of VF to asystole there comes a point at which the shock is very likely to produce postshock asystole. Under these conditions the patient might be better served if medications were administered before defibrillation.

New monitoring devices are under development that can estimate the duration of VF through median frequency analysis. These devices may supply rescuers with information to help decide between administration of a shock or a medication as the first therapy. This promising concept should not be misinterpreted. It does not resurrect the discredited concept of "sweetening up" or "coarsening" VF with medications. ***Rescuers should continue to place a higher priority on airway, ventilation, and early defibrillation than on administration of antiarrhythmics.***

Tracheal Administration of Resuscitation Medications

- Many ACLS providers use the memory aid **"A-L-E"** to recall **A**tropine, **L**idocaine, and **E**pinephrine—the most common resuscitation medications that can be given via the tracheal tube. Narcan can also be administered by tracheal route. If the ACLS provider frequently uses narcan during resuscitation, the alternative mnemonic **"L-E-A-N"** (**L**idocaine, **A**tropine, **E**pinephrine, **N**arcan) can be used.
- When equal amounts of the same drug are administered IV and tracheally, the serum concentration of drugs given by the tracheal route is much lower than the serum concentration given by the IV route.
- Tracheal doses of medications should be considerably higher than IV doses: in the range of 2 to 4 times the IV dose. For example, the tracheal dose of epinephrine is recommended to be at least 2 to 2.5 times the peripheral IV dose.

Why Only "*Consider*" Antiarrhythmics for VF and Pulseless VT?

Why does the VF/VT algorithm recommend that the ACLS provider only "consider" antiarrhythmics for VF? What type of evidence would be needed to make a firm statement that the use of antiarrhythmic agents improves the outcome of patients who remain in VF/VT after provision of several shocks, oxygen-rich ventilation through advanced airway devices, and continuing CPR? Experts agree that the following are needed:

- Clinical studies in humans (not animals or in vitro models)
- More than one double-blind, randomized, prospective, controlled clinical trial
- The end point or outcome of study needs to be as *long term* as possible, such as survival to 1 year or at least to hospital discharge. *Immediate outcomes* such as return of spontaneous circulation or *intermediate outcomes* such as "admission alive to hospital" or "survival to hospital admission" have much less power and meaning.

The current guidelines note that most antiarrhythmics have strong proarrhythmic effects and may actually make a patient's condition worse. If one ineffective or harmful drug is compared with another ineffective or harmful agent, the drug that is "less harmful" will appear to have a positive effect on outcomes.

- The magnitude of benefit of the antiarrhythmic must be clinically and not just statistically significant.

  The preferred way to express "magnitude of benefit" is now stated as "the number needed to treat." This concept refers to an easy, statistical determination of the number of people who need to be treated with one agent in order to have 1 more survivor in the treated group than in the control group. If more than 10 to 15 patients need to be treated with a new agent to produce 1 extra survivor, many experts would consider that drug—at most—of marginal value.

Extensive reviews by the *ECC Guidelines 2000* experts seldom located evidence meeting the above criteria. They found unsatisfactory support even for epinephrine and lidocaine as effective agents in cardiac resuscitation. There was insufficient scientific evidence to confirm the value of any antiarrhythmic for out-of-hospital VF/pulseless VT arrest. A major problem is that large, prospective, human clinical trials are expensive, difficult, and time-consuming.

Only one antiarrhythmic—amiodarone—has been evaluated in a prospective double-blind randomized controlled trial of study drug versus placebo for refractory out-of-hospital, human VF/VT arrest.

Despite elegant design and meticulous execution, the trial could show only an increase in the intermediate outcome of admission-to-hospital (or survival to hospital admission) following out-of-hospital refractory VF arrest. Amiodarone administration was not associated with improvement in the preferred long-term outcome of discharged-alive-from-hospital (survival to hospital discharge). Amiodarone in refractory VF arrest received only a Class IIb recommendation.

Providing Maintenance Antiarrhythmics After Return of Spontaneous Circulation

Once VF/pulseless VT converts to a spontaneous perfusing rhythm with the treatment outlined above, you will need to consider an IV infusion of an antiarrhythmic. If the patient develops a perfusing rhythm only to revert to VF/pulseless VT, continuous infusion of an antiarrhythmic is warranted. For recurrent VF/VT, amiodarone, lidocaine, or procainamide may be considered.

Amiodarone, lidocaine, or **procainamide** may be administered as follows:

- **Amiodarone (for recurrent VF/VT):** The maximum cumulative dose is 2.2 g over 24 hours. Begin with rapid infusion of 150 mg IV over the first 10 minutes (15 mg/min); then a slow infusion of 360 mg IV over the next 6 hours (1 mg/min); then a maintenance infusion of 540 mg IV over the next 18 hours (0.5 mg/min). Monitor for hypotension and bradycardia.
- **Lidocaine:** Loading dose of 1 to 1.5 mg/kg to a total of 3 mg/kg (if patient has not already received lidocaine during the arrest), followed by a continuous infusion of 1 to 4 mg/min.
- **Procainamide (for recurrent VF/VT):** infusion of 20 mg/min until the arrhythmia is suppressed, hypotension ensues, the QRS is prolonged by 50% from original duration, or a total of 17 mg/kg is infused. Under urgent conditions an infusion of up to 50 mg/min may be administered to a total of 17 mg/kg. The maintenance infusion is 1 to 4 mg/min.

Even if the victim has not yet been refibrillated, you may consider administration of an antiarrhythmic infusion (amiodarone, lidocaine, procainamide) to prevent recurrent VF/VT. Lidocaine may be infused in the setting of acute coronary ischemia for 6 to 24 hours *after* resuscitation from VF/pulseless VT (note that *prophylactic* lidocaine administration to patients with acute coronary ischemia is no longer recommended to *prevent* the development of VF/VT). If an antiarrhythmic was used successfully during resuscitation, consider administration of a continuous infusion of *that* agent without an initial loading dose. Such an infusion constitutes *secondary* prophylaxis; the initial arrhythmia was not prevented, but the intent of the antiarrhythmic infusion is to prevent additional arrhythmias.

Consider administration of **β-adrenoreceptor** blocking agents (particularly if blood pressure is adequate) to inhibit increased sympathetic tone and catecholamine excess in the setting of acute ischemia or infarction.

Critical Actions: Assessment and Management

The critical actions checklist that follows guides the management of a patient in VF/VT. Details of the ACLS scenarios will vary. Review this checklist until you understand the order and rationale for all the steps. For in-depth information about the new topics covered in Case 3, consult the *ECC Guidelines 2000* and the *ECC Handbook*. You will learn the details and practice the procedures in the course.

Do not try to memorize this checklist. It is designed to walk you through the Primary and Secondary Surveys in a case of VF/VT to help you see the underlying logic of this approach.

Equipment Available to the Rescuer

Conventional defibrillator/monitor

Equipment for airway management, IV access, and oxygen administration

Drugs for treating cardiac arrest

Critical Actions Checklist: ACLS Case 3
Witnessed Cardiac Arrest: Refractory VF/Pulseless VT

Scene Survey Steps	Assess: Do or Monitor	Manage: Do or Delegate
Recognize emergency and respond	***Rescuer and patient safety?*** ☐ Check for rescuer/patient safety ***Responsive?*** ☐ Stimulate for responsiveness (touch and talk; shake and shout)	***Unresponsive:*** ☐ Call out for help ☐ Activate an in-hospital or out-of-hospital-emergency response: — Hospital code plan — Phone 911; activate EMS; get AED (if lone * rescuer) ☐ "Glove-up" ☐ Position the victim ☐ Position yourself as rescuer
Primary ABCD Survey		
Airway	***Mouth and upper airway open and in position for ventilation?*** ☐ Look at head, neck, chin position ☐ Look in mouth	***Foreign body in mouth; head, neck, or chin out of position:*** ☐ Head tilt–chin lift or jaw thrust; reposition, reattempt ☐ Tongue-jaw lift, finger sweep; reattempt

Primary ABCD Survey (continued)		
Scene Survey Steps	**Assess: Do or Monitor**	**Manage: Do or Delegate**
Breathing	***Air movement?*** ☐ Look ☐ Listen ☐ Feel	***Not breathing—breathless:*** ☐ Use mouth-to-mouth breathing or ☐ Use noninvasive airway device (pocket face mask preferred) *or* ☐ Use a face shield if no alternatives ☐ Give 2 rescue breaths ☐ Observe for bilateral chest rise ☐ Use obstructed airway protocols if foreign-body airway obstruction is a possibility
Circulation	***Pulse?*** ☐ Check for a pulse, other? signs of circulation	***Pulse is absent***
Defibrillation	***Defibrillator/monitor is available*** ***Rhythm?*** ☐ Attach 3 monitor leads ☐ Recognize rhythm ***Rhythm after each shock?*** ☐ Check monitor	☐ Direct helper to begin CPR, stopping only at your direction when you need to assess, treat, or move the patient ***VF or pulseless VT:*** ☐ Deliver first shocks within 90 seconds of stopping CPR ☐ Use all safety precautions for defibrillation ☐ Deliver shocks of appropriate strength ☐ Check rhythm after each shock ☐ Use 3 stacked shocks ***VF or pulseless VT persists after 3 shocks***
Secondary ABCD Survey		
Airway	***Air movement?*** ☐ Check again — Look — Listen — Feel ***Placement of tracheal tube?*** ☐ Visualize tube tip passing through vocal cords ☐ Attach ventilation bag and confirm placement with end-tidal CO_2 ***If not confirmed go* to esophageal detector device** ☐ Listen for bilateral breathing	***Gurgling, noisy breathing:*** ☐ Suction airway ***No adequate, spontaneous breathing:*** ☐ Use abdominal thrust to remove obstruction according to obstructed airway protocols ☐ Prepare for intubation per protocol ☐ Get second rescuer to apply cricoid pressure ☐ Perform tracheal intubation ☐ Adjust position of tube until correct ☐ Secure tube ☐ Consider cervical-spine collar and backboard if transportation required

Secondary ABCD Survey (continued)		
Scene Survey Steps	**Assess: Do or Monitor**	**Manage: Do or Delegate**
Breathing	***Effective ventilation?*** ☐ **Look:** bilateral chest movement with ventilations? Moisture collects in tube with each breath? ☐ **Listen:** perform 5-point auscultation (over epigastrium, L-R axilla; L-R anterior chest; during hand ventilation) ☐ **Feel:** ventilation bag resistance? ***Secondary verification technique?*** ☐ End-tidal CO_2 detector? ☐ Esophageal detector device?	☐ Immediately remove tracheal tube if there is any question of esophageal intubation or other significant malposition ☐ Reposition and reverify tube placement if main bronchus intubation suspected ☐ Continue positive-pressure ventilation except during intubation and assessment ☐ Start supplemental O_2 ☐ Continue to assess airway and breathing while patient is intubated and until patient resumes spontaneous breathing
Other ACLS providers arrive		☐ Assign each team member to 1 or more of the following 4 activities: — Airway and intubation — Chest compressions — Monitoring and defibrillation — IV access; medication administration ☐ Oversee team to ensure necessary actions are taken
Circulation	***Advanced circulatory assessment?*** ☐ Attach ECG monitor leads ☐ Identify rhythm and rate ☐ Obtain blood pressure (BP) measurement (noninvasive) ☐ Determine best site for IV access ☐ Assess rhythm ☐ Assess rhythm between each shock ☐ Assess which drugs and dosages are indicated in this case ☐ Assess whether **sodium bicarbonate** is appropriate in this case	☐ Continue basic CPR (or tracheal ventilation plus chest compressions) except during shocks and rhythm assessment ☐ Establish peripheral IV access ☐ Provide rhythm-specific medications ☐ Provide vital sign–appropriate medication (rate and pressure control) ☐ Administer **epinephrine**—appropriate dose and schedule, ***or*** ☐ Administer **vasopressin** ☐ Give **epinephrine** by tracheal tube if IV access not yet available ☐ Establish peripheral IV access ☐ Administer appropriate IV fluid

Secondary ABCD Survey (continued)		
Scene Survey Steps	**Assess: Do or Monitor**	**Manage: Do or Delegate**
Circulation (continued)	***Assess rhythm***	***VF or pulseless VT continues:*** ☐ Deliver another 3 stacked shocks ***VF or pulseless VT continues:*** ☐ Start drug-shock-assess-CPR cycles for anti-arrhythmic medication: ☐ **Amiodarone** (correct dose-**shock**-assess-CPR) ☐ **Lidocaine** (correct dose-**shock**-assess-CPR) *then if appropriate* ☐ **Procainamide** (correct dose-**shock**-assess-CPR); *then* ☐ **Magnesium** sulfate (correct dose-**shock**-assess-CPR) ☐ Deliver **shocks** within 30 to 60 seconds after each drug is administered ☐ Give **sodium bicarbonate** (correct dose) whenever appropriate ☐ Troubleshoot problems if defibrillator malfunctions ***VF or pulseless VT continues:*** ☐ Add diagnosis (below) as a priority or ***Spontaneous perfusing cardiac rhythm returns:*** ☐ Go to "Postresuscitation Support" or ***If monitor shows a new rhythm (not VF/pulseless VT):*** ☐ Move to algorithm for that rhythm
Differential Diagnosis	***Consider possible reversible causes*** ☐ Consider 5 H's-5 T's* mnemonic (see Case 4: PEA) ☐ Gather relevant patient history ☐ Order indicated lab tests ***Reversible cause?*** ☐ Reassess ABCs, including — Assess rhythm — Assess if tracheal tube remains in place after shocks ☐ Gather relevant patient history ☐ Order appropriate laboratory tests	☐ Manage and treat any identified reversible cause of arrest ☐ Move to next algorithm according to suspected cause ☐ Take action to reverse any causes of refractory VF or pulseless VT

*Advanced providers may use 6 H's by adding hypo-/hyperglycemia and 6 T's by adding trauma.

Secondary ABCD Survey (continued)		
Scene Survey Steps	**Assess: Do or Monitor**	**Manage: Do or Delegate**
Postresuscitation Period	***Continue regular assessment:*** ☐ Vital signs (including pulse oximetry) ☐ Cardiac monitor/12-lead ECG ***Gather and review:*** ☐ Relevant history ☐ Physical findings ☐ Laboratory test results	☐ Continue positive-pressure ventilation except during assessment ☐ Arrange for further ventilatory support ☐ Continue or start antiarrhythmic medication ☐ Provide support to maximize cerebral perfusion

Personnel Available to Assist Rescuer

From the beginning you have one helper who knows CPR.

After the intubation attempt other ACLS providers arrive.

Unacceptable Actions: Perils and Pitfalls

Several rescuer actions will substantially compromise the effectiveness of the resuscitative effort. These should be identified and corrected by the instructor. Unacceptable actions include the following:

- Not performing CPR when required
- Not supporting ventilation for the nonbreathing patient with an appropriate device
- Not progressing to tracheal intubation
- Defibrillation errors, including failure to shock after each drug or failure to "clear" the patient before administering a shock
- Significant errors in drug selection or dose, particularly failure to consider contraindications for specific drug therapy

Read More About It

For details about the new topics covered in Case 3, see the following sections in the *ECC Guidelines 2000:*

- Page 112: Pharmacology I: Agents for Arrhythmias
- Page 129: Pharmacology II: Agents to Optimize Cardiac Output and Blood Pressure
- Page 136: Principles and Practice of ACLS
- Pages 147-150: Figure 3: VF/Pulseless VT
- Page 166: Postresuscitation Care

Supplemental Material for the ACLS Provider Course

Who Should Read Further?

The following material is not covered in the ACLS Provider Course, despite its obvious importance. A 2-day ACLS course is filled with presentations of new information and time for the provider to practice application of that information and demonstrate skills and acquistion of knowledge. These AHA-ACLS recommendations are provided to help healthcare providers taking the ACLS Provider Course for the first time. While lacking significant resuscitation experience, these providers still face the prospect of participating in and even being in charge of resuscitation events. These "novice" ACLS providers may include recent graduates of medical school who are entering a new residency, residency and fellowship graduates who are facing employment in nonacademic hospitals without 24-hour in-house physicians, or healthcare providers moving to a position where the frequency of resuscitation events and his or her level of responsibility are likely to increase. *Note:* These providers should also start looking for the nearest ACLS for Experienced Providers course!

Workbook Review

1. **A patient develops sudden VF arrest during evaluation for chest pain in an outpatient clinic. The patient has just received the first shock from the clinic AED. The monitor screen on the AED displays VF. What is the next action rescuers should take?**

   a. resume CPR for approximately 1 minute; then reanalyze the rhythm

   b. establish IV access for medication administration

   c. press the ANALYZE control on the AED to reanalyze the rhythm

   d. administer epinephrine 1 mg IV as soon as the IV is established

   Read more about it in the ECC Guidelines 2000, *page 129: "Epinephrine"; page 146: "Newly Recommended Agent: Vasopressin for VF/VT"; and pages 147-150: Figure 3: VF/Pulseless VT Algorithm and text*

2. **The patient in question 1 has failed to respond to 3 shocks (VF persists). Paramedics arrive, start an IV, and insert a tracheal tube, confirming proper placement. Which of the following drugs should this patient receive *first?***

   a. amiodarone 300 mg IV push

   b. lidocaine 1 to 1.5 mg/kg IV push

   c. procainamide 30 mg/min up to a total dose of 17 mg/kg

   d. epinephrine 1 mg IV push or vasopressin 40 U single dose

   Read more about it in the ECC Guidelines 2000, *page 129: "Epinephrine"; page 146: "Newly Recommended Agent: Vasopressin for VF/VT"; and pages 147-150: Figure 3: VF/Pulseless VT Algorithm and text*

3. **The patient in questions 1 and 2 remains in VF after epinephrine 1 mg IV and a fourth shock. You want to continue to administer epinephrine at appropriate doses and intervals if the patient remains in VF. Which epinephrine dose is *recommended* under these conditions?**

   a. give the following epinephrine dose sequence, each 3 minutes apart: 1 mg, 3 mg, and 5 mg

   b. give a single "high dose" of epinephrine: 0.1 to 0.2 mg/kg

   c. give epinephrine 1 mg IV, then in 5 minutes start vasopressin 40 U IV every 3 to 5 minutes

   d. give epinephrine 1 mg IV; repeat 1 mg every 3 to 5 minutes

   Read more about it in the ECC Guidelines 2000, *pages 129-130: "Epinephrine"; page 149: "New Class of Recommendation for Epinephrine and Lidocaine: Indeterminate"; and page 147: Figure 3: VF/Pulseless VT Algorithm*

4. Which of the following therapies is the *most important intervention* for VF/pulseless VT, with the greatest effect on survival to hospital discharge?

   a. epinephrine

   b. defibrillation

   c. oxygen

   d. amiodarone

   Read more about it in the ECC Guidelines 2000, *page 116: "VF/Pulseless VT"; and pages 147-150: Figure 3: VF/Pulseless VT Algorithm and text*

5. **The *ECC Guidelines 2000* recommend vasopressin as a new adrenergic-like agent for treatment of cardiac arrest. Which algorithms recommend vasopressin?**

   a. VF/pulseless VT

   b. asystole

   c. PEA

   d. bradycardia

   Read more about it in the ECC Guidelines 2000, *page 146: "Newly Recommended Agent: Vasopressin for VF/VT"*

6. **A 53-year-old man has suffered sudden VF arrest in the ED. He remains in VF after 3 "stacked" shocks, epinephrine, and a fourth shock. The team leader asks for amiodarone 300 mg IV. Which of the following statements is true about amiodarone for refractory VF?**

   a. Amiodarone is a Class IIb–recommended therapy for treatment of patients who have not responded to 3 stacked shocks, IV epinephrine, and a fourth shock

   b. Amiodarone is associated with better 1-year survival than that for any other therapy for people who remain in VF after 3 shocks, 1 mg epinephrine, and a fourth shock

   c. Amiodarone is not recommended for refractory VF

   d. Amiodarone should be administered as soon as an IV is available and at least 1 shock has failed to achieve defibrillation

   Read more about it in the ECC Guidelines 2000, *page 116: "VF/Pulseless VT"; page 120: "Amiodarone (IV)"; and page 148: Figure 3: VF/Pulseless VT*

(Continued on next page)

7. A 60-year-old man persists in VF arrest despite 3 stacked shocks at appropriate energy levels. Your code team, however, has been unable to start an IV or insert a tracheal tube. Therefore, administration of IV or tracheal medications will be delayed. What is the most appropriate immediate next step?

a. deliver additional shocks in an attempt to defibrillate

b. deliver a precordial thump

c. perform a venous cut-down to gain IV access

d. administer intramuscular epinephrine 2 mg

Read more about it in the ECC Guidelines 2000, *page 90: "Defibrillation"; and page 91: the paragraph beginning "The most important determinant of survival in adult VF is rapid defibrillation"*

8. A 75-year-old homeless man is in cardiac arrest with pulseless VT at a rate of 220 bpm. After CPR, 3 shocks in rapid succession, 1 mg IV epinephrine, plus 3 more shocks, the man continues to be in polymorphic pulseless VT. He appears wasted and malnourished. The paramedics recognize him as a chronic alcoholic known in the neighborhood. Since he remains in VT after 6 shocks, you are considering an antiarrhythmic. Which of the following agents would be *most appropriate* for *this* patient at *this* time?

a. amiodarone

b. procainamide

c. magnesium

d. diltiazem

Read more about it in the ECC Guidelines 2000, *page 116: "VF/Pulseless VT"; page 120: "Amiodarone (IV)"; page 123: "Magnesium"; and page 148: Figure 3: VF/Pulseless VT*

9. Which statement is true about the use of antiarrhythmics for patients with shock-refractory VF/pulseless VT?

a. antiarrhythmic agents are indicated because of the well-documented, long-term benefits of increasing 1-year survival for VF/VT victims

b. antiarrhythmic agents can replace the need for continued shocks if infused fast and early

c. antiarrhythmic agents reduce myocardial damage from continued shocks

d. in prospective, randomized trials, antiarrhythmic agents have not yet been found to improve survival to hospital discharge of patients with VF/pulseless VT

Read more about it in the ECC Guidelines 2000, *page 116: "VF/Pulseless VT"; and page 148: Figure 3: VF/Pulseless VT*

10. A 55-year-old man running in his first marathon collapses after 15 miles. Paramedics on the scene attempt defibrillation with an AED and report a pattern of "in-and-out" VF in which a perfusing rhythm resumes after 1 or more shocks but then VF recurs. Upon arrival in the ED the man continues to go into VF, respond briefly to a shock, then return to VF. Currently he has hypotensive tachycardia (BP = 80/50; HR = 120 to 140 bpm). What would be the most appropriate action to take to prevent VF from recurring?

a. institute transvenous pacing

b. search for and treat conditions that can be risk factors for recurrent VF, such as unstable angina, hypoxia, hypovolemia, hypoglycemia, and electrolyte disorders

c. administer epinephrine 1 mg IV every 3 to 5 minutes for at least 3 doses

d. begin a slow, prophylactic infusion of amiodarone 360 mg IV over 6 hours (1 mg/min) or procainamide 250 mg IV push every 3 minutes

Read more about it in the ECC Guidelines 2000, *pages 116-117: "VF/Pulseless VT"; page 120: "Antiarrhythmic Drugs and the Arrhythmias They Treat"; and pages 147-150: Figure 3: VF/Pulseless VT Algorithm and text*

Postresuscitation Care: Care of Patients Immediately After Cardiac Arrest

Key Learning Points

1. Postresuscitation care: the period between restoration of a spontaneous circulation and transfer of patient care to another healthcare provider who assumes responsibility.
   - In prehospital care this transfer usually occurs when emergency personnel deliver the resuscitated patient to an ED.
   - In the ED this transfer will be to the physician responsible for the intensive care service or the coronary care unit.
   - In general, postresuscitation care will last less than 30 minutes. Proper care in this period will make a critical difference in the eventual outcome, especially in neurologic function.
2. Patients display a wide spectrum of responses to resuscitation. On return of spontaneous circulation, patients may respond by becoming awake and alert with adequate spontaneous respirations and hemodynamic stability. Others will remain comatose with an unstable circulation and no spontaneous breathing.
3. Many will require 24 to 48 hours of invasive hemodynamic monitoring for optimal management after resuscitation. The ACLS course does *not* cover invasive hemodynamic monitoring because this topic more properly belongs in a discussion of critical care medicine.
4. Continue to use the ABCDs of the Primary and Secondary Surveys to organize your evaluations and therapy *(assessment and management)*. Your immediate goal is to provide cardiorespiratory support to optimize oxygenation and perfusion, particularly in the brain. All resuscitated patients require careful, repeated assessments to identify any additional problems with their cardiovascular, respiratory, or neurologic status.
5. Do *not* "apply the algorithms in reverse." That is, in the postresuscitation period do not "go back up" the tachycardia, bradycardia, and hypotension algorithms to treat postresuscitation tachycardia, bradycardia, and hypotension. As a general rule most postresuscitation arrhythmias should be left untreated for the immediate postresuscitation period.

The Postresuscitation Period: Critical Actions

Assess and Treat Using the Primary and Secondary ABCD Surveys

Airway

1. Secure the airway.
2. Confirm correct tracheal tube placement by *primary confirmation techniques* (visualize the tube passing through the cords, "5-point" auscultation, chest expansion) and a *secondary tube confirmation technique* (end-tidal CO_2 indicators, esophageal detector devices, capnography, chest x-ray).

Breathing

1. Administer 100% oxygen.
2. Supply positive-pressure ventilation through bag mask or appropriate mechanical ventilation.
3. Verify bilateral chest movement.
4. Check oxygen saturation levels; order arterial blood gas analyses (unless the patient is a candidate for fibrinolytic therapy).
5. Prepare for mechanical ventilation (unless the patient resumes immediate spontaneous respirations). Mechanical ventilation often requires paralysis and sedation. Knowledge and skills at this level are not provided or required in the ACLS Provider Course. See the *ECC Handbook* for supplemental information on rapid sequence intubation, tracheal intubation, and preintubation.
6. Check for potential complications from resuscitative efforts, such as pneumothorax, rib fractures, sternal fractures, and improper tracheal tube placement, and continue to monitor for tracheal tube dislodgment.

Circulation

1. Assess vital signs.
2. Start an IV line. Administer normal saline. Reserve glucose administration for patients with documented hypoglycemia.
3. Apply an ECG monitor, pulse oximeter, and automatic sphygmomanometer.
4. Insert bladder catheter; monitor urine output.
5. Insert nasogastric tube.
6. Consider administration of β-adrenergic blockers to treat the increased adrenergic stimulation that may follow an ischemic insult. Lidocaine may be infused in the setting of acute coronary ischemia for 6 to 24 hours after resuscitation from VF/pulseless VT (note that *prophylactic* lidocaine administration to patients with acute coronary ischemia is no longer recommended to prevent development of VF/VT).
7. If an antiarrhythmic agent was used *successfully* during the resuscitation

(ie, loading dose administered during resuscitation), consider initiation of a continuous infusion of that same agent without an initial loading dose. Such an infusion constitutes *secondary* prophylaxis; the initial arrhythmia was not prevented, but the intent of the antiarrhythmic infusion is to prevent additional arrhythmias.

8. Consider fibrinolytic therapy for patients with evidence of AMI on their postresuscitation 12-lead ECG, provided that resuscitation duration was not prolonged and there was minimal trauma, no central line placement, no arterial blood draw, and no other contraindications.

Differential Diagnosis

1. Search for any specific cause for the arrest. Review the 5 H's and 5 T's listed in the asystole and PEA algorithms.
2. Diagnose complications (rib fracture, hemopneumothorax, pericardial tamponade, intra-abdominal trauma, misplaced tracheal tube).
3. Order a portable chest radiograph if not already done.
4. Review the history, particularly the immediate prearrest period and current medications.
5. Perform a physical examination.
6. Order a 12-lead ECG.
7. Order serum electrolytes, including magnesium and calcium, and cardiac enzymes.

Other Actions

1. Change IV lines placed without proper sterile technique or those that cannot be maintained adequately.
2. Insert a nasogastric tube if there are no contraindications.
3. Insert a bladder catheter.
4. Treat aggressively any electrolyte abnormalities identified, particularly potassium, sodium, calcium, or magnesium.
5. Prepare the patient for transport to a special care unit. During transport the patient will require oxygen administration, ECG monitoring, a full supply of resuscitation equipment, and an adequate number of trained personnel.
6. Maintain mechanical ventilation and oxygenation along with ECG monitoring and blood pressure measurements.

Special Problems in the Immediate Postresuscitation Period

ACLS providers should monitor the patient closely in the immediate postresuscitation period. The following problems may develop:

- Hostile environment for the brain
- Hypotension
- Recurrent VF/pulseless VT in the postresuscitation period
- Postresuscitation tachycardias
- Postresuscitation bradycardia
- Postresuscitation premature ventricular contractions

Establish a Nonhostile Environment for the Brain

A healthy brain is the primary goal of all *cardiopulmonary-cerebral resuscitation (CP-CPR).* Every effort should be made to provide brain-oriented intensive care.

In the immediate postresuscitation period the most important action that ACLS providers can take to restore cerebral function is to *optimize the ABCs*—oxygenation and perfusion. This means providing well-oxygenated blood at a normal or slightly elevated mean arterial pressure. A growing body of evidence supports this concept of a "postresuscitation hypertensive bout." Initiate these specific actions in addition to maintaining oxygenation and blood pressure:

- Maintain normothermia; hyperthermia increases the oxygen requirements of the brain.
- Allow moderate hypothermia. This is not semantics. Evidence review performed for the *ECC Guidelines 2000* concludes that there is insufficient evidence to support induction of hypothermia in the postresuscitation period. However, if patients *are* hypothermic (moderately so) or become so in the postresuscitation period and are allowed to remain in that state, they have significantly better neurologic outcomes. Thus, mild hypothermia should not be corrected, but there is insufficient evidence to recommend that mild hypothermia be created.
- Control seizures; seizures increase cerebral oxygen requirements (consider phenobarbital, phenytoin, or diazepam).
- Elevate the victim's head approximately 30 degrees; this increases cerebral venous drainage and decreases intracranial pressure.

Hypotension

Even mild hypotension must be avoided because it can impair recovery of cerebral function. Assess both circulating fluid volume and ventricular function. The critically ill postresuscitation patient requires invasive hemodynamic monitoring. This monitoring includes intra-arterial assessment of blood pressure and may include evaluation of pulmonary artery pressure and cardiac output calculations using a pulmonary artery flow-directed catheter. A thorough presentation of invasive hemodynamic monitoring is beyond the scope of the ACLS Provider Course.

As a practical matter ACLS providers often have to deal with hemodynamic instability in the immediate postresuscitation period without invasive hemodynamic monitoring.

Clinicians should consider whether the instability arises from a problem with the cardiovascular system—a volume, pump, or rate problem.

- For volume problems, and often empirically, administer a fluid bolus of *250 to 500 mL of normal saline* unless you know with certainty that the patient has volume overload.
- If hypotension with or without signs of shock persists after 1 or 2 fluid boluses, then a trial of *inotropic (dobutamine) or vasopressor (dopamine, epinephrine, or norepinephrine)* therapy can be started.

Postresuscitation VF/Pulseless VT

VF/pulseless VT may recur in the immediate postresuscitation period after return of spontaneous circulation. Consider such recurrences as *recurrent* or *refractory* VF/pulseless VT.

- Consider administration of **β-adrenoreceptor** blocking agents (particularly if blood pressure is adequate) to inhibit increased sympathetic tone and catecholamine excess in the setting of acute ischemia or infarction.
- If the patient responded to an **antiarrhythmic** during resuscitation, consider administration of an infusion of that agent for 6 to 24 hours (if no contraindications).
- In patients with recurrent VF/pulseless VT, **antiarrhythmic agents** can facilitate and stabilize the return of circulation, so these patients are appropriate candidates to consider for antiarrhythmics.
- Consider administration of **procainamide** hydrochloride for recurrent VF/pulseless VT.
- Consider ***magnesium sulfate 1 to 2 g IV*** if the patient is likely to have hypomagnesemia (eg, patient is receiving chronic diuretic therapy, has chronic gastrointestinal problem, or is chronically malnourished).
- Defibrillate and administer drugs in the same *drug-shock, drug-shock pattern* used in the algorithm for VF/pulseless VT.

In addition, quickly review the ABCDs: airway security, breathing and ventilation, circulation, and differential diagnosis. Problems with poor ventilation, acid-base status, hypovolemia, drug ingestions, and electrolyte abnormalities will often be the culprits behind refractory or recurrent VF/pulseless VT. In this situation review of the ABCDs will produce better outcomes than additional pharmacologic interventions.

Postresuscitation Tachycardias

The rapid supraventricular tachycardias that may develop in the immediate postresuscitation period are best treated by *leaving them alone.* The hyperadrenergic state of cardiac arrest may cause the tachycardia, particularly if high doses of epinephrine were administered. Again, review the ABCDs. Thinking about the patient should take precedence over routine pharmacologic interventions.

If the blood pressure in a tachycardic, postresuscitation patient drops or fails to increase reasonably soon after resuscitation, then initiate the interventions listed in the stable (and unstable) tachycardia algorithms.

Postresuscitation Bradycardias

Poor ventilation and oxygenation play a major role in postresuscitation bradycardias. Clinicians should again attend to the ABCDs and rule out hypoxia or airway or ventilation problems before administering atropine or a chronotropic agent. A profound bradycardia associated with hypotension and hypoperfusion in the postresuscitation period is treated as directed in the bradycardia algorithm:

- Consider pacing, atropine, and catecholamine infusions.
- Consider insertion of a temporary transvenous pacemaker. Transcutaneous pacing may be superior to atropine for postresuscitation bradycardias, although there is insufficient data to support pacing as the first intervention.

Postresuscitation Premature Ventricular Contractions

Postresuscitation premature ventricular contractions may indicate problems with the Secondary ABCD Survey. Consider whether problems exist with the airway, breathing, or electrolytes. Watchful waiting while improved oxygenation takes effect is usually the most appropriate course of action. In addition, the high levels of catecholamines and acid-base status should soon return to more normal levels.

Pulseless Electrical Activity

Description

The PEA case focuses on assessing and treating patients with PEA. The case also presents the concept of ***search for reversible causes,*** which is the key to treating patients with PEA or asystole. *PEA refers to any semiorganized electrical activity that can be seen on the monitor screen although the patient lacks a palpable pulse.* This definition specifically excludes VF, ventricular tachycardia (VT), and asystole. PEA encompasses the broad range of electrical activity that hardly merits the term "rhythm" and that displays electrical activity but produces no clinically detectable pulse.

The term *electromechanical dissociation* (EMD) is now obsolete. EMD has always been an intrinsically illogical term, implying that somehow the ACLS provider can recognize a cardiac condition in which the conduction system appears to be working yet conduction is "dissociated" from the contractile function of the myocardium.

The state of EMD has never been definitively documented and has no real clinical usefulness. In the past the term *EMD* was used to describe patients who displayed electrical activity on the cardiac monitor but who lacked apparent contractile function because they had no detectable pulse. Two more accurate and descriptive terms for this electrical activity are *electrical activity without a pulse* or *pulseless electrical activity.* We prefer the term *pulseless electrical activity.*

What's New in the Guidelines...
Pulseless Electrical Activity

Revisions in the Treatment of the Patient With PEA

The *ECC Guidelines 2000* contain no revisions in the recommended treatments for pulseless electrical activity (PEA). As with asystole, the most important *therapy* for PEA continues to be to search for, identify, and reverse any treatable cause of asystole.

1. The overall therapeutic approach remains the same:
   - Perform effective *CPR*
   - Provide supplemental *oxygen*
   - Provide advanced airway control with *tracheal intubation* or alternative advanced airway devices
   - Administer IV *epinephrine*, *atropine*, and—when indicated—*sodium bicarbonate*
2. Although there is evidence to support *vasopressin* as a replacement for *epinephrine* in cardiac arrest associated with ventricular fibrillation (VF), evidence is lacking to establish equal effectiveness between *epinephrine* and *vasopressin* for cardiac arrest associated with asystole or PEA.

Revisions to the Approach to the Patient With PEA

The ACLS Subcommittee, with input from other experts, implemented several revisions to the ACLS Provider Course following publication of the *ECC Guidelines 2000.* The major learning objectives for Case 4: Pulseless Electrical Activity and Case 5: Asystole were revised. The learning objectives for the asystole case changed from *emphasis on a small number of potential therapies to reverse asystolic arrest to emphasis on appropriate therapies and support for asystole that represents the end of a person's life.* This allows us to use the asystole case to focus on ethical issues and end-of-life concerns, such as the criteria for not starting resuscitative efforts and for stopping such efforts.

(Continued on next page)

Before 1992 an even greater variety of confusing and redundant terms were used to describe this state of electrical activity and pulselessness. In addition to EMD, other obsolete terms that you may hear occasionally are *idioventricular rhythms, pulseless asystolic rhythms, bradyasystolic rhythms,* and *pseudo-EMD.* These terms make no valuable distinction beyond what is simply PEA, and their use should be avoided.

We can use Case 4: PEA to emphasize the concept of *"reversible causes."* No matter what the immediate or underlying cause, VF is always treated with shocks in an attempt to achieve defibrillation. The approach to asystole and PEA, however, is not so simple. The *ECC Guidelines 2000* recommend standard, nonspecific treatments for PEA and asystole, notably oxygen, epinephrine, atropine, and CPR. However, the ability to achieve an effective *resuscitation*, with return of a perfusing rhythm and spontaneous respirations, resides in the ability of the response team to *identify the cause* of PEA or asystole. When ACLS providers can identify a specific cause, they can provide a specific therapy.

Never make the mistake of thinking that treatment for PEA or asystole is limited to those therapies listed in the respective algorithms. *The treatment of these rhythm states is the treatment of the underlying cause.*

Because of the importance of searching for and treating reversible causes of PEA arrests, the algorithm includes a list of the most common reversible causes of PEA and asystole. Several memory aids by different authors and using different mnemonic devices are presented in the following sections. The specific memory aid adopted is of little consequence. The critical point is that all ACLS providers should adopt a system for always asking and reviewing the question "Why is *this* patient in cardiac arrest with PEA at *this* time?"

Approximately half of the new ACLS for Experienced Providers (ACLS-EP) Course is devoted to reversible causes of PEA and asystolic cardiac arrest. Toxicology and electrolyte abnormalities, 2 of the 4 major topics in the ACLS-EP course, are classic causes of PEA. The importance of this topic more than justifies the large amount of course time spent on it.

Settings and Scenarios

Setting: Prehospital, Unmonitored Patient

- EMTs arrive at the home of a 55-year-old man. His wife phoned 911 and reported that he had collapsed unconscious on the living room floor. He had previously complained of shortness of breath, which had progressed during the past 2 days (possible tension pneumothorax or hypoxia).
- EMTs arrive at the home of a 55-year-old man. His wife phoned 911 and reported that he had collapsed unconscious on the living room floor. He had complained of severe nausea, vomiting, diarrhea, and progressive weakness over the previous 2 days (possible hypovolemia or electrolyte imbalance).

Setting: Emergency Dept, Unmonitored Patient

- A 55-year-old man walks into the ED complaining of severe chest and abdominal pains. He is placed on a stretcher and begins to remove his clothes. Just as the nurse starts to attach the monitor leads, he falls back unconscious on the stretcher (possible hypovolemia from gastrointestinal bleeding or other causes or acute myocardial infarction [AMI]).
- A 37-year-old woman with a history of smoking has severe chest pain. Her only medication is oral contraceptives. She is found unresponsive (possible massive pulmonary embolus).
- A 30-year-old woman complains of chest pain 48 hours after a car crash in which she struck her chest on the steering wheel. She collapses in bed (possible pericardial tamponade, tension pneumothorax, or hypovolemia).

Setting: In-Hospital, Unmonitored Patient

- A 45-year-old woman is hospitalized to receive chemotherapy for breast cancer. A right subclavian central venous line was inserted for chemotherapy about 2 hours ago. You are called to her room because she is unresponsive (possible tension pneumothorax from the central line, pericardial tamponade from radiation or metastatic disease, or hypovolemia).
- A 25-year-old man with renal failure just began dialysis today and has collapsed in the hospital lobby (possible pericardial tamponade from uremia, acidosis from renal failure, hyperkalemia from renal failure, or hypovolemia from dialysis).
- A 67-year-old woman underwent surgery for a hip fracture 2 days ago. She is found in bed unresponsive from a possible pulmonary embolism or massive AMI.

Setting: Critical Care Unit, Monitored Patient

- A 55-year-old man has been admitted with AMI. He was resuscitated from a VF cardiac arrest last night and is in the critical care unit (CCU), on a monitor, with a subclavian vein central venous catheter in place. He is receiving nasal oxygen at 4 L/min. The nurse notices that he has become unresponsive (possible pericardial tamponade from CPR or tension pneumothorax from CPR or the central venous line).

- A 70-year-old man was intubated this morning for respiratory failure due to bilateral pneumonia. He is found lying in bed, unresponsive and pulseless (possible hypoxia, esophageal intubation, hypovolemia, or tension pneumothorax).

Learning and Skills Objectives

At the end of Case 4 you should be able to

1. Use the ACLS Approach (Primary and Secondary ABCD Surveys) to ensure careful assessment of the patient and stabilization of the critical systems: airway, breathing, and circulation.
2. Aggressively manage the airway. Hyperventilate the patient as quickly as possible because hypoventilation and hypoxemia are frequent causes of PEA. All ACLS team members and particularly the code team leader should monitor resuscitative efforts and at the same time focus on the **D**—*Differential Diagnosis*—of the Secondary ABCD Survey. All resuscitation team members can contribute by helping think about **D**—*Diagnosis.*
3. Use a memory aid to recite at least 10 possible causes of a PEA arrest.
4. Describe how to use the *rate* (too fast or too slow) and *width* of the QRS complexes (wide versus narrow) as clues to likely causes of the PEA.
5. Describe the sequence of treatments recommended in the PEA Algorithm.
6. Describe the physical and clinical signs of hypovolemia, pericardial tamponade, and tension pneumothorax.
7. Describe the *what?, how?, when?, why?,* and *watch out!* guides for fluid infusion.
8. Describe the indications for a resuscitation fluid bolus, which fluid to use, and the rate of administration.

Specific Skills to Learn

At the end of Case 4 you should be able to demonstrate

- How to assess for hypovolemia, pericardial tamponade, and tension pneumothorax
- How to manage fluid infusion, pericardiocentesis, and needle decompression of a pneumothorax

New Rhythms to Learn

At the end of Case 4 you should be able to identify PEA and its variations. You will learn that QRS complexes in PEA can be fast or slow, narrow or wide. Your treatment approach and ultimately the patient's prognosis may vary, based on fast versus slow and narrow versus wide complexes.

New Drugs to Learn

At the end of the case discussion you should be able to discuss indications and cautions for the use of the following drugs for the patient with PEA:

- Epinephrine
- Atropine
- Other medications, depending on the specific cause of the PEA arrest

See the *2000 Handbook of Emergency Cardiovascular Care for Healthcare Providers.*

A Walk Through the PEA Algorithm

Historically PEA has been known by a variety of different names:

- Electromechanical dissociation, or EMD
- Pseudo-EMD
- Idioventricular rhythms
- Ventricular escape rhythms
- Bradyasystolic rhythms
- Postdefibrillation idioventricular rhythms

As noted in the introduction, the term *pulseless electrical activity* seems to convey the meaning of the rhythm better than any of the terms above. You begin assessment and care of the patient with PEA in the same manner as you begin the management of every victim of cardiac arrest—with the Primary and Secondary ABCD Surveys.

Box 1: The Primary ABCD Survey

With the ACLS Approach you do the following:

Primary **A**BCD	Assess and manage (open) the airway
Primary A**B**CD	Assess and manage breathing (give rescue breaths)
Primary AB**C**D	Assess and manage the pulse (no pulse → no BP → start CPR)
Primary AB**C**D	Assess the rhythm → electrical activity present, thus → PEA
Primary ABC**D**	Assess for VF/VT → rhythm not shockable → defibrillation shocks not indicated

Box 2: The Secondary ABCD Survey and the PEA Algorithm

Note that Box 2 in the PEA algorithm includes the major steps of the Secondary ABCD Survey:

A: Place airway device as soon as possible

Proper airway management to ensure adequate oxygenation and ventilation is critical because hypoventilation and hypoxemia are frequent causes of PEA.

Pulseless Electrical Activity Algorithm.

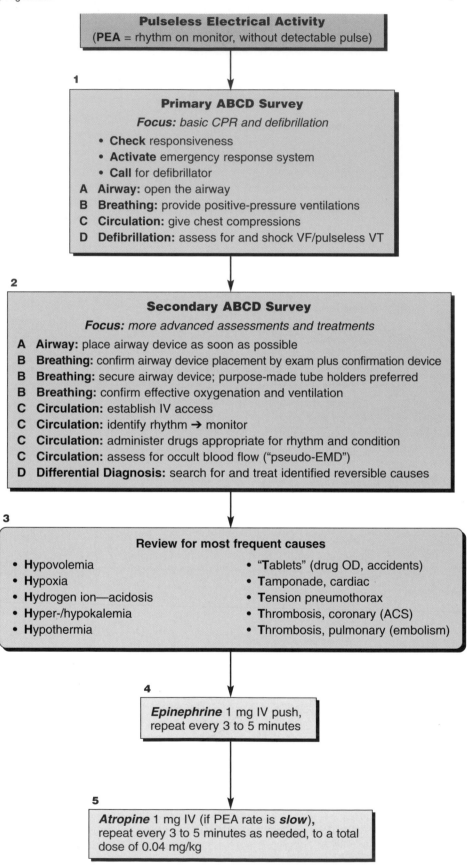

Pulseless Electrical Activity
(**PEA** = rhythm on monitor, without detectable pulse)

↓

1

Primary ABCD Survey

Focus: *basic CPR and defibrillation*

- **Check** responsiveness
- **Activate** emergency response system
- **Call** for defibrillator

A **Airway:** open the airway
B **Breathing:** provide positive-pressure ventilations
C **Circulation:** give chest compressions
D **Defibrillation:** assess for and shock VF/pulseless VT

↓

2

Secondary ABCD Survey

Focus: *more advanced assessments and treatments*

A **Airway:** place airway device as soon as possible
B **Breathing:** confirm airway device placement by exam plus confirmation device
B **Breathing:** secure airway device; purpose-made tube holders preferred
B **Breathing:** confirm effective oxygenation and ventilation
C **Circulation:** establish IV access
C **Circulation:** identify rhythm → monitor
C **Circulation:** administer drugs appropriate for rhythm and condition
C **Circulation:** assess for occult blood flow ("pseudo-EMD")
D **Differential Diagnosis:** search for and treat identified reversible causes

↓

3

Review for most frequent causes

- **H**ypovolemia
- **H**ypoxia
- **H**ydrogen ion—acidosis
- **H**yper-/hypokalemia
- **H**ypothermia
- "**T**ablets" (drug OD, accidents)
- **T**amponade, cardiac
- **T**ension pneumothorax
- **T**hrombosis, coronary (ACS)
- **T**hrombosis, pulmonary (embolism)

↓

4

Epinephrine 1 mg IV push,
repeat every 3 to 5 minutes

↓

5

Atropine 1 mg IV (if PEA rate is ***slow***),
repeat every 3 to 5 minutes as needed, to a total dose of 0.04 mg/kg

Secondary ABCD Survey

Focus: *more advanced assessments and treatments*

- A **Airway:** place airway device as soon as possible
- B **Breathing:** confirm airway device placement by exam plus confirmation device
- B **Breathing:** secure airway device; purpose-made tube holders preferred
- B **Breathing:** confirm effective oxygenation and ventilation
- C **Circulation:** establish IV access
- C **Circulation:** identify rhythm → monitor
- C **Circulation:** administer drugs appropriate for rhythm and condition
- C **Circulation:** assess for occult blood flow ("pseudo-EMD")
- D **Differential Diagnosis:** search for and treat identified reversible causes

B: Confirm airway device placement by clinical exam plus secondary confirmation device

Once correct placement of the tracheal tube or advanced airway device is confirmed (primary and secondary confirmation) and the tube or device is secured to prevent dislodgment, give 100% oxygen at 10 L/min by bag-mask device.

C: Establish IV access; identify the rhythm; administer fluids and volume as indicated

- Hypovolemia is a common cause of electrical activity without measurable blood pressure.
- Tachycardia with a narrow or normal-looking QRS complex is the classic rhythm seen with severe hypovolemia.
- In suspected hypovolemia give 500 mL normal saline (a *"medical"* resuscitation bolus) as quickly as possible.
- It is acceptable to administer an *"empiric medical bolus"* even without specific evidence of hypovolemia.

C: Assess for occult blood flow (the distinction here is *flow*, not *pressure* and not *heart rate*)

There are many reasons to assess blood flow and several ways to do it.

- Determine if there is a response to the ***medical bolus*** of normal saline.
- Identify patients with a greater probability of survival. Patients with detectable blood flow, measurable blood pressure, or good cardiac contractility are not truly in cardiac arrest. They should be identified and treated aggressively.
- A hand-held *Doppler ultrasound device* is the most sensitive way to detect the flow of blood with an associated *pressure* too low to be felt by palpation.
- *Continuous end-tidal CO_2 monitoring:* if a continuous or improving level of end-tidal CO_2 is detected, significant blood flow is indicated.
- *Transesophageal echocardiography* is being used with increased frequency during a cardiac arrest to detect subtle ventricular wall contractions, even if these contractions don't produce a measurable pulse. Some EDs use the continued presence of cardiac contractions as an indication for continued CPR and resuscitation. Lack of contractions has become an indication to stop resuscitative efforts.

Box 3: The "D" of the Secondary ABCD Survey: Consider Possible Causes (Differential Diagnosis)

Patients with PEA have poor outcomes. Rapid assessment and aggressive management offer the best chance of success. PEA is often associated with a reversible clinical state. If you can quickly identify the specific condition and treat it appropriately, you can often reverse the cardiac arrest. The need to search for a reversible cause is of paramount importance in any case of PEA and asystole.

In cases of PEA use the pattern of the electrical activity as a clue to guide treatment. The cardiac rhythm of the patient with PEA is not the primary target of treatment: the true target is **the cause** of PEA. Case 4 emphasizes the critical need to search for possible causes of PEA by using the characteristics of the PEA itself. You gather other clues as you use the ACLS Approach. Once you identify a possible cause, treat that cause (or combination of causes). In effect PEA is simply a clinical sign that will resolve once the primary cause is treated. For any case of PEA the major action—after ensuring that ventilation and circulation are stabilized—is to search for the possible causes.

How to Search for Causes of PEA and Treatments

Use information from the ECG, the history, and the physical exam to identify possible diagnoses. Table 1 combines (1) factors in the patient history and clinical examination that may identify reversible causes of PEA and (2) recommendations

Review for most frequent causes

- **Hypovolemia** (volume infusion)
- **Hypoxia** (oxygen, ventilation)
- **Hydrogen ion—*acidosis*** (buffer, ventilation)
- **Hyper-/hypokalemia** (CaCl plus others)
- **Hypothermia** (see Hypothermia Treatment Algorithm)
- **"Tablets"** (drug OD, accidents)
- **Tamponade, cardiac** (pericardiocentesis)
- **Tension pneumothorax** (needle decompression)
- **Thrombosis, coronary** (ACS), (fibrinolytics)
- **Thrombosis, pulmonary** (embolus), (bolus fibrinolytics, surgical evacuation)

TABLE 1. Conditions That Can Cause PEA (5 H's and 5 T's)[1]

Condition	Features of Electrical Activity	Historical/Physical Clues	Management
Hypovolemia	Narrow complex Rapid rate	History, flat neck veins	Volume infusion
Hypoxia	Slow rate (hypoxia)	Cyanosis, blood gases, airway problems	Oxygenation, ventilation
Hydrogen ion: acidosis	Smaller-amplitude QRS complexes	History of diabetes, bicarbonate-responsive preexisting acidosis, renal failure	Sodium bicarbonate, hyperventilation
Hyperkalemia or Hypokalemia	Both states cause wide-complex QRS *High potassium ECG:* ☐ T waves taller and peaked ☐ P waves get smaller ☐ QRS widens ☐ Sine-wave PEA *Low potassium ECG:* ☐ T waves flatten ☐ Prominent U waves ☐ QRS widens ☐ QT prolongs ☐ Wide-complex tachycardia	History of renal failure, diabetes, recent dialysis, dialysis fistulas, medications Abnormal loss of potassium; diuretic use	*Treat hyperkalemia:* Sodium bicarbonate Glucose plus insulin Calcium chloride Kayexalate/sorbitol Dialysis (long-term) Possible albuterol *Hypokalemia:* rapid but controlled infusion of potassium; add magnesium if cardiac arrest
Hypothermia	J or Osborne waves	History of exposure to cold, central body temperature	See Hypothermia Treatment Algorithm
Tablets: Drug overdose (tricyclics, digoxin, β-blockers, calcium channel blockers) Accidents	Various effects on ECG; predominantly prolonged QT interval	Bradycardia, history of ingestion, empty bottles at the scene, pupils, neurologic exam	Drug screens, intubation, lavage, activated charcoal, lactulose per local protocols, specific antidotes and agents per toxidrome
Tamponade: cardiac tamponade	Narrow complex Rapid rate	History, no pulse with CPR, vein distention	Pericardiocentesis

Condition	Features of Electrical Activity	Historical/Physical Clues	Management
Tension pneumothorax	Narrow complex Slow rate (hypoxia)	History, no pulse with CPR, neck vein distention, tracheal deviation, unequal breath sounds, difficulty ventilating patient	Needle decompression
Thrombosis, coronary: ACS	Abnormal 12-lead ECG: Q waves ST-segment changes T waves, inversions	History, ECG, enzymes	Thrombolytic agents; see AMI cases
Thrombosis, pulmonary (massive embolism)	Narrow complex Rapid rate	History, no pulse felt with CPR, distended neck veins	Pulmonary arteriogram, surgical embolectomy, thrombolytics

[1]Modified with permission from Cummins RO, Graves JR. *ACLS Scenarios: Core Concepts for Case-Based Learning.* St Louis, MO: Mosby Lifeline; 1996.

for management. The possible causes of PEA are presented as the **5 H's** and the **5 T's,** which are combined with clues from the ECG, history, and physical examination.

Memory Aids for Causes of PEA

PEA is associated with many conditions. Memorize a list of possible causes so that you can review the list quickly when faced with a cardiac arrest patient with PEA. Several authors, many of them ACLS instructors, have recognized the need for easily remembered lists of some of these causes. You can also devise a personal system for memorizing the list of causes. Several examples of memory aids follow.

1. The 5 H's and 5 T's Approach[2]

The 5 H's and 5 T's are presented in Table 2.

2. Hypoxia Comes First

Another listing—"hypoxia comes first"—is really not a memory aid but simply a listing according to frequency and ease of reversal (Table 3).

3. Causes of EMD: The Mnemonic "MATCH-HHH-ED"

This mnemonic (see Table 4) has the advantage of spelling something that resembles a word, which helps recall the 5 causes that fit with "MATCH." The total list, however, is not arranged in order of frequency or importance.

4. The Primary and Secondary ABCD Surveys

For uniformity we recommend referring to the ***Primary and Secondary ABCD Surveys.*** For each component of these 2 surveys you can list causes that may

TABLE 2. The 5 H's and 5 T's*

5 Causes That Start With "H"	5 Causes That Start With "T"
Hypovolemia	Tablets (drug overdose)
Hypoxia	Tamponade (cardiac)
Hydrogen ion (acidosis)	Tension pneumothorax
Hyperkalemia/hypokalemia	Thrombosis (coronary)
Hypothermia	Thrombosis (pulmonary)

*Note: Advanced providers may use 6 H's by adding hypo-/hyperglycemia and 6 T's by adding trauma.

[2]Kloeck W, Cummins RO, Chamberlain D, Bossaert L, Callanan V, Carli P, Christenson J, Connolly B, Ornato J, Sanders A, Steen P, et al. The Universal ACLS Algorithm: an advisory statement by the Advanced Life Support Working Group of the International Liaison Committee on Resuscitation. *Resuscitation.* 1997;34:109-111.

TABLE 3. Sequential Recall of Causes of EMD[3]

Hypoxia

Hypovolemia

The Obstructive 3 (3 P's)

- Pneumothorax (tension)
- Pericardial tamponade
- Pulmonary emboli, air emboli, amniotic fluid emboli

The Miscellaneous 3:

- Electrolyte and metabolic disturbance
- Massive hypothermia
- Drugs and toxins

[3]Hughes S, McQuillan PJ, Baskett P. Sequential recall of causes of electro-mechanical dissociation (EMD). *Resuscitation.* 1998;37:51.

TABLE 4. "MATCHHHHED" Causes of EMD[4]

M—Myocardial infarction, myocardial injury-ischemia
A—Acidosis
T—Tension pneumothorax
C—Cardiac tamponade
H—Hypothermia
H—Hyperkalemia/hypokalemia
H—Hypoxia
H—Hypovolemia
E—Embolism (pulmonary, air, amniotic fluid)
D—Drug overdose, toxins

[4] Rosenberg D, Levin E, Myerburg RJ. A mnemonic for the recall of causes of electro-mechanical dissociation (EMD). *Resuscitation.* 1999;40:57.

play a role in either the original arrest or persistence of cardiac arrest. The box below provides a detailed list for reviewing possible causes of a PEA arrest. This table uses the **ABCD** mnemonic of the 2 ACLS surveys. This technique can also be used during an arrest of any cause.

ECG Clues

Use all available clues to sort quickly through the possible causes of PEA. One clue is the type of electrical activity in the monitored complexes. To many the term *PEA* refers to the broad, slurred, disorganized electrical activity that in no way resembles a normal P wave–QRS complex. The ECG, however, may include normal complexes or other characteristics that suggest the cause of the problem.

In many disease processes the "pulseless" state is due to volume and pump causes *external* to the heart. For example, massive pulmonary edema, tension pneumothorax, and pericardial tamponade are lethal processes that start with a normally beating heart. Similarly, during exsanguination or life-threatening hypovolemia, the QRS complexes maintain a normal appearance.

Reassess the monitored rhythm and note the rate and width of the QRS complexes (see Tables 4 and 5). If possible and with-

PEA Arrest: "Hunting for Reversible Causes"

Step 1: Troubleshoot
Recheck the Primary and Secondary ABCD Survey

Airway:
- Airway is open and air is moving easily through airway adjuncts
- Tracheal tube, if in place, is open and unobstructed

Breathing:
- Bilateral, symmetric chest expansions with ventilations
- Ventilation is provided at correct rate and force

Circulation:
- CPR chest compressions are adequate in rate, force, depth, location
- IV access established correctly
- Medications administered properly
- Monitor used correctly (leads connected, correct control settings)

Step 2: Differential Diagnosis
Review the Secondary "D" by asking "What else could be causing this PEA?"

Airway *(problems lead to* ***hypoxia****):*
- Tube in the wrong place, the esophagus or right main bronchus
- Tube obstructed or kinked
- Foreign-body aspiration
- Anaphylaxis (angioedema), producing laryngospasm or glottic edema
- Craniofacial trauma, laryngeal or tracheal disruption

Breathing *(problems lead to* ***hypoxia****):*
- Preexisting mechanical abnormalities of the chest wall (scoliosis, emphysema, congenital)
- ***Tension pneumothorax*** from resuscitative efforts
- Bronchospasm as in acute asthma or exacerbation of chronic obstructive pulmonary disease (COPD)

Circulation:
- ***Hypovolemia***
- *Tamponade:* ***pericardial tamponade*** *from resuscitative efforts*
- *Thrombus:* ***pulmonary embolus***
- *Hypoxia:* ***prolonged hypoxia*** causing cardiac failure
- *Thrombus:* ***massive AMI***
- *Electrolyte* ***disturbances (potassium, calcium, magnesium)***
- Tablets: ***drug overdoses*** of many types: cyclic antidepressants, aspirin, b-blockers, or calcium channel blockers
- Anaphylaxis (angioedema)
- ***Trauma: occult trauma—cardiac tamponade, hypovolemia, exsanguination***
- Illicit drugs: cocaine, heroin, cyanide poisoning (from fires from synthetics)
- Carbon monoxide poisoning
- Anesthetic agent toxicity

out interrupting CPR for more than a few seconds, obtain a 12-lead ECG. Several types of PEA classified by ***width*** of QRS complexes and ***rate*** of associated electrical activity can provide valuable clues about possible causes of PEA (Table 5).

Hypovolemia, a very common cause of primary PEA, initially produces the classic physiologic response of a rapid, *narrow-complex tachycardia,* with increased diastolic and decreased systolic pressures. As loss of volume continues, blood pressure drops further, eventually becoming undetectable, but the narrow QRS complexes and rapid rate continue (ie, PEA). Alerted by the rhythm, clinicians can discover the cause of hypovolemia. Providing prompt treatment can then reverse the pulseless state simply by correcting the hypovolemia. Common nontraumatic causes of hypovolemia include occult internal hemorrhage, severe dehydration, cardiac tamponade, tension pneumothorax, and massive pulmonary embolism.

Box 4: Initial Treatment of PEA: Epinephrine

> ***Epinephrine*** 1 mg IV push, repeat every 3 to 5 minutes

Epinephrine is administered every 3 to 5 minutes during cardiac arrest.

Box 5: Atropine in PEA

> ***Atropine*** 1 mg IV (if PEA rate is ***slow***), repeat every 3 to 5 minutes as needed, to a total dose of 0.04 mg/kg

Atropine for Treatment of Relative Bradycardia

Bradycardia has traditionally been defined as *normal sinus rhythm at a rate of less than 60 bpm in an adult.* ***"Relative bradycardia"*** indicates that the heart rate is too slow for the clinical condition. A relative bradycardia is present if the heart rate is slow and shock (hypotension) is present. For example, a pale, diaphoretic man with a blood pressure of 90/60 mm Hg and a heart rate of 80 bpm has a relative bradycardia, because 80 bpm is too slow for a blood pressure of 90/60 mm Hg—the patient should be tachycardic. This person would be a candidate for atropine.

Informal surveys suggest that many ACLS providers consider atropine one of the standard agents for treating PEA without reference to the electrical activity rate. There is little evidence to indicate whether this helps or harms the patient. Until specific evidence accumulates otherwise, follow the ACLS recommendation of limiting atropine to absolute or relative bradycardia. The shorter dosing interval (every 3 minutes) is possibly helpful (Class IIb) in cardiac arrest.

Shock Index and Relative Bradycardia

As an informal gauge of relative bradycardia, some clinicians teach use of the heart rate in relation to blood pressure. The ratio of systolic blood pressure to heart rate yields the "shock index." (Some articles invert the numerator and denominator and define the index as heart rate divided by systolic blood pressure.) A normal systolic pressure of 120 mm Hg divided by a typical heart rate of 80 bpm gives a normal index greater than 1 (specifically 1.5). Most clinicians would consider a systolic blood pressure of 110 mm Hg and a heart rate of 120 bpm acceptable when each vital sign is considered separately. The shock index, however, is less than 1. Such a value at least signals the need for a more in-depth examination.

TABLE 5. Classification of PEA Rhythms by Rate and QRS Width

Rate of Complexes	Width of Complexes	
	Narrow More likely to have noncardiac cause; low volume, low vascular tone	***Wide*** More often due to cardiac cause; also drug and electrolyte toxicities
Fast (>60 bpm)	■ Sinus (P wave) EMD ■ Pseudo-EMD ■ PSVT	■ VF ■ VT
Slow (<60 bpm)	■ EMD ■ Pseudo-EMD ■ Postdefibrillation ■ Idioventricular rhythms	■ Bradyasystolic rhythms ■ Idioventricular rhythms ■ Ventricular escape rhythms

Specific Treatments

Drugs and Electrolytes

Cardiac toxicity from drug overdoses is a common cause of PEA. Approach these patients with great optimism because the period of toxicity may be very brief. In these situations the myocardium is healthy, but a temporary cardiac disturbance has caused clinical death. Numerous case reports confirm the success of many specific limited interventions with one thing in common—they buy time.

These treatments support a viable level of blood flow to the brain and heart while awaiting correction of specific electrolyte abnormalities or the diminution of toxic blood levels of drugs or poisons. Treatments that can provide this level of support include prolonged basic CPR (case reports have documented successful recovery after 6 hours of CPR), intra-aortic balloon pumping, cardiopulmonary bypass, renal dialysis, specific drug antidotes (digibind, glucagon, bicarbonate), transcutaneous pacing, and delayed treatment of profound electrolyte disturbances (potassium, magnesium, calcium, acidosis).

"Pseudo-PEA"

In some PEA cases, especially patients in shock and those with marked peripheral vasoconstriction, the victim seems "pulseless" on physical examination, but the ventricles are contracting and moving blood in forward flow. Careful assessment (eg, with Doppler ultrasound or transesophageal echocardiography) may reveal this arterial blood flow. Echocardiography may indicate surprisingly good cardiac contractility. These patients need specific interventions based on the cause of the cardiovascular compromise. Review Box 3 and Table 2 for lists of possible causes and appropriate treatments.

Critical Actions: Assessment and Management

See the Critical Actions Checklist.

Unacceptable Actions: Perils and Pitfalls

Remember that you have a limited window of time to identify and treat reversible causes of PEA. If you fail to identify cardiac arrest or fail to identify reversible causes, you are missing an opportunity for successful resuscitation. ACLS providers can be led astray in a number of areas:

- Not assessing the patient carefully. The rhythm complexes can "look so good" on the monitor screen that the pulse check is never completed, delaying recognition of the pulseless state.
- Not considering the different possible causes of PEA: "If you don't think about it, you won't recognize it." As simple as the idea is, the memorized list of causes to consider is the best way to keep from overlooking an obvious cause with an easy resolution. Keep these lists available in the clinical setting so that you are not forced to rely on memory during a hectic resuscitation.
- Treating with epinephrine only. Recognize the concepts of absolute and relative bradycardia as indications for atropine. Excessive parasympathetic tone may be easily reversed.
- Not troubleshooting ventilation/intubating the patient. Hypoxia and asphyxia affect heart rate in a sequence: first tachycardia, then, with progressive damage, profound bradycardia ending with asystole.
- Not giving a volume infusion. It cannot hurt; it treats occult hypovolemia, a common cause of PEA. Many experts have recommended "empiric fluid challenge" as a standard part of the PEA Algorithm.
- Defibrillation. Never shock an organized or regular rhythm. The smallest chance of resuscitation will be lost.
- Not performing chest compressions. The rhythm complexes look good, but without a peripheral pulse the victim needs CPR.

Critical Actions Checklist: ACLS Case 4 Pulseless Electrical Activity		
Scene Survey Steps	**Assess: Do or Monitor**	**Manage: Do or Delegate**
Start Primary ABCD Survey		
Airway and Breathing	☐ *Check airway location* ☐ *Rule out pneumothorax* ☐ *Evaluate oxygenation: is pulmonary embolus present?*	☐ Primary and secondary confirmation of airway ☐ Check breath sounds, oxygenation, ventilation, chest expansion ☐ Evaluate oxygenation and ventilation
Circulation	*Truly "pulseless"?*	Doppler ultrasound Echocardiography
Defibrillation	*Rhythm?* ☐ Assess the rhythm with AED or defibrillator/monitor ☐ Recognize that the rhythm is not VF, VT, or asystole	*Rhythm other than VF or VT or asystole?* ☐ Continue CPR
Start Secondary ABCD Survey: Use the PEA Algorithm		
Circulation drugs	*Assess context of resuscitation:* ☐ Renal dialysis? ☐ Diabetes? ☐ Rehabilitation clinic (emboli)? ☐ Bleeding disorder, anti-coagulants? ☐ Needle marks, drug abuse? ☐ Under psychiatric care?	Empiric use of specific agents: ☐ NS boluses? ☐ Calcium chloride? ☐ Naloxone? ☐ tPA?
Differential diagnoses	*Reversible cause?* ☐ Use a system to review possible causes: — 5 H's and 5 T's — MATCHHHHED — "HYPOXIA 1st" ☐ Don't limit your thinking ☐ Gather and review clues: — Relevant history — Physical findings — X-ray, echocardiographic findings — Laboratory results	☐ Be able to list the various possible causes of PEA and their clues and treatments. ☐ Act aggressively to identify and treat possible causes of PEA. ☐ Persist until you have identified a cause or the resuscitative effort is terminated. ☐ Longer CPR? ☐ Cardiopulmonary bypass? ☐ Intra-aortic balloon pump?

Workbook Review

1. **You are called to assist in the attempted resuscitation of a patient who is demonstrating PEA. As you hurry to the patient's room, you review the information you learned in the ACLS course about management of PEA. Which one of the following statements about PEA is *true?***
   - **a.** chest compressions should be administered only if the patient with PEA develops a ventricular rate of less than 50 bpm
   - **b.** successful treatment of PEA requires identification and treatment of reversible causes, such as the 5 H's and 5 T's
   - **c.** atropine is the drug of choice for treatment of PEA, whether the ventricular rate is slow or fast
   - **d.** PEA is rarely caused by hypovolemia, so fluid administration is contraindicated and should not be attempted

   Read more about it in the ECC Guidelines 2000, *pages 150-152: Figure 4: Pulseless Electrical Activity and PEA Algorithm*

2. **You are called to the ED to assist in the attempted resuscitation of a patient in pulseless cardiac arrest from unknown causes. When the patient arrives in the ED, chest compressions are being performed, and the patient is receiving ventilations through a tracheal tube placed by EMS personnel in the field. The patient is transferred to a gurney; you confirm that chest compressions are producing palpable femoral pulses, but no pulses are palpable between administered compressions. The patient is attached to a cardiac monitor that confirms the presence of organized QRS complexes. What is the *first* thing you should assess in an attempt to identify a reversible cause of cardiac arrest in this patient?**
   - **a.** check tracheal tube placement with primary and secondary techniques and evaluate breath sounds to rule out tension pneumothorax
   - **b.** check arterial blood gases
   - **c.** check serum electrolytes to rule out imbalances
   - **d.** obtain a serum sample to identify drug overdose

   Read more about it in the ECC Guidelines 2000, page *151: PEA Algorithm, Secondary ABCD Survey*

3. **You are participating in the attempted resuscitation of a 62-year-old woman who collapsed suddenly at her home 3 weeks after cardiovascular surgery for aortic and mitral valve replacement. She recently began taking anticoagulants. Chest compressions are being performed, a tracheal tube is in place (proper placement was confirmed using primary and secondary confirmation techniques), and the patient is receiving 100% oxygen. Ventilation is producing bilateral chest expansion and adequate breath sounds. The ECG reveals narrow QRS complexes with a rate of 80 bpm, but no pulses are present. Ultrasound reveals no cardiac tamponade. Which of the following sequences of therapy is most appropriate for this patient?**
   - **a.** atropine 1 mg IV every 3 to 5 minutes to a total dose of 0.04 mg/kg, followed by vasopressin 40 U IV single dose
   - **b.** sodium bicarbonate 1 mEq/kg every 3 to 5 minutes for empiric treatment of hyperkalemia
   - **c.** epinephrine 1 mg, followed by a fluid bolus and search for reversible causes
   - **d.** send blood for coagulation screening profile, and send the patient for immediate CT scan to rule out intracranial hemorrhage

   Read more about it in the ECC Guidelines 2000, *pages 150-152: Figure 4: Pulseless Electrical Activity and PEA Algorithm, particularly page 152: top paragraph, right column*

4. **You are participating in the attempted resuscitation of a patient with PEA. The patient has been intubated (with tube position confirmed) and is receiving 100% oxygen and effective ventilation with bilateral breath sounds and good chest expansion. Epinephrine 1 mg was administered 2 minutes ago. PEA continues, with a ventricular rate of 45 bpm. While you search for reversible causes of the PEA, which of the following therapies would now be appropriate?**
   - **a.** monophasic defibrillation up to 3 times at 200 J, 200 to 300 J, and 360 J, or biphasic defibrillation at approximately 150 J
   - **b.** synchronized cardioversion
   - **c.** epinephrine 10 mL of 1:10 000 solution IV bolus
   - **d.** atropine 1 mg IV

   Read more about it in the ECC Guidelines 2000, *pages 150-152: Figure 4: Pulseless Electrical Activity and PEA Algorithm*

5. **For which of the following patients with PEA is sodium bicarbonate therapy (1 mEq/kg) most likely to be *most* effective?**
   - **a.** the patient with hypercarbic acidosis and tension pneumothorax treated with decompression
   - **b.** the patient with a brief arrest interval
   - **c.** the patient with documented severe hyperkalemia
   - **d.** the patient with documented severe hypokalemia

   Read more about it in the ECC Guidelines 2000, *pages 150-152: Figure 4: Pulseless Electrical Activity and PEA Algorithm, particularly page 152: top left column, sodium bicarbonate. Information about treatment of hyperkalemia is presented on page 217: "Life-Threatening Electrolyte Abnormalities; Hyperkalemia."*

Asystole: The Silent Heart Algorithm

Description

Case 5 focuses on the assessment and management of *asystole.* Asystole is a cardiac arrest rhythm associated with no discernable electrical activity on the ECG ("flat line"). Asystole is rarely associated with a positive outcome. Successful resuscitation of a person in asystolic cardiac arrest is rare, happening only when rescuers stop, think, and ask *"Why did **this** person have **this** cardiac arrest at **this** time?"* Only if the cause of asystole is identified and treated in a timely fashion will there be any reasonable possibility of survival.

A large percentage of asystolic patients do not survive. Asystole occurs almost exclusively in severely ill persons. Often this rhythm represents the terminal rhythm of patients whose organs have failed and whose condition has deteriorated. Cardiac function has diminished until cardiac electrical and functional activity finally stops. The person has died.

In such scenarios resuscitation fades as a high-priority action. Prolonged efforts are unnecessary, futile, often unethical, and ultimately dehumanizing if not demeaning. The asystole case provides the most appropriate place to discuss and understand ethics, when *not* to start resuscitative efforts, and indications for terminating resuscitative attempts.

What's New in the Guidelines... Asystole

Revisions in the Treatment of Asystole

The *ECC Guidelines 2000* contain no revisions in the recommended *treatments* for asystole. The single most important therapy for asystole continues to be search for, identify, and reverse any treatable cause.

1. The overall treatment approach remains consistent with that of previous guidelines:
   - Effective *CPR*
   - Supplemental *oxygen*
   - Advanced airway control with *tracheal intubation*
   - Occasional *transcutaneous pacing*
   - IV medications *epinephrine, atropine,* and when indicated, *sodium bicarbonate.* (In rare situations, such as asystolic heart transplants, *isoproterenol* may be indicated.)
2. The evidence is lacking to establish equal effectiveness between *epinephrine* and the recently approved adrenergic-like agent *vasopressin.* There is evidence to support vasopressin as a replacement for epinephrine in cardiac arrest associated with ventricular fibrillation (VF) but not for cardiac arrest associated with asystole or pulseless electrical activity (PEA).

Revisions in the Concept of Asystole

A series of dramatic revisions in the ACLS Provider Course have been incorporated into the *ECC Guidelines 2000.* The major focus of the asystole case changed from *learning the few things you can try to reverse asystolic arrest* to *learning the care you can provide when you realize that asystole is usually the end of a person's life.* New, important, and long-overdue guidelines have followed from this enriched perspective. They include these specific new recommendations:

(Continued on next page)

Settings and Scenarios

Setting: Prehospital

You are a paramedic responding to a 911 call about an unconscious/unresponsive 18-year-old woman. The woman was discovered unconscious after she returned to her room "to take a little nap." There were reports that she had been feeling "down" and "depressed." She is not breathing. You begin rescue breathing and find that she has no pulse or other signs of circulation. Begin management of this patient.

Setting: Emergency Dept, Monitored Patient

Relatives have brought a 64-year-old woman into the Emergency Department after she collapsed in the hospital parking lot. Hospital personnel have started CPR, but no ACLS intervention has been initiated. You overhear a relative say the woman was on her way to her last oncology clinic appointment.

Setting: In-Hospital, Unmonitored Patient

A 48-year-old woman is spending her first day in a step-down postoperative unit after undergoing bilateral knee replacements 1 week ago. Her family reports that she was trying to stand beside her bed when she suddenly fell to the floor unconscious. She has not responded to stimulation.

Setting: Critical Care Unit, Monitored Patient

A 55-year-old patient is admitted to the critical care unit (CCU) with an acute myocardial infarction. The monitor alarm sounds, and the screen shows progressive bradycardia. When the nurse responding to the cardiac monitor enters the room she finds the patient unresponsive.

- In support of an end-of-life decision made by a terminally ill patient, rescuers should be alert to any communications or expressions made by the patient before the arrest that indicate that he or she has decided against any resuscitative attempts ("do not attempt resuscitation")
- To preserve the dignity of the patient and the patient's loved ones at the end of the patient's life, Emergency Departments, in-hospital code teams, and EMS responders should adopt the new AHA criteria for stopping resuscitative efforts much sooner than currently practiced.
- To prevent inappropriate prolongation of CPR and resuscitative efforts for the many without denying the small possibility of meaningful survival for the few: *stop resuscitative efforts for all arrest victims who, despite successful deployment of advanced interventions, continue in asystole for more than 10 minutes with no potential reversible cause.*
- To enable EMS professionals to participate effectively and with dignity in the end of a patient's life, EMS systems should develop supportive protocols that
  - Allow EMS personnel to provide end-of-life comfort and care but free them from an obligation to attempt resuscitation should the victim develop cardiac arrest
  - Allow death certification at the scene (out of hospital) via on-line medical control
  - Reduce the futile transport of pulseless patients to local Emergency Departments after failed field resuscitative attempts
  - Allow EMS personnel to leave the victim's body at the scene.
- To enable Emergency Department and critical care unit personnel to provide the therapeutic benefits of *having the patient's family present at resuscitative attempts,* Emergency Departments, in-hospital code teams, and EMS responders should give thoughtful consideration to this new concept.

The international coalition of experts and clinicians assembled by the AHA in September 1999 and February 2000 were so firmly committed to these new guidelines that many of the recommendations are stated explicitly in the Asystole Algorithm.

Learning and Skills Objectives

Major Learning Points

At the end of Case 5 you should be able to

1. Verify that the flat line seen on the ECG monitor is indeed "true asystole" (an electrically silent heart) and not another rhythm (eg, fine VF) masquerading as a flat line or an operator error that creates a flat line (ie, "asystole") on the monitor screen when in fact another rhythm is present.
2. Use the ACLS Approach (the Primary and Secondary ABCD Surveys) for a patient in asystole.
3. Discuss the relative merits of adequate ventilation—not IV buffer therapy—as the mainstay of acidosis treatment.
4. Describe why successful resuscitation in asystole requires identification of a treatable cause. The team leader must rapidly and energetically focus on the differential diagnosis of asystole.

5. State the most common *reversible* conditions associated with asystole. *(Reversible causes of asystole are not limited to the list below.)* Note that these conditions are the same conditions that should be identified or ruled out when PEA develops.

- 5 H's:
  1. Hypovolemia
  2. Hypoxia
  3. Hydrogen ion—acidosis
  4. Hyperkalemia/hypokalemia
  5. Hypothermia
- 5 T's
  1. "Tablets"
  2. Tamponade, cardiac
  3. Tension pneumothorax
  4. Thrombosis, coronary (acute coronary syndrome [ACS])
  5. Thrombosis, pulmonary (embolism)
- Keep in mind that these conditions do not directly cause the rhythm to convert to asystole. Instead, asystole occurs in association with the clinical deterioration of these conditions.

6. Recognize that asystole usually represents a confirmation of death rather than a "rhythm" to be treated. Describe the criteria that clinicians should follow for terminating resuscitative efforts.

Specific Skills to Learn

At the end of Case 5 you should be able to

1. Provide airway maintenance and ventilation, because adequate ventilation is the mainstay of care for asystole while trying to identify the reversible cause.

2. Conduct a rapid "secondary D" (assessment of asystole and its causes).

3. Recognize indications for terminating resuscitative efforts.

New Rhythms to Learn

- Asystole versus slow PEA
- False asystole
- Occult VF

New Drugs to Learn

Epinephrine, sodium bicarbonate, atropine. See the *ECC Handbook* and Chapter 3, ACLS Skill 7.

The Asystole Algorithm

Box 1: Primary ABCD Survey

Box 1 provides you with a reminder that you need to follow the **ACLS Approach of the Primary and Secondary ABCD Surveys.** To complete the Primary ABCD Survey you need to perform the following:

Airway: open and manage the airway

Breathing: give rescue breaths

Heart rate: check for a pulse; no central pulse found

Rhythm: note the absence of any electrical activity on the monitored rhythm

- The critical feature of a patient in asystole is the absence of any cardiac electrical activity as recorded on body-surface electrodes.
- This "electrical silence" appears on the monitor as a completely flat ("isoelectric") tracing.
- A few variations of "asystole" have been observed. They include (1) "P-wave asystole," in which persistent atrial activity exists without any ventricular response and (2) "agonal" or "idioventricular" electrical complexes that appear at a rate of less than 6 per minute (every 10 seconds).*

Defibrillation: recognize that the patient did not have a shockable rhythm; no one administers defibrillatory shocks.

*Researchers studying the epidemiology of out-of-hospital cardiac arrest rhythms have arbitrarily drawn the line between PEA and "asystole with a few complexes." More than 10 complexes per minute is defined as PEA, and fewer than that is defined as asystole.

1

Primary ABCD Survey

Focus: *basic CPR and defibrillation*

Rapid scene survey: *is there any evidence that personnel should* ***not*** *attempt resuscitation (eg, DNAR order, signs of death)?* ***(Note 2)***

- **Check** responsiveness
- **Activate** emergency response system
- **Call** for defibrillator

A **Airway:** open the airway
B **Breathing:** provide positive-pressure ventilations
C **Circulation:** give chest compressions
C **Confirm** true asystole ***(Note 1)***
D **Defibrillation:** assess for VF/pulseless VT; shock if indicated

Note 1: **Confirm true asystole**

- Check lead and cable connections
- Monitor power on?
- Monitor gain up?
- Verify asystole in another lead?

Note 2: DNAR patient?

- Do not start/attempt resuscitation?
- Any indicators of DNAR status? Bracelet? Anklet? Written documentation?
- Clinical indications that resuscitative efforts are not an appropriate or indicated intervention? If no, continue resuscitative efforts

Asystole: The Silent Heart Algorithm.

Asystole

↓

1

Primary ABCD Survey

Focus: *basic CPR and defibrillation*

Rapid scene survey: *is there any evidence that personnel should* ***not*** *attempt resuscitation (eg, DNAR order, signs of death)?*

- **Check** responsiveness
- **Activate** emergency response system
- **Call** for defibrillator

A **Airway:** open the airway
B **Breathing:** provide positive-pressure ventilations
C **Circulation:** give chest compressions
C **Confirm** true asystole
D **Defibrillation:** assess for VF/pulseless VT; shock if indicated

↓

2

Secondary ABCD Survey

Focus: *more advanced assessments and treatments*

A **Airway:** place airway device as soon as possible
B **Breathing:** confirm airway device placement by exam plus confirmation device
B **Breathing:** secure airway device; purpose-made tube holders preferred
B **Breathing:** confirm effective oxygenation and ventilation
C **Circulation:** confirm true asystole
C **Circulation:** establish IV access
C **Circulation:** identify rhythm → monitor
C **Circulation:** give medications appropriate for rhythm and condition
C **Circulation:** assess for occult blood flow ("pseudo-EMD")
D **Differential Diagnosis:** search for and treat identified reversible causes

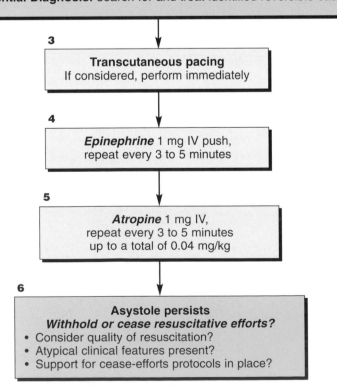

↓

3

Transcutaneous pacing
If considered, perform immediately

↓

4

Epinephrine 1 mg IV push,
repeat every 3 to 5 minutes

↓

5

Atropine 1 mg IV,
repeat every 3 to 5 minutes
up to a total of 0.04 mg/kg

↓

6

Asystole persists

Withhold or cease resuscitative efforts?

- Consider quality of resuscitation?
- Atypical clinical features present?
- Support for cease-efforts protocols in place?

Box 2: The Secondary ABCD Survey

Airway

- Place an advanced airway.
- Verify correct position with primary and secondary tube confirmation techniques.
- Secure the airway device to prevent dislodgment.
- Continue to monitor tube position throughout the resuscitative effort.

Do Not Shock Asystole

Some clinicians have argued for "shock asystole" protocols. These protocols include shocking asystole, using the rationale that "empiric shocks to asystolic hearts may help," "shocking asystole cannot make the rhythm any worse," or "if you administer a shock you may convert patients with undetected fine VF and give them a chance to survive." There is no valid data in human adults to support this rationale. In 1993 a Nine City Study Group published an analysis of 77 asystolic patients who received initial countershock compared with 117 who received standard therapy.* The countershock group had worse short-term and long-term outcomes.

Shocks can be harmful. Electrical shocks can produce a "stunned heart" and profound parasympathetic discharge. Such shocks to an asystolic heart would more likely eliminate any possibility of return of spontaneous cardiac activity. The ACLS Subcommittee has reviewed this question many times and considers empiric shocking of asystole a Class III recommendation (no evidence to support and possibly harmful).

*Martin DR, Gavin T, Bianco J, Brown CG, Stueven H, Pepe PE, Cummins RO, Gonzalez E, Jastremski M. Initial countershock in the treatment of asystole. *Resuscitation.* 1993; 26:63-68.

Secondary ABCD Survey

Focus: *more advanced assessments and treatments*

- A **Airway:** place airway device as soon as possible
- B **Breathing:** confirm airway device placement by exam plus confirmation device
- B **Breathing:** secure airway device; purpose-made tube holders preferred
- B **Breathing:** confirm effective oxygenation and ventilation
- C **Circulation:** confirm true asystole
- C **Circulation:** establish IV access
- C **Circulation:** identify rhythm → monitor
- C **Circulation:** give medications ***(Note 3)*** appropriate for rhythm and condition
- C **Circulation:** assess for occult blood flow ("pseudo-EMD")
- D **Differential Diagnosis:** search for and treat identified reversible causes

Note 3: Sodium bicarbonate 1 mEq/kg. Indications for use include overdose with tricyclic antidepressants; alkalinization of urine in overdoses; tracheal intubation and long arrest intervals; and upon return of spontaneous circulation if long arrest interval. Ineffective or harmful in hypercarbic acidosis.

- This treatment sequence is virtually identical to the treatment sequence for patients with slow-rate PEA.

Breathing

- Supply positive-pressure ventilation with a bag mask or appropriate mechanical ventilation.
- Verify bilateral chest movement.
- Check blood oxygenation with a pulse oximeter; order arterial blood gas analyses.
- Arrange for mechanical ventilation (unless the patient resumes immediate spontaneous respirations).
- Check for potential complications in breathing caused by resuscitation, such as pneumothorax, rib fractures, sternal fractures, and improper airway placement. Proper airway management and adequate ventilation are critical for maintaining acid-base balance in any cardiac arrest. Conditions to rule out can be remembered with the mnemonic DOPE: **D**isplacement of tube, **O**bstruction of tube, **P**neumothorax, or **E**quipment failure.

Circulation

Confirm that the flat line is not a result of operator error, which is a more common cause of a flat ECG than fine VF. (*Note:* One good clue to the possibility of operator error is a pulse in "asystolic" patients.) Be sure to check the following:

- Ensure proper connection of the monitor cable to the patient.
- Verify proper connection of the monitor cable to the defibrillator.
- Ensure that the power switch is ON.

Differential Diagnoses

Memory Aids for the Causes of Asystole

The possible reversible causes of asystolic and PEA cardiac arrest are the same, which means you can use the same memory aids. An example is the memory aid *"The 5 H's and 5 T's Approach."*

Box 3

Transcutaneous pacing *(Note 4)*
If considered, perform immediately

Note 4: To be effective, ***transcutaneous pacing*** must be performed early and combined with drug therapy. Evidence does not support routine use of transcutaneous pacing for asystole.

The Flat Line Protocol

ACLS providers should recognize that asystole is a specific diagnosis. A flat line, however, is not. The term *flat line* is nonspecific and could apply to several possible conditions of which true asystole is only one. The other "diagnoses" are really technical and operational problems that must be identified. Some of these diagnoses are not applicable to all defibrillators. A third cause of a flat line is derived from the so-called "VF-has-a-vector" theory. This well-known theory—which lacks significant confirmation in human studies—states that VF may appear as a flat line in any lead that records at 90 degrees to VF waves moving through the myocardium with a specific vector.

These problems should be identifiable during the flat line protocol and include ruling out the following conditions (none should be present if the diagnosis of asystole is made):

- Power to monitor or defibrillator OFF
- Batteries "dead"
- Monitor gain too low
- Monitor cable not connected to patient, 3-lead connector, or monitor

Upon seeing a flat line on either an in-hospital or out-of-hospital monitor, you should conduct the flat line protocol:

Is the rhythm asystole?	*Flat Line Protocol*
Assess rhythm with defibrillator/monitor	Check power to both defibrillator and monitor (some devices have separate POWER ON controls for the defibrillator and monitor).
Recognize non-VF	Check all connections: device ➔ cables, cables ➔ patient, device ➔ paddles, paddles ➔ patient.
Recognize flat line	Check GAIN or SENSITIVITY setting on defibrillator/monitor. If low or off, all rhythms will appear as a flat line.
Recognize that flat line has a differential diagnosis	Check LEAD SELECT setting: for paddles? three-lead cable? lead I? II? III?
Identify asystole (after flat line protocol)	If on LEAD SELECT, do quick check for a rhythm in each lead (vector of VF concept).
	If on PADDLES, do 90-degree rotation to check for vector of VF (upper right sternum paddle to upper left sternum; left apex paddle to right lower sternal border).
	If using adhesive electrode pads, do not attempt to remove the pads and reattach them at 90-degree rotations. Instead, connect 3-lead limb leads.
	Note: A totally blank monitor screen means "NO POWER." All current-generation defibrillator/monitors can operate from sealed, lead-acid batteries (usually) or direct-line power supplied through high-grade power cords plugged into a 120- to 240-volt power source. When unplugged from line power—for example, responding to a "code"—the defibrillator/monitor automatically switches to the internal batteries as the source of current.
	An unfortunate and surprisingly common error occurs when the unit is not plugged back in or if the power cord is inadvertently disconnected. If used for routine monitoring, the batteries will steadily discharge until rhythm display is successful, but the batteries will not support multiple rapid charges and discharges by the defibrillator. These events can have tragic outcomes.

The 5 H's and 5 T's Approach*†

5 Reversible Causes That Start With "H"	5 Reversible Causes That Start With "T"
Hypovolemia	Tablets (drug overdoses)
Hypoxia	Tamponade (cardiac)
Hydrogen ion (acidosis)	Tension pneumothorax
Hyperkalemia/hypokalemia	Thrombosis—heart (AMI)
Hypothermia	Thrombosis—lungs (pulmonary embolus)

Note: Not all of the above would cause rapid conversion to asystole, but asystole may occur as a "pass-through" rhythm in a condition that is unremitting and deteriorating.

A more detailed approach to these causes, including clinical clues and suggested treatments, is provided in Case 4: PEA, in Table 1: Conditions That Can Cause Pulseless Electrical Activity and the box PEA Arrest: Hunting for Reversible Causes.

*Advanced providers may use 6 H's by adding hypo-/hyperglycemia and 6 T's by adding trauma.

†Kloeck W, Cummins RO, Chamberlain D, Bossaert L, Callanan V, Carli P, Christenson J, Connolly B, Ornato J, Sanders A, Steen P, et al. The universal ACLS algorithm: an advisory statement by the Advanced Life Support Working Group of the International Liaison Committee on Resuscitation. *Resuscitation.* 1997;34:109-111.

Transcutaneous Pacing for Asystole

Transcutaneous cardiac pacing (TCP) stimulates the heart externally through the skin and muscles of the chest wall, causing the heart to contract and maintain cardiac output. TCP is a short-term intervention performed through large pacing electrodes positioned on the patient's chest and back. Details of TCP are presented at the end of Case 7: Bradycardia.

Defibrillators With TCP Mode

Many defibrillator manufacturers have incorporated TCP capabilities into their devices. This option has emerged as a valuable intervention for clinical situations involving symptomatic bradycardia without cardiac arrest. The *1992 ECC Guidelines* introduced a strong recommendation for use of TCP in cases of symptomatic bradycardia without cardiac arrest. For asystole, however, this recommendation was only Class IIb. The *ECC Guidelines 2000* continue to make both the same positive recommendations and the same cautions and caveats in the Asystole Algorithm as in previous versions of the guidelines.

TCP Must Be Initiated Early

Reports of success with TCP in the treatment of asystole are rare and anecdotal. To have any chance of effectively treating asystole, TCP must be performed early—as soon as possible after the start of asystole. Clinical experience and one prospective, randomized clinical trial have shown that pacing is ineffective in prehospital settings. The AHA does not recommend routine pacing for out-of-hospital asystolic cardiac arrest.

Identification of Potential Pacing-Responsive Victims

The *1992 ECC Guidelines* considered the use of TCP for asystole acceptable, mainly because of occasional anecdotes of its temporary success for in-hospital arrest, Emergency Department use, and out-of-hospital arrest witnessed by ACLS-skilled personnel. TCP advocates theorized that patients in full cardiac arrest for no more than 5 minutes should be able to respond briefly to a pacing stimulus.

Cohorts of asystolic patients who are pacing responsive should exist. They might consist of people who suddenly develop a bradyasystolic arrest, Stokes-Adams attack, asystole due to vagal discharge, or myocardial stunning after a defibrillation shock. Patients in asystole caused by a drug overdose may also be responsive to pacing. In these patients the myocardium should be healthy and normal, but the toxic agents have disturbed the heart's conduction system. Early pacing with direct stimulation of the myocardium (rather than pharmacologic stimulation of the conduction system) can produce life-sustaining heart contractions for a limited time. TCP buys time while awaiting correction of drug-induced rhythm disturbances, electrolyte abnormalities, acidosis, or hypoxia.

Patients most commonly develop asystole after a defibrillation attempt in the presence of a healthcare provider. These patients in postshock asystole are better candidates for pacing because of a short arrest-to-pacing interval. Even in this situation, however, the experienced clinician will select only those patients for whom pacing has some chance of success. In general these will be patients with witnessed asystole for whom pacing can be initiated in less than 1 to 2 minutes.

The entity informally referred to as *P-wave asystole* occurs most often as a sequela of sudden, severe hypoxia. Theoretically these patients should be capable of responding to TCP stimuli. But no published reports of success exist, although it is unclear whether this represents a nonexistent entity, a failure rate of 100%, or simply clinical absence of the publishing imperative.

Additional Points About TCP for Asystolic Arrest

- Continue CPR chest compressions during pacing. Forego compressions if the paced complexes appear to produce a measurable pulse. (The failure rate of TCP for asystole is high; do not deprive the victim of the benefits of CPR.)
- Administer drugs (epinephrine and atropine) independent of TCP.
- For asystole start at the maximum energy output of the pacing device.
- Periodically turn the pacer off to eliminate pacing artifact, and examine the ECG. Look for promising ECG features such as P waves or QRS complexes. More commonly, however, the asystolic rhythm will have converted to VF or VT. Although the outcome of VF/pulseless VT is definitely superior to that of asystole, it also requires specific emergency therapy.

Box 4: Epinephrine in Asystole

Remember, every cardiac arrest victim should receive epinephrine except victims who respond to interventions before rescuers achieve IV access or VF patients who receive vasopressin. By producing marked vasoconstriction, epinephrine increases diastolic blood pressure, blood flow to the brain, and some blood flow to the heart, specifically the coronary arteries.

Epinephrine 1 mg IV push, repeat every 3 to 5 minutes ***(Note 5)***

Note 5: Epinephrine: The recommended dose is 1 mg IV push every 3 to 5 minutes. If this approach fails, higher doses of epinephrine (up to 0.2 mg/kg) may be used but are not recommended. Unlike persistent VF/VT, evidence is lacking to support routine use of ***vasopressin*** in treatment of **asystole.**

Epinephrine and Sodium Bicarbonate for Asystole

The recommended dose of **epinephrine** is 1 mg IV push every 3 to 5 minutes. High-dose epinephrine (0.1 mg/kg IV push every 3 to 5 minutes) is not recommended for routine use but can be considered if 1-mg doses fail (Class IIb).

A dose of **sodium bicarbonate** equal to 1 mEq/kg is definitely helpful (Class I) in the asystolic patient known to have preexisting hyperkalemia, in a known overdose with tricyclic antidepressants, and to alkalinize urine in drug overdoses (Class IIa). See the footnotes to the Asystole Algorithm for other lower-class recommendations for sodium bicarbon-

If the initial dose fails, continue to repeat epinephrine 1 mg IV every 3 to 5 minutes. The *1992 ECC Guidelines* accepted the use of higher doses of epinephrine in either escalating doses (1, 3, 5 mg), intermediate doses (5 mg per dose rather than 1 mg per dose), or high doses based on body weight (up to 0.2 mg/kg). By the year 2000, however, a growing body of indirect evidence suggested that high-dose epinephrine therapy might be harmful. Although high-dose epinephrine appears to be better at "restarting the heart," this is not equivalent to "restarting the head." In patients resuscitated from cardiac arrest there was a negative correlation between the total amount of epinephrine administered and cerebral function in the postresuscitation period. In the *ECC Guidelines 2000* higher doses of epinephrine are considered a Class IIb recommendation: acceptable but not recommended, because of weak supporting evidence and some evidence suggesting harm.

Atropine 1 mg IV ***(Note 6)***, repeat every 3 to 5 minutes up to a total of 0.04 mg/kg

Note 6: Atropine: use the shorter dosing interval (every 3 minutes) and the higher dose (0.04 mg/kg) in asystolic arrest

Box 5: Atropine in Asystole

Atropine is recommended in asystolic cardiac arrest based on an unconfirmed assumption. Some clinical experts have argued that excessive vagal or parasympathetic tone might play a role in stopping both ventricular and supraventricular pacemaker activity. Little direct evidence supports this assumption. Avoid atropine in cases in which the lack of cardiac activity has a clear explanation, such as hypothermic arrest.

The dosing of atropine can vary by amount (0.03 to 0.04 mg/kg) and interval (every 3 to 5 minutes). In practice most clinicians use the more aggressive approach of 1 mg of atropine every 3 minutes until 0.04 mg/kg has been infused. Evidence for the effectiveness of this approach is only fair (Class IIb).

Asystole persists
Stop resuscitative efforts?
- Consider quality of resuscitation? ***(Note 7)***
- Atypical clinical features present? ***(Note 8)***
- Clinical/management support in place? ***(Note 9)***

Box 6: Asystole Persists

Termination of Resuscitation Attempts

"Do Not Start"

Well-accepted criteria exist for not starting resuscitative efforts: a valid DNAR order, clear expression of a patient's self-determination, obvious signs of death. When none of these criteria is apparent, resuscitative efforts should start rapidly,

"Yes" to the questions in Notes 7 and 8 complies with recommended criteria to stop resuscitative efforts.

Note 7: Review resuscitation quality: adequate trial of BLS? ACLS?

- Effective ventilation performed via tracheal tube?
- VF shocked if present?
- IV epinephrine? IV atropine?
- Reversible causes ruled out or corrected?
- Continuous and documented asystole for more than 5 to 10 minutes after all of the above have been accomplished?

Note 8: Reviewed for atypical clinical features?

- Not a victim of drowning or hypothermia?
- No reversible therapeutic or illicit drug overdose?

Note 9: Clinical/management support in place?

- Field personnel under formal medical control can be authorized to stop efforts in the field **(Class IIa).**
- For patients meeting the above criteria ➔ urgent field-to-hospital transport with continuing CPR – **Class III** (harmful; no benefit)

proceed aggressively and effectively, and terminate sensitively.

Asystole as Confirmation of Death

As an ACLS provider you will see asystole most frequently in 2 situations:

- As a terminal rhythm in a resuscitation attempt that started with another rhythm
- As the first identified rhythm when responding to an emergency

In either of these scenarios asystole most often represents a confirmation of death rather than a "rhythm" to be treated or a patient who can be resuscitated if the attempt persists long enough. Persistent asystole represents extensive myocardial ischemia and damage from prolonged periods of inadequate coronary perfusion. Such a status has a grim prognosis.

Criteria for Stopping Resuscitative Efforts

Know the criteria for stopping resuscitative efforts set by your prehospital care system or wherever you provide professional services. Stop resuscitative efforts if there is no response after successful initiation of standard interventions, provided that this is not at variance with local policies and that cessation is approved by an authorized physician.

Stopping Efforts in the Field Without Transport of Patients Needing Continued CPR

If these criteria *(no response to full ACLS interventions)* are met in an out-of-hospital setting, resuscitative efforts should stop—either under existing physician-authorized protocols or after direct voice contact with the on-line medical control physician. Extensive evidence confirms that with rare exceptions (eg, hypothermia, electrocution), there is *no physiological value to transporting patients in asystolic cardiac arrest* to an ED or a hospital.

If patients fail to respond to the standard interventions listed above in the out-of-hospital setting, it is futile to think there might be a response in the ED. Since publication of the *1992 ECC Guidelines,* the AHA has recommended stopping resuscitations in the field and instituting no-transport protocols for patients receiving continuing CPR. The major caveat to this recommendation has been that an effective survivor support program must be in place. EMS systems need to provide "24/7" on-call coverage by trained bereavement personnel. These personnel may be from a community-wide chaplains' panel or may include designated healthcare personnel, shift supervisors, or even ride-along staff with specific assigned roles to help survivors.

In addition, a procedure for legal death certification should be in place, with clear directions and support for handling a death at home.

Common Criteria for Termination of ACLS Efforts

- Acceptable basic CPR provided
- VF eliminated
- Advanced airway device placed successfully
- Airway device confirmed and secured
- Oxygen and end-tidal CO_2 monitored to ensure proper oxygenation and ventilation achieved
- IV access established
- Intervention maintained for 10 minutes or longer
- All rhythm-appropriate drugs administered
- Family/friends updated on patient's condition
- Concepts of programs to support family presence during resuscitation attempts discussed

Family Presence at Resuscitation Attempts

Allowing—even encouraging—family presence at resuscitation attempts is an emerging clinical practice. Interviews with family members and survivors confirm a positive and prolonged effect of this experience. Everyone needs to "say goodbye" and obtain closure on the death of a loved one. There are obvious limits to this practice. Variable levels of staff resistance must be overcome. An impressive body of evidence, however, documents a strong therapeutic effect of these programs. This is a good thing to do.

Cessation of Efforts in the Prehospital Setting

How long should resuscitative efforts continue? The *ECC Guidelines 2000* do not state a specific time limit beyond which rescuers can never have a successful resuscitation. Cardiac arrests in special situations such as hypothermia, electrocution, and drug overdoses are exceptions to any rules. Special situations call for common sense and clinical judgment.

It is inappropriate, futile, and ethically unacceptable to routinely continue prehospital resuscitative efforts and require ambulance transport and ongoing CPR for all patients. Likewise, it is inappropriate for clinicians to routinely apply rules for stopping resuscitative efforts without thinking about the particular clinical situation. Medical directors of prehospital care systems must develop criteria by which emergency personnel, in coordination with medical control physicians, can cease efforts in the field to resuscitate patients with asystole. Chapter 4: The Human Dimension of CPR and ACLS: Human, Ethical, and Legal Issues provides a more detailed discussion of these issues. Cessation of efforts in the prehospital setting, following system-specific criteria and under direct medical control, should be standard practice in all EMS systems.

Critical Actions: Assessment and Management

The critical actions checklist identifies steps in the Primary and Secondary ABCD Surveys for identifying asystole, stabilizing the patient, identifying and treating the cause(s), and knowing when to end resuscitative efforts.

Do not try to memorize the table. Review the checklist until you understand the order and rationale for all the steps. For in-depth information, see "Read More About It."

Equipment

Conventional defibrillator/monitor

Transcutaneous pacemaker

Oxygen

Advanced airway devices

Equipment to review IV access

Personnel

Other ACLS providers will respond to your call for help in a layered response:

- Rescuer 1 to help with CPR
- Rescuer 2 to manage airway and use an advanced airway device
- Rescuer 3 to monitor the patient and operate the AED
- Rescuer 4 to start an IV and administer medications

Unacceptable Actions: Perils and Pitfalls

- Neglecting to use the ACLS Approach
- Late use of TCP (use early or not at all)
- Failing to recognize the presence of underlying treatable VF
- Neglecting to run through the flat line protocol (eg, diagnosing *asystole* in only one lead)
- Deficiencies in repeated, focused assessments of patient
- Neglecting to consider what could be causing this victim's *asystole*. This means taking a moment to consider a range of causes of asystole.
- Neglecting to assess the victim's response to infusion of fluids
- Deficiencies in repeated evaluation of airway placement and adequacy of ventilations
- Deficiencies in quality of CPR

Read More About It

For details about the new topics covered in Case 5 and related topics, see the following sections in the *ECC Guidelines 2000:*

- Part 2: Ethical Aspects of CPR and ECC
- Part 6: Advanced Cardiovascular Life Support, Section 7: Algorithm Approach to ACLS Emergencies
- Part 6: ACLS, Section 7B: Understanding the Algorithm Approach to ACLS
- Part 6: ACLS, Section 7C: A Guide to the International ACLS Algorithms: Figure 5: Asystole: The Silent Heart Algorithm and Notes

Critical Actions Checklist: ACLS Case 5
Asystole

This critical actions checklist is limited to actions specific for asystole. To avoid unnecessary repetition, this checklist does not repeat all assessment and management steps of the Primary and Secondary ABCD Surveys. Remember that these steps must always be performed for all patients.

Scene Survey Steps	Assess: Do or Monitor	Manage: Do or Delegate
Start Primary ABCD Survey: Use Asystole Algorithm		
Airway	***Air movement?*** ☐ Check again for open airway: — Look — Listen — Feel ☐ Placement of advanced airway? — Look — Listen — Feel	***Ensure open airway:*** ☐ Position before intubation ☐ Suction as needed
Breathing	☐ Recognize importance of ventilatory support ☐ Frequently reassess ABCs, including placement of airway	☐ Provide oxygenation and ventilation after securing airway ☐ Start ventilating patient ☐ Administer supplemental oxygen
Circulation	***Rhythm?*** ☐ Reassess rhythm ☐ Confirm asystole in more than 1 lead ☐ If ECG is still flat, check attachments and settings ☐ Assess usefulness of TCP for this patient ☐ Assess usefulness of sodium bicarbonate for this patient ***If ECG rhythm changes:*** ☐ Check pulse ☐ If pulse returns, check blood pressure, perfusion	***Rhythm is asystole:*** ☐ Continue chest compressions ☐ Obtain peripheral IV access ☐ Administer appropriate fluid ☐ Monitor access with proper technique ☐ If indicated, start TCP as soon as possible ☐ Administer epinephrine and atropine in correct dosages ☐ If indicated give sodium bicarbonate

Primary ABCD Survey (continued)		
Scene Survey Steps	**Assess: Do or Monitor**	**Manage: Do or Delegate**
Defibrillation	***Rhythm?*** ☐ Assess rhythm with defibrillator/ monitor ☐ Recognize non VF ☐ Recognize flat line ECG ☐ Recognize the potential differential diagnosis of flat line ECG ☐ Identify asystole (after flat line protocol)	***Manage flat line protocol:*** ☐ Check power to both defibrillator and monitor (some devices have separate controls for POWER ON) ☐ Check all connections: device to cables, cables to patient, device to paddles, paddles to patient ☐ Check GAIN or SENSITIVITY on defibrillator/monitor for appropriate setting ☐ Check setting of LEAD SELECT—paddles? 3-lead cable? lead I? II? III? ☐ If set on LEAD SELECT, do a quick check for a rhythm in each lead (vector of VF concept) ☐ If set on PADDLES, do 90-degree rotation to check for vector of VF (upper right sternum paddle to upper left sternum; left apex paddle to right lower sternal border) ☐ If using electrode pads for monitoring, attach leads ☐ Continue CPR
Start Secondary ABCD Survey: Use Asystole Algorithm		
Airway	***Air movement?*** ☐ Check again for open airway: — Look — Listen — Feel *Placement of advanced airway?* — Look — Listen — Feel	***Ensure open airway:*** ☐ Position before intubation ☐ Suction as needed
Breathing	☐ Recognize importance of ventilatory support ☐ Frequently reassess ABCs, including placement of airway	☐ Provide oxygenation and ventilation after securing airway ☐ Start ventilating patient ☐ Administer supplemental oxygen

Secondary ABCD Survey (continued)

Scene Survey Steps	Assess: Do or Monitor	Manage: Do or Delegate
Circulation	***Rhythm?*** ☐ Reassess rhythm ***If ECG rhythm changes:*** ☐ Check pulse ☐ If pulse returns, check blood pressure, perfusion	***Rhythm is asystole:*** ☐ Continue chest compressions ☐ Administer epinephrine and atropine in correct dosages ☐ If indicated give sodium bicarbonate
Differential Diagnosis	***Reversible cause?*** ☐ Consider possible reversible causes (5 H's and 5 T's)*: — Hypovolemia — Hypoxia — Hydrogen ion—acidosis — Hyperkalemia (other electrolytes) — Hypothermia — Tablets: drug overdose — Tamponade, cardiac — Tension pneumothorax Thrombosis, AMI — Thrombosis: pulmonary embolus ***Don't limit your thinking*** ☐ Gather and review the clues: — Relevant history — Physical findings — X-ray, echocardiographic findings — Laboratory test results ☐ Assess whether to continue resuscitative effort: — Know criteria for stopping resuscitative efforts in the hospital, EMS system, or lay response settings	**A. ACLS Course activity** Be able to list reversible causes of asystole and describe their management. **B. Clinical activity** ***If you are the team leader:*** ☐ Take aggressive action to identify and treat reversible causes of asystole ☐ Ask team members for their thoughts about the resuscitation ☐ When appropriate, stop the effort ***If you are a team member:*** Contribute your observations and insights at the appropriate time

*Advanced providers may use 6 H's by adding hypo-/hyperglycemia and 6 T's by adding trauma.

Workbook Review

1. **Which of the following potential causes of prehospital asystole is most likely to respond to immediate treatment?**
   - **a.** prolonged cardiac arrest
   - **b.** prolonged submersion in warm water
   - **c.** drug overdose
   - **d.** blunt multisystem trauma

   Read more about it in the ECC Guidelines 2000, *page 154: Notes for Figure 5: Asystole Algorithm; and page 227: "Prolonged CPR and Resuscitation." Issues to be considered before termination of resuscitative efforts are also presented on page 14: "Criteria for Terminating Resuscitative Efforts." Prognostic factors associated with poor outcome following submersion are presented on page 233: "Definitions, Classifications, and Prognostic Indicators." The outcome of cardiac arrest associated with trauma is presented on page 244: "Cardiac Arrest Associated With Trauma."*

2. **Which of the following is the correct *initial* drug and dose for treatment of asystole?**
   - **a.** epinephrine 2 mg IV
   - **b.** atropine 0.5 mg IV
   - **c.** lidocaine 1 mg/kg IV
   - **d.** epinephrine 1 mg IV

   Read more about it in the ECC Guidelines 2000, *pages 152-154: Figure 5: Asystole: The Silent Heart Algorithm and notes*

3. **Paramedics have arrived with an asystolic 42-year-old man who was found unconscious, breathless, and pulseless in the hallway of his apartment. CPR is ongoing. The patient is intubated. He has bilateral breath sounds and equal and adequate chest expansion. IV access has been successfully established, with fluid infusion at a "keep open" rate. The patient's vital signs are as follows: PaO_2 = 85 mm Hg; $PaCO_2$ = 32 mm Hg; pH = 7.3; serum potassium = 4.5 mEq/L; core body temperature = 37°C. In this scenario, which is the most likely reversible cause to consider before stopping the resuscitation attempt?**
   - **a.** tracheal tube in the esophagus
   - **b.** drug overdose
   - **c.** tension pneumothorax
   - **d.** hypothermia

   Read more about it in the ECC Guidelines 2000, *pages 153-154: Figure 5: Asystole Algorithm and notes; and page 227: "Prolonged CPR and Resuscitation"*

4. **You are considering transcutaneous pacing for a patient in asystole. Which of the following candidates would be most likely to respond to such a pacing attempt?**
   - **a.** the patient in asystole who has failed to respond to 20 minutes of BLS and ACLS therapy
   - **b.** the patient in asystole following blunt trauma
   - **c.** the patient in asystole following a defibrillatory shock
   - **d.** the patient who has just arrived in the ED following transport and CPR in the field for persistent asystole after submersion

   Read more about it in the ECC Guidelines 2000, *pages 153-154: Figure 5: Asystole Algorithm and notes; and page 244: "Cardiac Arrest Associated With Trauma."*

5. **Which of the following should be checked as part of the flat line protocol to confirm the presence of asystole and rule out operator or monitoring error as the reason for the isoelectric ECG?**
   - **a.** check power switch, all connections between the monitor and patient, monitor/defibrillator battery, sensitivity or gain, and lead choice
   - **b.** obtain a 12-lead ECG
   - **c.** press the SYNCHRONIZE button on the cardioverter/defibrillator
   - **d.** administer a trial defibrillatory shock to rule out occult VF

   Read more about it in the ECC Guidelines 2000, *page 154: "Confirm True Asystole"; and page 93: "'Occult' Versus 'False' Asystole." This information is also presented in the box "The Flat Line Protocol" in Case 5.*

6. **You are in the ED assisting in a resuscitation attempt for a normothermic patient who was transported in asystolic cardiac arrest. You are providing a trial of BLS and ACLS. The patient has been successfully intubated, and you have confirmed proper tube placement. IV access has been obtained. Which of the following interventions would be most likely to have the greatest therapeutic effect at this time?**
   - **a.** ask the family if they would like to be present during the resuscitation attempt
   - **b.** administer escalating doses of epinephrine
   - **c.** administer fibrinolytics to treat a possible myocardial infarction
   - **d.** administer an empiric defibrillatory shock of 200 J

   Read more about it in the ECC Guidelines 2000, *pages 153-155: Figure 5: Asystole Algorithm and notes; pages 14-15: "Criteria for Terminating Resuscitative Efforts"; page 19: "Family Presence During Resuscitation Attempts"; and page 93: "'Occult' Versus 'False' Asystole"*

Acute Coronary Syndromes: Patients With Acute Ischemic Chest Pain

Description

The ACLS provider must have basic knowledge about the immediate assessment and stabilization of patients who are experiencing an ACS. All victims in the ACS scenarios present with signs and symptoms of an ACS, probably an AMI. The initial 12-lead ECG is used in all ACS cases to classify patients into 1 of 3 clinical categories, each with different assessment and management needs. ACLS providers should focus particular attention on patients with the most critical ACS: significant ST-segment elevation.

Additional scenarios are available to challenge experienced providers. These scenarios develop the learning objectives applicable to patients with ST-segment depression or non-diagnostic ECG. They focus on treatment with conventional agents such as β-adrenoreceptor blocking agents and new agents, including low-molecular-weight heparin (LMWH) and glycoprotein (GP) IIb/IIIa inhibitors.

Update: The Acute Coronary Syndromes From 1992 to 2000

Reperfusion therapy has been the most significant treatment added to the emergency care of cardiac patients in the past 2 decades. Patients with acute chest pain should be evaluated as potential candidates for fibrinolytic therapy or coronary angiography with catheter-based (angioplasty or stent) treatment. CHF is the leading cause of in-hospital death in

What's New in the Guidelines...

Acute Coronary Syndromes

The text provides a review of the past decade's developments in the assessment and treatment of patients with an acute coronary syndrome (ACS). This period was guided by 3 sets of ACLS Guidelines. The major new recommendations in the *ECC Guidelines 2000* include the following:

- Greater use of prehospital electrocardiography by urban and suburban EMS units
- Conservative support for the use of prehospital fibrinolysis under certain circumstances. Specifically prehospital fibrinolytic therapy is recommended when a physician is present or transport time is 60 minutes or longer.
- Patients with cardiogenic shock and large AMIs with congestive heart failure are best served by rapid triage to facilities that can provide invasive interventions. When possible, this triage should occur in the prehospital setting, bypassing hospital facilities that lack advanced diagnostic and treatment capabilities.
- Provide a percutaneous coronary intervention (PCI)—either angioplasty or intracoronary stenting—for patients less than 75 years of age with ACS and signs of shock
- Consideration of a PCI (either angioplasty or stenting) when fibrinolytics are contraindicated and potential benefit from reperfusion exists
- To reduce risk of hemorrhage, use of a heparin dose lower than the dose recommended in previous guidelines (current dose: bolus of 60 U/kg, followed by infusion of 12 U/kg per hour; *maximum bolus* of 4000 U and *maximum infusion* of 1000 U/h for patients weighing more than 70 kg)

patients with ACS who survive to hospital admission. Early reperfusion limits infarct size and reduces the impact of muscle loss. This beneficial effect can be captured only in the first few hours after the onset of MI. Emphasize the need to reduce the major factors associated with delayed reperfusion: patient denial and misinterpretation of symptoms, delay to EMS call, delay in EMS triage, and delay in hospital door-to-drug or door-to-balloon times.

New Recommendations: 1994 to 1997

After publication of the *1992 ECC Guidelines,* the ACLS Subcommittee began converting the ACLS Provider Course from a subject-based to a case-based learning experience. When case-based teaching began in 1994, the ACS case (No. 6) focused on the important theme of eliminating barriers to fibrinolytic therapy. At that time the major barrier to this therapy was the lack of timely actions by patients and their families in seeking care and prolonged "ED door–to-drug times" in hospitals and Emergency Departments. The 1994 recommendations included the following:

- A public education campaign known as Heart Attack Alert to promote rapid recognition of the signs and symptoms of AMI and the importance of EMS involvement in early evaluation and treatment
- Rapid, organized assessment and treatment in the ED to shorten the "door-to-drug" time as much as possible and to significantly reduce or eliminate delays associated with 12-lead ECG interpretation and early decision making about fibrinolytic therapy
- Knowledge and use of the critical emergency medications (oxygen, nitroglycerin, morphine, aspirin, fibrinolytic agents, β-blockers, heparin, lidocaine) and the reperfusion intervention of coronary angioplasty

New Recommendations: 1997 to 2000

The growth of evidence supporting the efficacy of reperfusion therapy led to extensive revision of recommendations for treatment of ACS and stroke in the 1997 edition of the *ACLS Textbook.* New recommendations emphasized the importance of rapid recognition and early reperfusion, including new insights gleaned from reperfusion studies.

AMI was recognized as part of a broader spectrum of disease requiring a new nomenclature and a more comprehensive name: *acute coronary syndromes* (see Figure 1). Patients with ACS were classified on the basis of their initial ECG as demonstrating one of the following: *Q-wave MI, non–Q-wave MI,* and *unstable angina*. Initial patient management was based on this classification. Under the same classification system a new Ischemic Chest Pain Algorithm expanded the focus to include all patients presenting with chest pain.

Understanding the classification system and therapy associated with each clinical syndrome was a major goal of the 1997 *ACLS Textbook* revisions. ACLS provider courses focused on treatment of ST elevation, again emphasizing the need for early reperfusion for selected patients. Advanced providers were taught additional strategies for treatment of high-risk patients with unstable angina. All providers were trained to avoid the use of fibrinolytic therapy in ACS patients with ST depression. Although rupture of a lipid-laden plaque is the inciting event in both ST elevation and ST depression, fibrinolytics provide no benefit for ACS patients with ST depression and often pose a risk of harm.

The following triage scheme provides performance goals for all providers:

- Patients with ischemic-type chest pain should have an ECG performed within 10 minutes of EMS or ED presentation.
- ACC/AHA 2002 guidelines recommend triage of patients into 3 groups based on analysis of the 12-lead ECG and ST-segment deviation:
  - ST-segment elevation ≥0.5 mm or new-onset bundle branch block
  - ST-segment depression ≥1 mm (or transient ST-segment elevation)
  - Nondiagnostic ECG (ST-segment depression less than 0.5 mm or T-wave abnormalities) or normal ECG

New Recommendations: 2000

By the year 2000 more than 750,000 ACS patients worldwide had participated in randomized clinical trials. This experience has led to even more diagnostic and treatment recommendations, including new fibrinolytic agents for clinical use for patients with ST-segment elevation. In addition, accumulating evidence confirmed the benefits of *triple pharmacotherapy* for high-risk patients with ST-segment depression:

- Aspirin (antiplatelet agent) *plus*
- GP IIb/IIIa platelet inhibitors *and*
- Unfractionated heparin (UFH) *or* LMWH

The most important new recommendations are presented below.

New Recommendations for ST-Elevation AMI

The major new recommendations for patients with acute ST-elevation AMI include the following:

- The use of prehospital 12-lead ECGs in urban and suburban EMS systems—prehospital ECGs give receiving hospitals advance notification of the arrival of a patient with AMI with ST elevation, thereby speeding the administration of fibrinolytic agents when the patient arrives in the ED.

FIGURE 1. Acute Coronary Syndromes. Patients with coronary atherosclerosis may develop a spectrum of clinical syndromes representing varying degrees of coronary artery occlusion. These syndromes include unstable angina, non–Q-wave MI, and Q-wave MI. Sudden cardiac death may occur with each of these syndromes.

A **Unstable plaque.** Rupture of a lipid-laden plaque with a thin cap is the most common cause of an ACS. The majority of these plaques are not hemodynamically significant before rupture. An inflammatory component is present in the subendothelial area and further weakens and predisposes the plaque to rupture. Blood flow velocity, turbulence, and vessel anatomy may be important contributing factors. Superficial erosion of a plaque occurs in a small percentage of patients.

B **Plaque rupture.** After rupture a monolayer of platelets covers the surface of the ruptured plaque (platelet adhesion). Additional platelets are recruited (platelet aggregation) and activated. Fibrinogen cross-links platelets, and the coagulation system is activated with thrombin generation.

C **Unstable angina.** A partially occluding thrombus produces symptoms of ischemia, which are prolonged and may occur at rest. At this stage the thrombus is platelet-rich. Therapy with antiplatelet agents such as aspirin and GP IIb/IIIa receptor inhibitors is most effective at this time. Fibrinolytic therapy is *not* effective and may paradoxically accelerate occlusion by the release of clot-bound thrombin, which further activates platelets. An intermittently occlusive thrombus may cause myocardial necrosis, producing a non–Q-wave MI.

D **Microemboli.** As the clot enlarges, microemboli may originate from the distal thrombus and lodge in the coronary microvasculature, causing small elevations of cardiac troponins, new sensitive cardiac markers. These patients are at highest risk for progression to MI. This process is known as minimal myocardial damage.

E **Occlusive thrombus.** If the thrombus occludes the coronary vessel for a prolonged period, a Q-wave MI occurs. This clot is rich in thrombin; early/prompt fibrinolysis or direct PCI may limit infarct size if performed sufficiently early.

Natural History of Coronary Artery Disease: Evolution to the Major Acute Coronary Syndromes

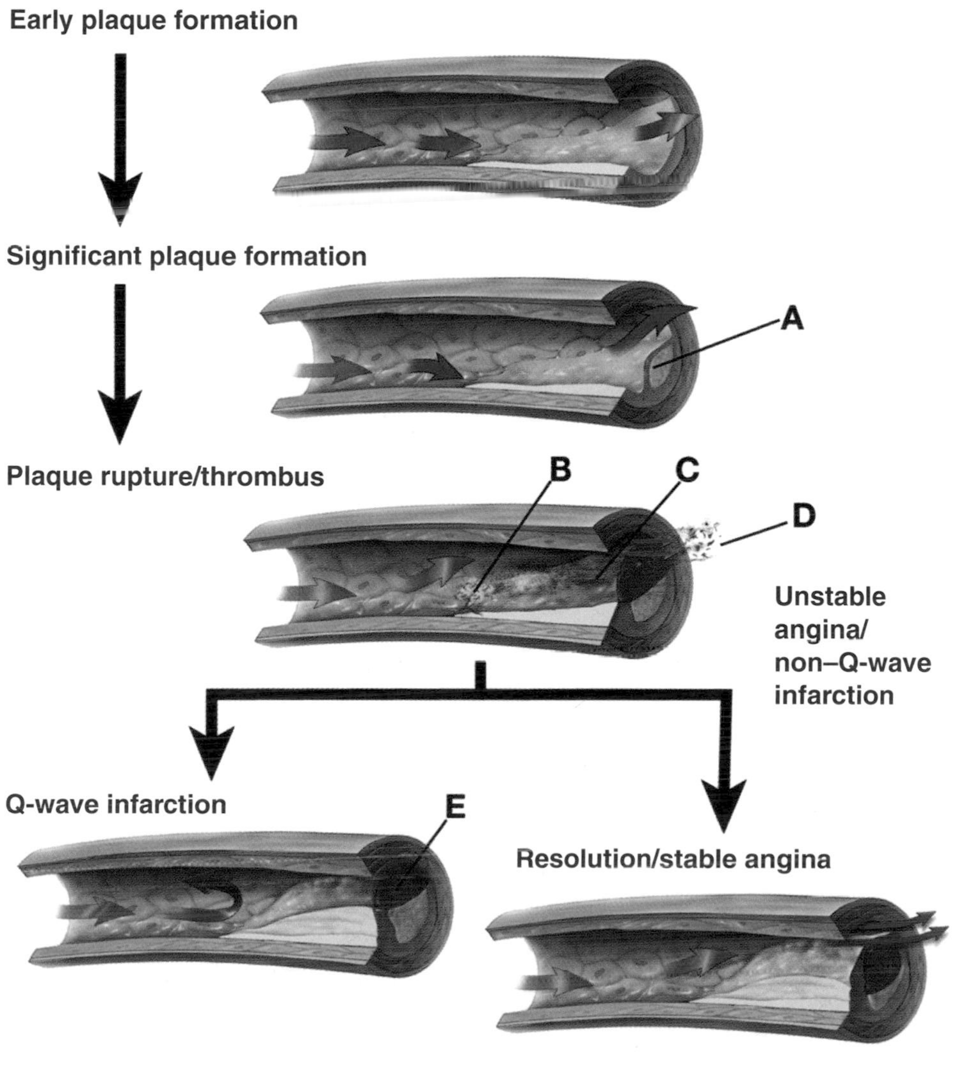

- The use of a prehospital checklist by EMS personnel to identify indications and contraindications for fibrinolytic therapy for patients with ischemic-like chest pain. The checklist helps EMS personnel determine a patient's eligibility/ineligibility for this therapy before arrival in the ED. Although EMS personnel cannot make the treat/no treat decision, this checklist could shorten the time to reperfusion.
- The potential use of prehospital fibrinolytic therapy if a physician is present in the prehospital setting and is qualified to interpret 12-lead ECGs and risk-stratify candidates for fibrinolytic treatment *or* if the average transport time to the closest appropriate facility is more than 1 hour
- The need to identify patients with cardiogenic shock or heart failure due to a large AMI and transport them to facilities with interventional specialists—facilities capable of PCI and coronary artery bypass graft (CABG)
- The acknowledgment that PCIs and fibrinolytic therapy can be *equivalent* therapies when the following conditions are met:
  - PCI (balloon dilation) can be performed within 90±30 minutes
  - PCI operators are highly experienced
  - The PCI center performs a large number of procedures each year
  - The PCI center achieves normal flow rate in more than 90% of cases without emergency CABG, stroke, or death
- PCI is favored for patients in cardiogenic shock who are less than 75 years of age
- The use of EMS protocols that direct AMI patients with a blood pressure ≤100 mm Hg ***and*** heart rate ≥100 bpm to interventional facilities capable of PCI and CABG if transport time is less than 30 to 45 minutes
- The use of the adjunct therapies aspirin and β-blockers with the same indications and contraindications as before
- The use of heparin as an adjunct therapy with fibrin-specific lytics (eg, alteplase, reteplase, and tenecteplase) and for all patients undergoing direct or adjunctive PCI
- The use of a lower dose of heparin than previously recommended in an effort to reduce the risk of intracerebral hemorrhage. The ACC/AHA Committee on Management of Acute Myocardial Infarction concurs with these reductions. Give heparin as a **60 U/kg bolus,** then a **12 U/kg per hour** infusion. (The previous recommendation called for an 80 U/kg bolus and an 18 U/kg per hour infusion.) In the *ECC Guidelines 2000* the maximum heparin bolus is 4000 U with a maximum infusion of 1000 U/h for patients weighing more than 70 kg.
- The use of ACE inhibitors for patients with CHF, large anterior MI, or an ejection fraction less than 40%

New Recommendations for ST-Depression AMI and Unstable Angina

Data from the numerous fibrinolytic trials suggest that ST depression is a high-risk indicator for coronary events. Recent trials confirm that mortality and morbidity rates in these patients rival those for ST-elevation MI, despite therapy with aspirin and heparin.

- Agents that inhibit **GP IIb/IIIa receptors** are approved for blocking the final common pathway of platelet aggregation (specifically the short-acting agents *eptifibatide* and *tirofiban*). These agents improve prognosis in patients at high risk due to ST depression, positive cardiac markers, and refractory ischemia.
- **GP IIb/IIIa receptor inhibitors** are also recommended for patients undergoing PCIs. Administration during the intervention reduces the incidence of complications.
- A large number of clinical trials have compared **LMWHs** with **UFH.** The trials noted *enoxaparin* as superior to UFH and easier to administer without rebound angina. The safety and efficacy of LMWHs used with GP IIb/IIIa inhibitor therapy appears promising but in late 2000 remained under investigation.
- Use *triple antithrombotic therapy* (aspirin, GP IIb/IIIa inhibitors, and UFH[1] or LMWH) as the most effective treatment for ST-depression AMI and high-risk unstable angina positive troponin release). Clopidogrel was added to the ACC/AHA recommendations in 2002 for use in specific instances in addition to aspirin.

Settings and Scenarios

Setting: Prehospital

Patient 1

EMT-Ps receive a 911 call for severe chest pain. They evaluate a 55-year-old man who is at home with dramatic, severe (10 of 10) substernal chest pain. He reports most of the classic signs and symptoms of an AMI, including left-arm pain radiation, jaw radiation, nausea, diaphoresis, and a profound sense of impending doom *(angor animi).* Describe the assessments and treatments that should be performed in this at-home scenario before transport to the ED.

Setting: Emergency Department

Patient 2

At home a 55-year-old man begins to experience "severe chest pain." He states he is having severe (10 of 10) substernal chest pain, plus most of the classic signs and symptoms of an AMI, including left-arm pain radiation, jaw radiation, nausea, diaphoresis, and a profound sense of *angor animi* (impending doom). He refuses to let his wife call 911. The two of them use the family car to make a difficult journey to the nearest ED. Describe the immediate assessments and treatments that the ED staff should perform in the first 10 minutes after the man's arrival.

---

[1]Many experts predict LMWHs will replace UFH based on clinical trials in progress in 2000-2001.

Patient 3

A 60-year-old woman with long-standing hypertension presents with gradually increasing substernal chest and interscapular back pain over the past 2 hours. The pain radiates to her back, between her shoulder blades, and into her left arm. She grades the pain as 4 of 10 at onset, increasing to 7 of 10 over 45 minutes. When the pain increased to 7 of 10 she asked her husband to drive her to the ED. She complains of weakness and slight nausea, but she is not short of breath.

Setting: General Hospital

Patient 4

A 75-year-old woman is being evaluated in the rheumatology clinic. While there she develops gradual onset of substernal chest pressure, some nausea, and slight diaphoresis. She is referred to the ED for further evaluation. Her vital signs are as follows: HR = 90 bpm; BP = 140/90 mm Hg; resp = 15 breaths/min; temperature = 37.2°C.

Optional Cases for Experienced Providers

Patient 5

This patient is a 55-year-old man with a long history of hypertension and coronary artery disease. One year ago he was admitted to another hospital for a similar chest pain episode that was diagnosed as an AMI. He has been taking an ACE inhibitor as well as a long-acting β-blocker for the past year.

Patient 6

You are evaluating a 68-year-old woman in the ED. She has a history of stable, exertional angina (4 blocks, 2 flights of stairs) treated with b-blockers and isosorbide dinitrate. She also takes a daily aspirin. She presents to the ED stating that her chest pain began quickly as she walked across the room. After 20 minutes the pain was relieved when she rested and took 3 nitroglycerin tablets SL. She usually gets relief by resting only or resting and taking just 1 nitroglycerin tablet.

Patient 7

An obese, hypertensive, 40-year-old woman with a 10-year history of insulin-dependent diabetes presents to the general medical clinic for "chest and back discomfort." She describes vague, interscapular discomfort, which started about 4 hours ago. She complains of nonspecific anterior chest sensations that are more of an "ache" than a specific pain. The discomfort is in her epigastric region and is not related to exercise or activity. She continues to smoke half a pack of cigarettes each day. Her father and uncle died in their early 40s of coronary artery disease, and her younger brother has angina.

Learning and Skills Objectives

At the end of Case 6 you should be able to

1. **Discuss the ACS (Figure 2) as a continuum of related disease processes.** These processes include
   - **Stable angina:** a flow/demand imbalance between reduced blood flow through narrow coronary arteries and the demand placed on the heart. Angina may be chronic, acute, or unstable.
   - **Unstable angina:** symptoms of angina that are new or increasing or that occur at rest or with no exertion. The symptoms are usually due to platelet aggregation in narrowed coronary arteries with chronic atherosclerotic occlusion, which leads to atypical chest pain, which leads to spontaneous disaggregation.
   - **Non–Q-wave infarction:** platelet aggregation, which leads to thrombus formation, which leads to release of cell markers, which leads to spontaneous or iatrogenic thrombolysis, resulting in brief and usually incomplete coronary occlusion
   - **Q-wave infarction:** platelet aggregation, which leads to thrombus formation, which allows the blockage to persist, which leads to infarction, usually from a complete and sustained occlusion. Spontaneous lysis occurs often but too late to salvage heart muscle.
2. **Describe and demonstrate classification of ACS based on the 12-lead ECG as follows:**
   - **ST-segment elevation** (injury) or new-onset (or presumably new-onset) left bundle branch block (LBBB) usually signifies extensive muscle involvement in infarct
   - **ST-segment depression or T-wave inversion** (ischemia)
   - **Nondiagnostic or normal ECGs:** many of these patients have unstable angina
3. **Apply the Ischemic Chest Pain Algorithm** (Figure 4) as a systematic approach to the timely assessment and treatment of patients with ischemic chest pain or suspected ACS. Describe how the algorithm focuses the ACLS provider on identification of the subset of patients who qualify for acute reperfusion therapy and use the algorithm to describe the assessment and management of a patient described in a scenario.
4. **Discuss the one mechanical intervention (PCI) and 10 pharmacologic agents that may be used in the management of the patient with ACS.** Faced with a patient with a suspected ACS, the ACLS provider should consider the 10 agents listed below. Providers are expected to learn the *why?* (actions), *when?*

FIGURE 2. Overlapping relationships of the acute coronary syndromes.

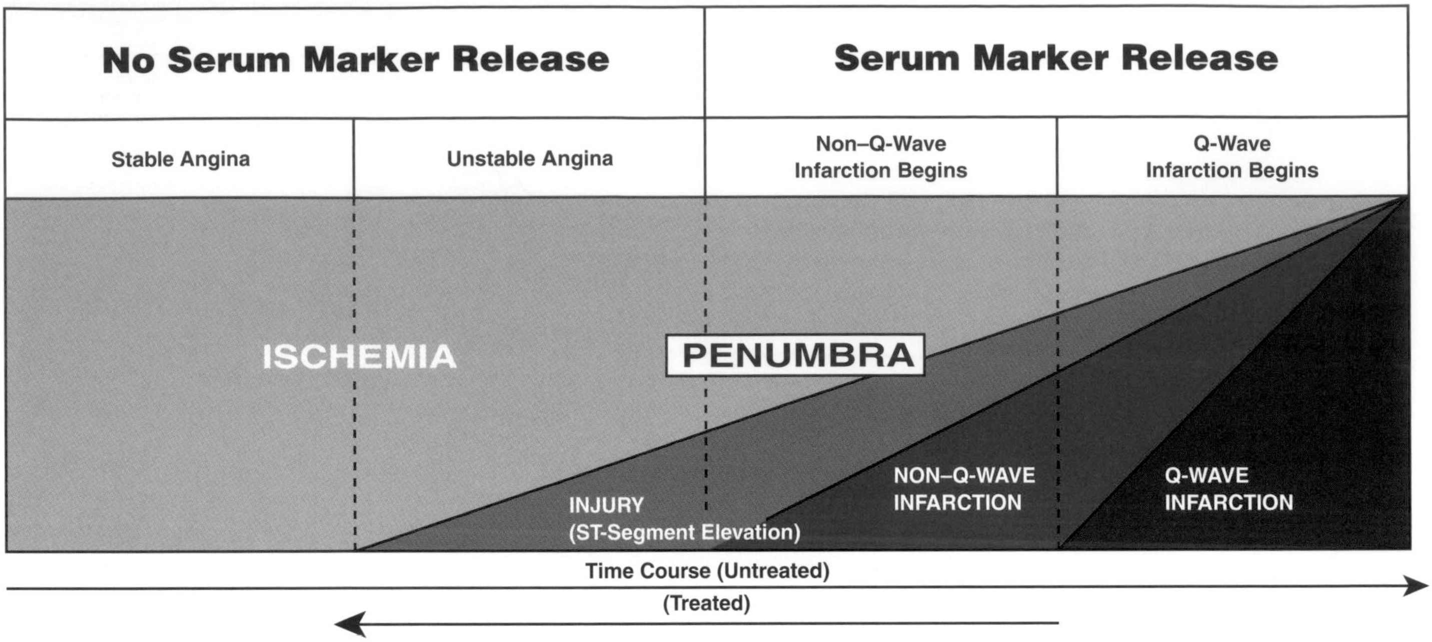

Schematic drawing showing the overlapping relationships of the acute coronary syndromes. The areas of ischemia and injury represent compromised but salvageable tissue in zones of reduced blood flow. In this zone, called the *penumbra,* the blood supply is inadequate to maintain normal myocardial functions. The penumbra is viable up to several hours from the primary onset of arterial occlusion. The myocardium in the penumbra dies (infarcts) if not salvaged by reperfusion strategies such as fibrinolytic agents or angioplasty.

(indications), *how?* (dosing), and *watch out!* (contraindications and precautions) for the following interventions:

- Primary PCI
- Morphine
- Oxygen
- Nitroglycerin
- Aspirin
- Heparin (UFH, LMWH)
- GP IIb/IIIa receptor inhibitors
- β-Blockers
- Fibrinolytic agents
- ACE inhibitors

5. Demonstrate *infarct localization:* how to recognize *infarct-injury-ischemia* on the ECG (Figure 3), how to locate the related anatomy on the heart of the infarct-injury-ischemia, and then identify the specific coronary artery that supplies that area.

The anatomic areas to recognize are

- Anterior myocardium
- Inferior myocardium
- Septal myocardium
- Lateral myocardium
- Right ventricle
- BBBs (to recognize the significance of new from old)

6. Describe the arrhythmias and complications most likely to develop, given the anatomic localization:

- Heart failure with large anterior infarcts
- Bradycardia and heart blocks with inferior infarcts
- Cardiac rupture with small first infarcts (usually patients with hypertension and left ventricular hypertrophy, often lateral MI; may be reduced with early β-blocker therapy)

7. Discuss the *patient* actions that have the greatest effect on ACS morbidity and mortality. The actions are *early recognition by the patient* that he or she is experiencing significant symptoms and early *decision making by the patient* to seek an evaluation for the symptoms and signs.

8. Describe the prehospital and ED team approach to rapid triage of all patients with ischemic-type chest pain that will minimize door-to-drug intervals. This team approach will ensure that the interval from when the patient arrives at the ED door to when a reperfusion strategy starts is within 30 minutes (door-to-drug) and 90 minutes (door-to-balloon).

9. Identify the clinical decision maker about use of fibrinolytics in the ED, EMS system, or coronary care unit where you work.

FIGURE 3. Relationship of 12-lead ECG to coronary artery anatomy.

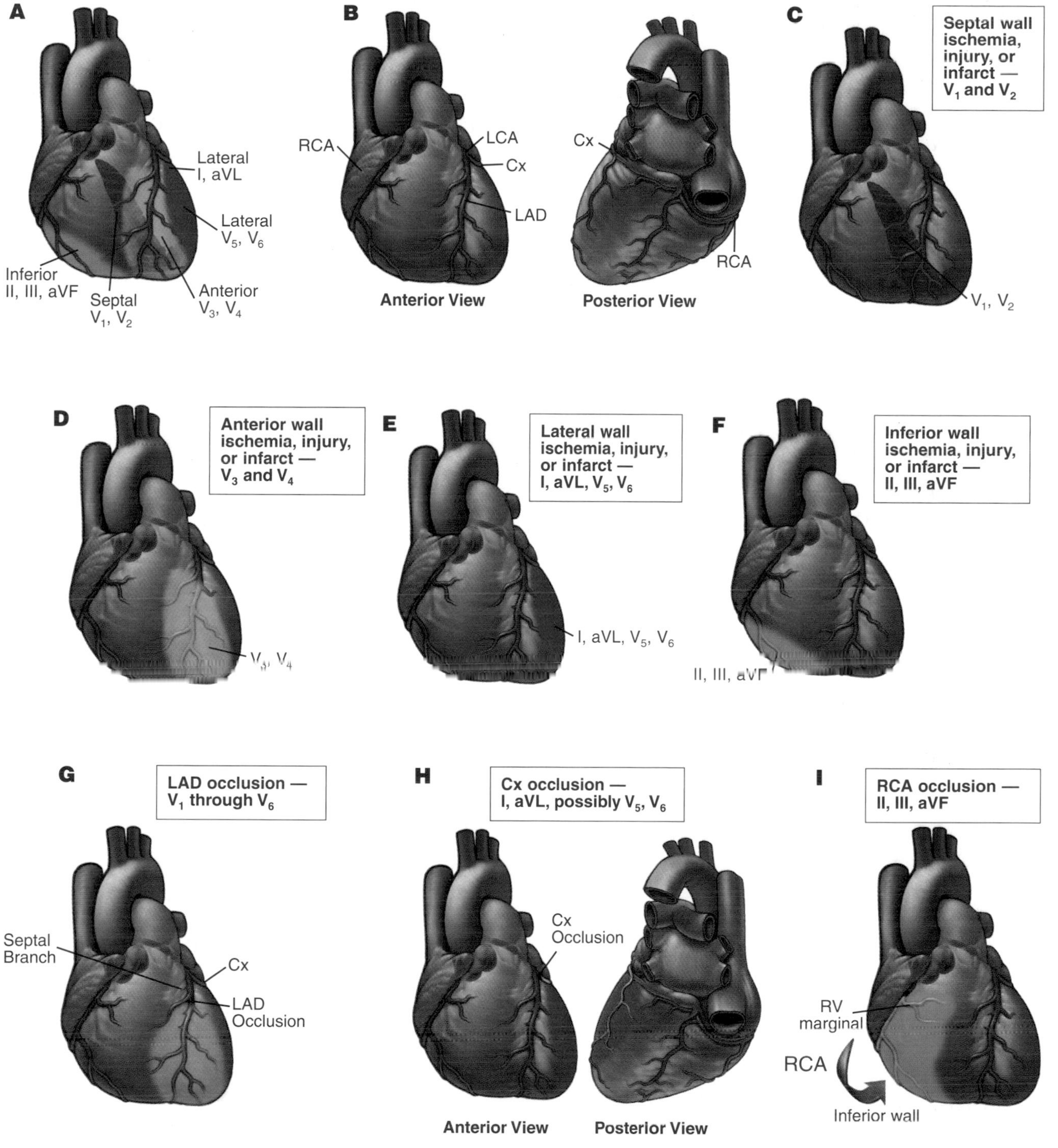

I lateral	aVR	V_1 septal	V_4 anterior
II inferior	aVL lateral	V_2 septal	V_5 lateral
III inferior	aVF inferior	V_3 anterior	V_6 lateral

Localizing ischemia, injury, or infarct using the 12-lead ECG: relationship to coronary artery anatomy.

10. Describe the AHA-recommended ED plan for *immediate assessment* and *general treatment* of the patient with chest pain suggestive of ischemia. This plan should include directions for who will perform these tasks, when, and where:

- Checking vital signs
- Determining oxygen saturation
- Starting an IV
- Having a 12-lead ECG device on-site at all times
- Obtaining the initial ECG in less than 10 minutes from arrival, based on a standing order
- Obtaining a brief, targeted history and physical examination that focuses on indications and contraindications for fibrinolytic therapy. A standard checklist is very helpful; see the *ECC Handbook* for a typical chest pain checklist.
- Rapidly deciding on the patient's eligibility and appropriateness for acute reperfusion therapy with either PCI or fibrinolytic therapy.
- Giving orders for initial cardiac marker levels. The troponin serum markers appear useful for diagnosis, prognosis, and risk stratification.
- Giving orders for chest x-rays, electrolyte and coagulation studies, and consultations as needed.

A Walk Through the Ischemic Chest Pain Algorithm

The Ischemic Chest Pain Algorithm (Figure 4) provides general guidelines that may not apply to all patients. Two critical pieces of information for classifying patients are missing at the time of initial evaluation. First, the ACLS provider at the patient's bedside lacks information about the evolution of the ECG in regard to Q-wave development over time. Second, the ACLS provider lacks information about the levels of serum cardiac markers that will be reached over time. The evolution of both the ECG and serum markers provides important information to classify the patient in terms of infarction or high-risk unstable angina.

The algorithm uses clinical tools known to have prognostic value, such as the initial ECG classification (ST elevation, ST depression, or normal/nondiagnostic), initial clinical features (heart failure, hypotension), and serum marker status at presentation (troponins, CK-Mb levels). ACLS providers will recognize that *the algorithm seeks to identify the subset of patients eligible and most likely to benefit from acute reperfusion therapy and those most likely to respond to aggressive fibrinolytic treatment.* Time will be required to reach a definitive classification for other patients.

Chest pain suggestive of ischemia

Box 1: Chest Pain Suggestive of Ischemia

You must begin prompt and targeted evaluation of every patient with initial complaints that suggest the possibility of an ACS. *The single most common symptom of infarction is retrosternal chest discomfort.* This discomfort may be perceived as more of a pressure than actual pain. Additional heart attack warning signs may include

- Uncomfortable pressure, fullness, squeezing, or pain in the center of the chest lasting several minutes (usually more than 15 minutes)
- Pain spreading to the shoulders, neck, arms, or jaw, or pain in the back or between the shoulder blades
- Chest discomfort with lightheadedness, fainting, sweating, nausea, or shortness of breath
- A global feeling of distress, anxiety, or impending doom

The clinician must consider the likelihood that the presenting condition is an ACS or one of its potentially lethal mimics. The most important conditions other than ACS that may cause acute chest pain or discomfort are

- Aortic dissection
- Acute pericarditis with effusion and tamponade
- Acute myocarditis
- Spontaneous pneumothorax
- Pulmonary embolism
- Esophageal rupture

An ACLS provider should continue to think of these alternative diagnostic possibilities while proceeding with the management outlined in the rest of the algorithm.

Immediate assessment (<10 minutes)
- Measure vital signs (automatic/standard BP cuff)
- Measure oxygen saturation
- Obtain IV access
- Obtain 12-lead ECG (physician reviews)
- Perform brief, targeted history and physical exam; focus on eligibility for fibrinolytic therapy
- Obtain initial serum cardiac marker levels
- Evaluate initial electrolyte and coagulation studies
- Request, review portable chest x-ray (<30 minutes)

Box 2: Immediate Assessment (<10 minutes)

Every EMS system and every ED must establish a protocol approach for patients who present with chest pain and suspected AMI. Such protocols and intervals to therapy should be evaluated on a regular basis to minimize times to therapy.

Prehospital Care

EMS and dispatch systems should have a trained and dedicated staff to respond to

FIGURE 4. Ischemic Chest Pain Algorithm.

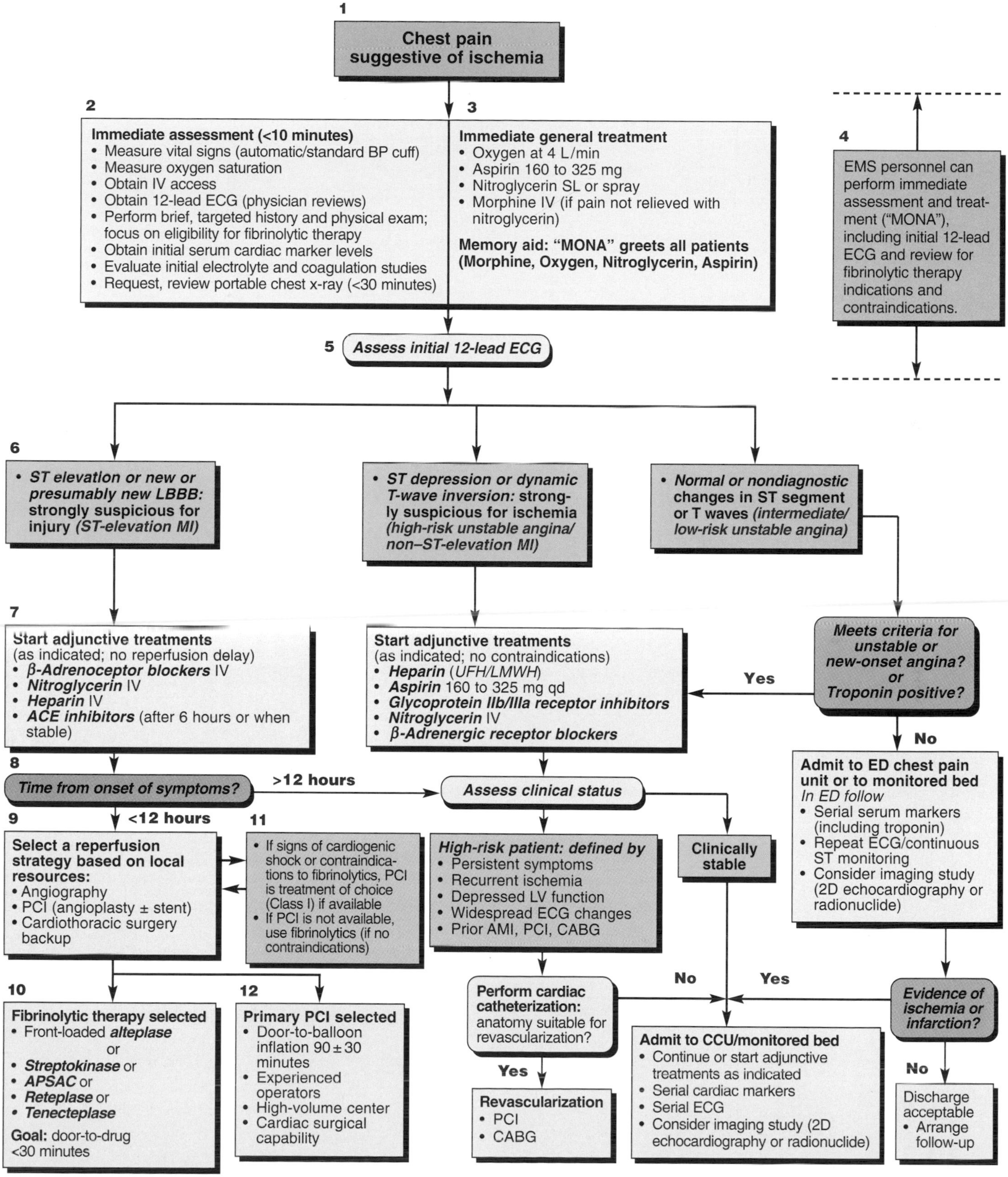
1
Chest pain suggestive of ischemia
2
Immediate assessment (<10 minutes)
• Measure vital signs (automatic/standard BP cuff)
• Measure oxygen saturation
• Obtain IV access
• Obtain 12-lead ECG (physician reviews)
• Perform brief, targeted history and physical exam; focus on eligibility for fibrinolytic therapy
• Obtain initial serum cardiac marker levels
• Evaluate initial electrolyte and coagulation studies
• Request, review portable chest x-ray (<30 minutes)
3
Immediate general treatment
• Oxygen at 4 L/min
• Aspirin 160 to 325 mg
• Nitroglycerin SL or spray
• Morphine IV (if pain not relieved with nitroglycerin)
Memory aid: "MONA" greets all patients (Morphine, Oxygen, Nitroglycerin, Aspirin)
4
EMS personnel can perform immediate assessment and treatment ("MONA"), including initial 12-lead ECG and review for fibrinolytic therapy indications and contraindications.
5
Assess initial 12-lead ECG
6
• ST elevation or new or presumably new LBBB: strongly suspicious for injury (ST-elevation MI)
• ST depression or dynamic T-wave inversion: strongly suspicious for ischemia (high-risk unstable angina/non–ST-elevation MI)
• Normal or nondiagnostic changes in ST segment or T waves (intermediate/low-risk unstable angina)
7
Start adjunctive treatments (as indicated; no reperfusion delay)
• β-Adrenoceptor blockers IV
• Nitroglycerin IV
• Heparin IV
• ACE inhibitors (after 6 hours or when stable)
Start adjunctive treatments (as indicated; no contraindications)
• Heparin (UFH/LMWH)
• Aspirin 160 to 325 mg qd
• Glycoprotein IIb/IIIa receptor inhibitors
• Nitroglycerin IV
• β-Adrenergic receptor blockers
Meets criteria for unstable or new-onset angina? or Troponin positive?
Yes
No
Admit to ED chest pain unit or to monitored bed
In ED follow
• Serial serum markers (including troponin)
• Repeat ECG/continuous ST monitoring
• Consider imaging study (2D echocardiography or radionuclide)
8
Time from onset of symptoms?
>12 hours
Assess clinical status
9
<12 hours
Select a reperfusion strategy based on local resources:
• Angiography
• PCI (angioplasty ± stent)
• Cardiothoracic surgery backup
11
• If signs of cardiogenic shock or contraindications to fibrinolytics, PCI is treatment of choice (Class I) if available
• If PCI is not available, use fibrinolytics (if no contraindications)
High-risk patient: defined by
• Persistent symptoms
• Recurrent ischemia
• Depressed LV function
• Widespread ECG changes
• Prior AMI, PCI, CABG
Clinically stable
10
Fibrinolytic therapy selected
• Front-loaded alteplase
or
• Streptokinase or
• APSAC or
• Reteplase or
• Tenecteplase
Goal: door-to-drug <30 minutes
12
Primary PCI selected
• Door-to-balloon inflation 90 ± 30 minutes
• Experienced operators
• High-volume center
• Cardiac surgical capability
Perform cardiac catheterization: anatomy suitable for revascularization?
No
Yes
Revascularization
• PCI
• CABG
Admit to CCU/monitored bed
• Continue or start adjunctive treatments as indicated
• Serial cardiac markers
• Serial ECG
• Consider imaging study (2D echocardiography or radionuclide)
Yes
Evidence of ischemia or infarction?
No
Discharge acceptable
• Arrange follow-up

This algorithm provides general guidelines that may not apply to all patients. Carefully consider proper indications and contraindications.

cardiac emergencies. BLS providers can provide CPR; use an AED; support airway, oxygenation, and ventilation; and if local protocol permits, administer aspirin and nitroglycerin in the out-of-hospital setting. For further information about EMS prehospital care for ACS, refer to Box 4: EMS care.

In-Hospital ED Care

Clinicians use the term *door-to-drug interval* to refer to the interval from the patient's arrival in the ED to determination of eligibility for reperfusion therapy and start of fibrinolytic agents. Professional staff in EDs should aim for a goal of no more than 30 minutes to assess the patient, determine eligibility, and start reperfusion treatment for patients with evidence of coronary thrombosis. ED personnel should also consider the availability of interventional facilities. High-volume interventional suites with skilled personnel should be able to achieve a door-to-balloon time of less than 90 minutes for the large majority of patients. To help meet this goal, the items listed under immediate assessment should be performed whenever possible in less than 10 minutes.

Defined EMS and ED protocols should cover both assessment and the start of immediate general treatment. Some tasks may be accomplished in the prehospital setting and reported to the ED to reduce evaluation time in the ED. Team members should have predetermined roles that include these tasks:

- Measurement of vital signs, including oxygen saturation (the "fifth vital sign")
- Attachment of a cardiac monitor
- Initiation of 1 or 2 IV infusion lines
- Drawing of initial blood studies while the IV lines are being started. Cardiac markers, electrolytes, and coagulation studies can be drawn and labeled but not necessarily sent for laboratory processing in these initial 10 minutes.
- Portable chest x-rays are generally indicated and should be included for most patients, if not immediately then soon.

One member of the emergency team must be identified as the person to obtain the initial 12-lead ECG. This person should be under standing orders to obtain a 12-lead ECG for all patients triaged for chest pain and suspected of having an ACS. **The 12-lead ECG is at the center of the decision pathway in the management of patients with ischemic chest pain. Delays in obtaining the12-lead ECG must be eliminated.** All EDs should have a dedicated electrocardiograph device and should not depend on a device from another location in the facility.

Immediate general treatment
- Oxygen at 4 L/min
- Aspirin 160 to 325 mg
- Nitroglycerin SL or spray
- Morphine IV (if pain not relieved with nitroglycerin)

Memory aid: "MONA" greets all patients (Morphine, Oxygen, Nitroglycerin, Aspirin)

Box 3: Immediate General Treatment

Four agents are now routinely recommended for patients with ischemic-type chest pain unless allergies or contraindications exist:

- **Oxygen** at 4 L/min. Use a mask or nasal cannula. O_2 saturation should be maintained at more than 90%.
- **Aspirin** PO. The routine use of aspirin (160 to 325 mg) is strongly recommended for all patients with AMI or ACS (Class I), especially those who receive fibrinolytic therapy and PCIs.
- **Nitroglycerin** SL or IV for continuing chest discomfort if systolic blood pressure is greater than 90 mm Hg and no other contraindications are present. If chest discomfort continues, follow administration of nitroglycerin with morphine.
- **Morphine** IV. Use small (2 to 4 mg) IV doses of morphine sulfate, repeated at 5-minute intervals as needed for patients who do not have complete pain relief from nitroglycerin. Meperidine is an acceptable alternative to morphine. Pain relief is a high priority.

ACLS instructors use the phrase *"MONA greets all patients"* as a memory aid to help ACLS providers remember this list of immediate treatments. Unless contraindicated, MONA **(morphine, oxygen, nitroglycerin, aspirin)** is recommended for all 3 subsets of patients suspected of having ischemic chest pain: those with ST elevation, those with ST depression, and those with nondiagnostic ECG changes. The major contraindications to nitroglycerin and morphine are hypotension, particularly hypotension from a right ventricular infarction. The major contraindication to aspirin is aspirin sensitivity.

EMS personnel can perform immediate assessment and treatment ("MONA"), including initial 12-lead ECG and review for fibrinolytic therapy indications and contraindications.

Box 4: EMS Systems

In the United States only about 50% of all patients with ischemic chest pain arrive at the ED after calling 911 and receiving EMS care and transport. Major educational initiatives are under way to increase the percentage of people who recognize the warning signs of possible heart attack and call 911. EMS personnel can easily and appropriately start much of the initial assessment and immediate general treatment.

Half of all deaths caused by AMI occur in the prehospital setting as the result of VF or pulseless VT. Every emergency vehicle that responds to cardiac arrest should carry a defibrillator with staff skilled in its use.

EMS personnel follow standing protocols and can contact medical control physicians as needed. They start IV lines, measure vital signs and oxygen saturation, and obtain a targeted history. The

ECC Guidelines 2000 recommend that EMS personnel use a chest pain checklist to determine the patient's eligibility for fibrinolytic therapy and obtain an initial 12-lead ECG to alert base EDs when chest pain patients have ST elevation. This is a Class IIa recommendation in the *ECC Guidelines 2000.* Multiple studies have shown that obtaining prehospital 12-lead ECGs speeds diagnosis and shortens time to fibrinolysis in eligible patients. EMS personnel start the "MONA" treatments and transmit initial 12-lead ECGs by cellular or landline telephone. Computerized ECG interpretation, available on field 12-lead ECGs, can be read orally to the receiving ED.

Fibrinolytics should be administered at the earliest possible moment after the onset of symptoms of ischemic-type chest pain. The potential benefit of administration of fibrinolytics in the prehospital setting has been addressed in several prospective clinical trials. Positive benefit from starting fibrinolytics in the field are significant only in settings in which prehospital transport time is more than 60 minutes or when prehospital administration of fibrinolytics "beats" in-hospital administration by 60 to 90 minutes. In rural settings transport times can often exceed 60 minutes. In such circumstances several studies have shown prehospital fibrinolytic therapy to be "safe and effective." This is true, however, only when a knowledgeable physician can review the prehospital 12-lead ECG (usually by telemetry or telephonic transmission) and can combine that review with a patient-specific risk assessment. For this reason the *ECC Guidelines 2000* recommend out-of-hospital fibrinolytic therapy only when a physician is present or out-of-hospital transport time is 60 minutes or longer.

Continued improvement in ED triage, driven by a "time is muscle" approach, can achieve routine door-to-needle times of 30 minutes or less. This "fast-track" approach has offset the value of prehospital fibrinolytic therapy, which may not be much faster than taking the chest pain patient straight to the ED. To a large extent recent reductions in the interval between the start of chest pain and the start of fibrinolytic agents have come from the "alerting function" of the prehospital 12-lead ECG. Most EMS systems therefore should focus on early identification of patients with ACS (including obtaining the 12-lead ECG) and rapid transport with prearrival notification to the ED. The ED should focus on rapid evaluation, determination of eligibility, and rapid administration of fibrinolytics.

Assess initial 12-lead ECG

Box 5: Assess Initial 12-Lead ECG

Today the 12-lead ECG (Figure 3) stands at the center of decision making for the care of the patient with ACS. For patients suspected of having AMI and ischemia, a 12-lead ECG should be obtained and reviewed by the responsible clinician as quickly as possible, within 10 minutes of arrival at the ED unless special circumstances intervene. The AHA Committee on Emergency Cardiovascular Care, the National Heart Attack Alert Program, and the ACC/AHA Task Force on Practice Guidelines, Committee on the Management of Acute Myocardial Infarction, all place the highest priority on being able to classify patients into 1 of 3 ECG classification groups:

- ST-segment elevation
- ST depression or T-wave inversion
- Nondiagnostic or normal ECG

During medical observation in suggestive clinical circumstances, obtain repeat ECGs (serial or continuous ECGs or ST-segment monitoring). If a patient's serial ECG changes from characteristics of one group to those of another, eg, from nondiagnostic ECG to ST elevation, change the therapeutic approach to follow the new classification.

- ***ST elevation or new or presumably new LBBB:*** **strongly suspicious for injury** ***ST-elevation AMI***

Box 6: ST Elevation or New or Presumably New LBBB

This group of chest pain patients receives major clinical attention because these patients are the only patients who benefit from acute reperfusion therapy. Many trials of reperfusion therapy over the last decade confirm the unequivocal value of fibrinolytic therapy or the combination of acute angiography plus a reperfusion intervention (angioplasty/stent) for this group of patients.

The clinician must search for ST elevation that is *≥0.1 mV (1 mm on ECG calibrated to 10 mm/1 mV) in 2 or more anatomically contiguous leads.* The clinician should also search for new or presumably new LBBB (BBB that obscures ST-segment analysis).

Fibrinolytic therapy is a Class I recommendation if the patient is less than 75 years of age and the time to therapy is 12 hours or less from onset of symptoms. Patients more than 75 years of age also benefit from fibrinolytic therapy, but because of the increased risk of stroke and the smaller number of patients studied, this is a Class IIa recommendation. A careful risk-benefit assessment is necessary. For example, treatment of a large anterior infarction presenting within 2 to 3 hours of onset of pain has the potential to yield much greater benefits than treatment of a small, inferior, uncomplicated infarction presenting 6 to 8 hours after onset of pain. Many clinicians would elect not to treat the latter patient with fibrinolytics.

ST-segment elevation must be measured correctly (see Figure 5):

- Measure at 0.04 second (1 mm) after the J point. The J point is the position of juncture (angle change) between the QRS complex and the ST wave.

- The baseline for this measurement has been the PR segment. But a baseline drawn from the *end* of the T wave to the *start* of the P wave is considered to be more accurate.

Exceptions to the ST-Segment Elevation Rule

Patients with posterior infarction or with tall, hyperacute T waves may be eligible for fibrinolytic therapy even though they do not present with ST-segment elevation or new LBBB. Fibrinolytic therapy is appropriate for these patients, especially if ischemic chest pain continues unabated or recurs after initial treatment:

Infarct Localization

Clinicians who evaluate 12-lead ECGs for ST changes should develop the ability to estimate the location and extent of the infarction, ischemia, or injury and identify the affected coronary artery. In particular, clinicians responsible for the decision to give fibrinolytic agents must understand the concept of anatomically contiguous leads.

The *ACLS Reference Textbook* provides more details on this topic, and the illustrations in Figure 4 assist with infarct localization. Infarct localization helps identify those patients who will benefit the most from fibrinolytic therapy and helps predict specific complications that are more likely to develop from specific infarct locations (eg, RV infarction).

In particular, all patients with inferior injury or infarction should receive a right precordial lead ECG as soon as the inferior abnormalities are recognized. The ECG will help identify patients with possible RV infarction. These patients have a higher in-hospital mortality rate, and if dysfunction is present they require the support of RV filling pressure for cardiac output.

Patients with RV infarction should not in general receive nitroglycerin, morphine, or diuretics. If clinically significant RV infarction is present (jugular venous distention and clear lungs, hypotension or marginal BP), nitrates and vasodilators are contraindicated.

FIGURE 5. How to measure ST-segment deviation. **A,** Inferior MI. ST segment has no low point (it is coved or concave). **B,** Anterior MI.

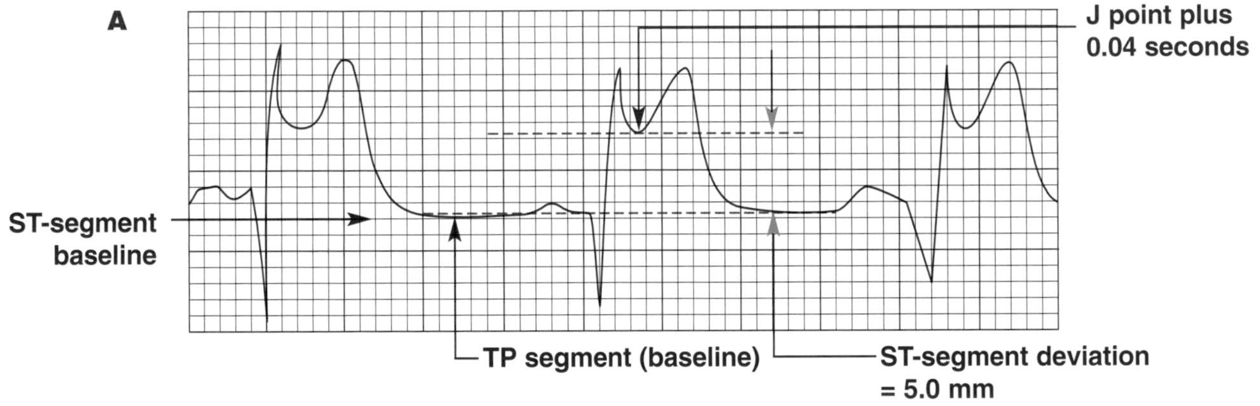

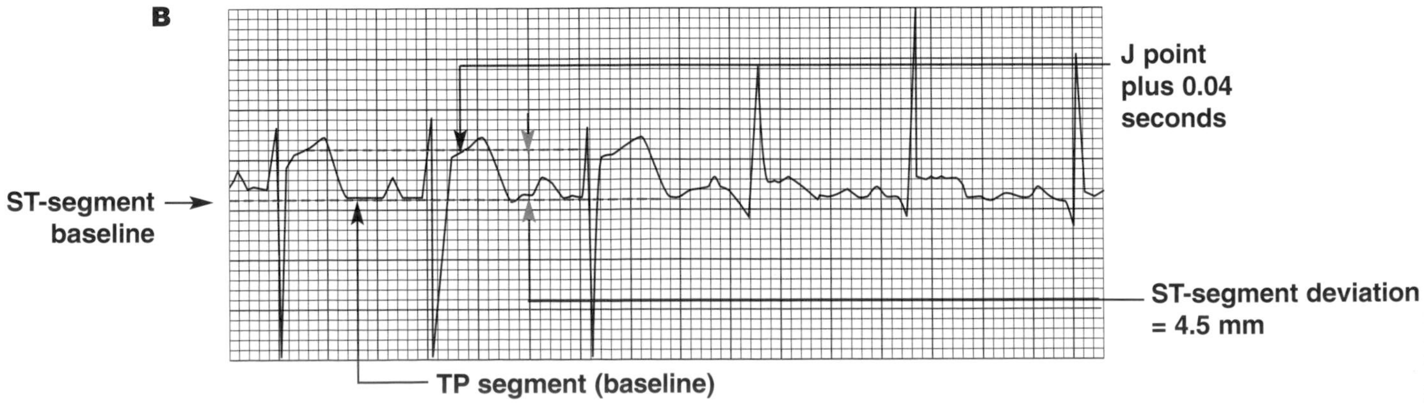

- ***Posterior current of acute injury.*** Occlusions of the circumflex artery, the posterior descending artery, or the posterolateral branch of the right coronary artery can each produce a posterior LV infarction. This may be manifested only by marked ST-segment *depression* confined to leads V_1 through V_4.
- ***Tall, hyperacute T waves.*** In the earliest phases of acute infarction the ECG may show only giant, hyperacute T waves, without ST-segment elevation.

New or Presumably New LBBB

BBBs interfere with ST-segment analysis and can obscure the ECG diagnosis of MI—LBBB more so than RBBB. Clinicians consider new LBBB to be the more serious of the 2 types of BBB. LBBBs are caused by occlusion of the left anterior descending (LAD) branch of the left coronary artery. LAD occlusion causes loss of a large amount of myocardium, including myocardium perfused by both branches of the left bundle (the left anterior and left posterior division). Patients with new LBBB have lost a lot of myocardium; LV failure will develop and may be the cause of death. Early reperfusion is of paramount importance for these patients.

RBBBs are most often caused by occlusion of a branch of the right coronary artery. In general, RBBB does not obscure the ability to interpret the ECG for ischemic and injury changes. RBBB obscures only the terminal 0.04 second of the QRS complex. ST-segment changes due to acute ischemia can often but not always be delineated in the appropriate clinical setting. New RBBB in the clinical setting of ischemic-type chest pain is associated with increased mortality and is an indication for fibrinolytic therapy.

Determination of "new or presumably new" BBB requires copies or reports of previous ECGs. Often these tracings are difficult to obtain. With an inability to determine old versus new LBBB comes a dependence on clinical judgment and assessment of the risks and benefits of fibrinolytic therapy. In this situation most clinicians let the story of onset of symptoms and degree of severity weigh heavily in the final choice of therapy. The more it appears that the pain and associated signs and symptoms are due to an AMI, the more likely the LBBB is to be new.

Known Preexisting LBBB: Difficult to Read New Ischemic Changes

Some studies have identified ECG criteria for reading ischemic changes in patients with preexisting LBBB. The sensitivity and specificity of these criteria remain under review. The management of these patients, particularly in decisions about the best reperfusion strategy, should be undertaken in consultation with a cardiologist.

Start adjunctive treatments
(as indicated; no reperfusion delay)
- ***β-Adrenoceptor blockers*** IV
- ***Nitroglycerin*** IV
- ***Heparin*** IV
- ***ACE inhibitors*** (after 6 hours or when stable)

Box 7: Start Adjunctive Treatments

Patients with acute ischemic pain and ST elevation or new LBBB who have not yet received **aspirin** and **nitroglycerin** should receive these agents immediately. If pain persists after administration of nitroglycerin and oxygen, pain control with IV **morphine** becomes a major priority.

In addition, clinicians should consider administration of the following adjunctive treatments:

- β-Adrenoceptor blocking agents (β-blockers)
- Nitroglycerin IV
- Heparin IV

β-Adrenoceptor Blocking Agents (β-Blockers)

β-Blockers have many positive effects. They can

- Increase myocardial salvage in the anatomic area of the infarct-related artery by reducing the size of the ischemic penumbra or shadow
- Prevent extension of infarction by reducing oxygen consumption and demands on threatened, ischemic myocardium
- Reduce short- and long-term mortality rates in survivors of AMI
- Reduce the incidence of VF and "electrical storm"

Recommended Use of β-Blockers for Patients With ST-Segment Elevation

- All patients without a contraindication to β-adrenoceptor blocker therapy if treated within 12 hours of onset of infarction (Class I). This means that β-blockers are given not only as an adjunct to fibrinolytic agents but also as agents with independent benefit.

Contraindications to β-Blocker Therapy

β-Adrenoreceptor blocking agents are contraindicated for the following conditions:

- HR <60 bpm (HR <50 bpm absolute)
- Systolic BP <100 mm Hg (absolute)
- Moderate (relative Class IIb) or severe (absolute Class III) LV failure
- Signs of peripheral hypoperfusion/shock (absolute Class III)
- PR interval >0.24 second (relative)
- Second- or third-degree block (absolute)
- Severe chronic obstructive pulmonary disease (relative)
- History of asthma (relative)
- Severe peripheral vascular disease (relative)

Nitroglycerin IV

Although IV nitroglycerin has been extensively studied in large clinical trials, its precise role in management of AMI patients with ST-segment elevation has not been established. In particular, the value of routine administration of IV nitroglycerin to patients also receiving fibrinolytic therapy is indeterminate. Recent large clinical trials (GISSI-3, ISIS-4) have not shown a mortality reduction for IV, topical, or long-acting nitrates.

Nevertheless, nitroglycerin is beneficial for dilation of the coronary arteries adjacent to sites of recent plaque disruption and for positive hemodynamic effects on the peripheral arteries and venous capacitance vessels.

Recommended Use of Nitroglycerin

The ACC/AHA Practice Guidelines make the following recommendations:

- Nitroglycerin IV is Class I therapy for the first 24 to 48 hours in patients with AMI complicated by any of the following:
  - — CHF
  - — Large anterior infarction
  - — Persistent or recurrent ischemia
  - — Hypertension
- IV nitroglycerin infusion should be started early in the patients noted above, but this infusion should not delay start of reperfusion strategy (see "Precautions" below). Nitroglycerin infusion is generally continued for 24 to 48 hours. Nitrate tolerance may develop within this time period, and a nitrate-free interval is recommended in patients who have indications for continued therapy. A switch to topical or long-acting nitrates with a nitrate-free interval after 24 hours is recommended.
- For AMI patients without hypotension, bradycardia, or tachycardia, IV nitroglycerin is considered acceptable but only possibly helpful (Class IIb).

Precautions in the Use of Nitroglycerin

The following *precautions* should be noted when considering use of nitroglycerin for patients with ACS:

- Avoid systemic hypotension because this will worsen myocardial ischemia and perfusion.
- Limit any fall in systolic blood pressure to no lower than 110 mm Hg if the patient is normotensive and to 25% of baseline systolic pressure if the patient is hypertensive. In any event avoid a drop in systolic blood pressure below 100 mm Hg.
- Use pain as a way of titrating the infusion rate of nitroglycerin when indicated for ischemia.
- Use a target blood pressure as above when used for hypertension, CHF, or other indications.
- Do not use nitroglycerin as a substitute for narcotic analgesics to achieve pain control: patients will often require both.
- Exercise extreme caution in the use of nitroglycerin in patients who may have RV infarction. These patients are particularly sensitive to nitroglycerin, diuretics, morphine, and any vasodilators. At highest risk for RV infarction are patients with ECG changes of inferior injury: ST-segment elevation in the inferior leads (II, III, aVF). These patients may experience profound hypotension because the infarction compromises RV function. Vasodilators are contraindicated in the presence of clinically significant RV infarction.
- Avoid use of nitroglycerin in patients who have taken sildenafil (Viagra™) within 24 hours. Sildenafil is a phosphodiesterase inhibitor that increases cyclic GMP, which in turn mediates vascular smooth muscle relaxation. Nitrate-mediated vasodilation is markedly increased when administered with sildenafil. Refractory hypotension and death have been reported.

Heparin IV for Patients With ST-Segment Elevation

Heparin is an anticoagulant that indirectly inhibits thrombin. It is a useful adjunct to fibrin-specific fibrinolytic therapy, and recommendations for its use will be determined by the fibrinolytic agent chosen.

Recommended Use of Heparin

Heparin administration is effective and recommended for the following patients:

- Patients receiving fibrin-specific lytics (eg, tPA, reteplase, tenecteplase)
- Patients for whom the planned reperfusion strategy is direct or adjunct PCI (Class I)

Precautions for Heparin Therapy

The precautions for use of heparin therapy include the following:

- Same contraindications as for fibrinolytic therapy:
  - — Active bleeding
  - — Recent intracranial, intraspinal, or eye surgery
  - — Severe hypertension
  - — Bleeding disorders
  - — Gastrointestinal bleeding
- Sensitivity to heparin may be decreased when it is used concomitantly with IV nitroglycerin. Higher doses may be needed to achieve the anticoagulation end point. Risk of bleeding is increased if nitroglycerin is stopped and heparin is continued.

ACE Inhibitors

Early oral therapy with ACE inhibitors reduces mortality and CHF associated with MI. This reduction occurs whether or not fibrinolytic agents are used, especially when ACE inhibitors are given within the first 12 to 24 hours after the onset of symptoms. In clinical trials ACE inhibitors have been particularly helpful for patients with larger or anterior AMIs and with CHF without hypotension. These drugs help prevent adverse LV remodeling, delay progression of heart failure, and decrease sudden death and recurrent MI. Although these agents are placed in an algorithm box ahead of "Select a reperfusion strategy," they are not administered in the first 6 hours after an AMI. In fact, ACE inhibitors are an *adjunctive* therapy usually started in the coronary care unit after administration of fibrinolytics. *The highest priority should be on instituting definitive reperfusion therapy at the earliest possible time after the onset of symptoms of infarction.*

Recommended Use of ACE Inhibitors for Patients With ST-Segment Elevation

ACE inhibitors are recommended for the following:

- When suspected AMI is associated with ST-segment elevation in 2 or more anterior precordial leads
- When LV ejection fraction of less than 40% develops during AMI
- When patients with AMI develop clinical signs of heart failure due to systolic pump dysfunction

Precautions:

- In general, ACE inhibitors are not started in the ED but within the first 12 to 24 hours, after fibrinolytic therapy has ended and blood pressure has stabilized.

Precautions are listed in the *ECC Handbook*.

> ***Time from onset of symptoms?***

Box 8: Time From Onset of Symptoms

Onset of symptoms is defined as the beginning of continuous, persistent discomfort that led the patient to call 911, come to the ED, or otherwise seek help. Frequently, however, patients will present with a "stuttering" or "on-off" pattern of pain, thus making the time of the onset of symptoms difficult to determine. In general, for *onset time* use the time of the experience that prompted the patient to seek care.

Patient delays in decision making after the onset of symptoms continue to present a major barrier to realizing the full benefits of reperfusion therapy. *The key to reperfusion therapy is that the earlier therapy begins, the better the outcome.* The greatest benefit in survival and LV function occurs when therapy is provided within the first 3 hours of symptom onset.

Studies have shown, however, that significant survival benefit occurs up to at least 12 hours after onset of symptoms. Because management for the 2 groups is different, the Ischemic Chest Pain Algorithm attempts to divide patients into 2 groups: those with onset of symptoms less than 12 hours before evaluation and those with onset of symptoms more than 12 hours before evaluation.

> **Select a reperfusion strategy based on local resources:**
> - Angiography
> - PCI (angioplasty + stent)
> - Cardiothoracic surgery backup

Box 9: Select a Reperfusion Strategy

A reperfusion strategy should be selected on the basis of local resources. Fibrinolytic therapy is a Class I intervention if

- Clinical complaints are consistent with ischemic-type pain
- ST elevation ≥1 mm is identified in at least 2 anatomically contiguous leads
- There are no contraindications (see contraindications in the *ECC Handbook*)
- Patient is less than 75 years of age

Patients More Than 75 Years of Age

For patients more than 75 years of age, fibrinolytic therapy drops to a Class IIa intervention. The risks of complications of fibrinolytic therapy (primarily intracranial hemorrhage), increase in this age group, but so does the risk and mortality rate of AMI. These patients should still be treated with fibrinolytic agents even though the relative benefit of therapy is reduced. A careful risk-benefit assessment, however, is needed to carefully evaluate the increased risk of intracerebral hemorrhage compared with the treatment benefit. PCI may be a better alternative in some patients at increased risk for hemorrhage.

Time to Therapy Is More Than 12 Hours

The algorithm indicates that patients presenting more than 12 hours after the onset of symptoms are no longer candidates for an immediate reperfusion strategy. Clinical studies indicate only a small benefit of either fibrinolytic therapy or primary PCI for these patients. Sometimes, however, patients may give a story of long duration (more than 12 hours), but on presentation they still have pain and ST elevation. It is reasonable to conclude that there is continuing ischemia with viable myocardium at risk. Fibrinolytic therapy is therefore considered a Class IIb intervention (may offer some benefit) for this specific group of patients who display continuing ischemic pain plus extensive ST elevation. These patients may also be better evaluated and treated with PCI if available in a timely manner.

> **Fibrinolytic therapy selected**
> - Front-loaded ***alteplase***
>
> or
> - ***Streptokinase*** or
> - ***APSAC*** or
> - ***Reteplase*** or
> - ***Tenecteplase***
>
> **Goal:** door-to-drug <30 minutes

Box 10: Fibrinolytic Therapy Selected

At the end of the year 2000 both primary PCI and fibrinolytic therapy were considered Class I interventions for acute developing MI. Some experts, however, think primary PCI is superior to fibrinolytic agents alone. See the ACC/AHA Practice Guidelines and the *ACLS Reference Textbook* for more on this issue.

As of August 2000 the following 5 fibrinolytic agents have been approved, are in common use, and are available for treatment of acute ST-segment elevation MI (see the *ECC Handbook* for more details).

Tissue Plasminogen Activator (tPA): Alteplase

The GUSTO-1 study and other recent clinical trials suggest that **alteplase,** given as an accelerated infusion ***and*** combined with IV **heparin,** is currently the most effective therapy to achieve early coronary reperfusion. Although this is described as the "most effective" regimen, only slightly more than 50% of patients achieve normal flow associated with reduced mortality (TIMI grade III flow). This benefit is achieved at the cost of a small but definite increase in intracerebral hemorrhage. Alteplase also is much more expensive than streptokinase and carries a greater risk of intracranial hemorrhage. The cost-benefit ratio favors alteplase when patients present early with large areas of damage and low risk of brain hemorrhage (eg, a young patient with a large MI).

The recommended accelerated infusion dose of alteplase is

- 15 mg IV bolus
- Then 0.75 mg/kg over the next 30 minutes (not to exceed 50 mg)
- *Then 0.5 mg/kg over the next 60 minutes (not to exceed 35 mg)*

Recent trial data also shows that excessive anticoagulation with UFH is associated with increased risk of intracerebral hemorrhage. To improve the safety profile of tPA, the ACC/AHA Guidelines have been modified to *reduce* the dose of heparin used in combination with fibrin-specific lytics. Give UFH to patients weighing more than 70 kg as an initial bolus of 60 U/kg, not to exceed a 4000-U bolus; then administer 12 U/kg per hour, not to exceed 1000 U/h. An activated partial thromboplastin time (aPTT) of 50 to 70 seconds is then maintained by a heparin administration protocol. LMWH has not been tested for efficacy, and the risk for intracerebral hemorrhage is unknown. Use only UFH until clinical trial data for LMWH is known.

Streptokinase

Streptokinase is the agent of choice for patients with a greater relative risk of brain hemorrhage and a smaller potential for benefit (those patients with longer times from onset of symptoms and smaller areas of myocardial injury). In ISIS-3 an accelerated tPA regimen had a small but significant excess of hemorrhagic stroke, but there were 9 fewer deaths or disabling strokes per 1000 patients treated with tPA. Avoid reuse of streptokinase for at least 2 years (preferably indefinitely). Prior exposure within 5 days to 2 years is a contraindication to re-administration. This is because of a high prevalence of potentially neutralizing antibodies and a risk of anaphylaxis. The standard dose is 1.5 million IU in a 1-hour infusion.

Reteplase, Recombinant (Retavase)

Reteplase is a double-bolus fibrinolytic agent approved for clinical use in the United States in 1996. Retavase is a deletion mutation of tPA. The GUSTO-III trial documented equivalence in efficacy to tPA. Retavase has the advantage over current treatment regimens in that it is administered as a double bolus. Bolus administration has the advantages of simplified administration and no requirements for infusion pump. Retavase dosing is not based on weight. The regimen is a double dose for all patients:

- 10 U IV plus a 10-U IV bolus over 2 minutes, 30 minutes apart

Heparin and **aspirin** should be administered conjunctively because all clinical trials have been conducted with conjunctive heparin and aspirin administration. An infusion pump is not required, and administration is complete in 30 minutes.

Anistreplase (Eminase) (Anisoylated Plasminogen Streptokinase Activator Complex [APSAC])

Eminase is a combination of streptokinase and plasminogen. Eminase was the first bolus lytic developed. The anisoylated modification allowed for slow release of the streptokinase-plasminogen complex and bolus administration. This positioned APSAC for use in the prehospital setting. In Europe a number of important trials used this concept for prehospital administration. In the GREAT trial a 50% reduction in 3-month mortality was observed. The EMIP study reduced by about 1 hour the time to fibrinolytic administration.

Eminase is administered as a 30 U bolus over 4 to 5 minutes. Eminase shares a side-effect profile with streptokinase. In ISIS-3 eminase had more allergy side effects and intracerebral hemorrhage complications than streptokinase. The use of tPA and reteplase has significantly reduced the use of eminase.

TNKase (Tenecteplase)

TNKase is the newest fibrinolytic agent, approved by the Food and Drug Administration (FDA) in 2000. Like tPA, TNKase is based on the natural enzyme tissue plasminogen activator (tPA), the same as alteplase. Streptokinase, in contrast, is based on a bacterial enzyme, which acts indirectly by forming a complex with naturally occurring plasminogen. "Synthetic" tPA is made by recombinant methods (rtPA). TNKase was formed by substituting key amino acids in rtPA, in contrast to Retavase, which is a deletion mutation. These are small but significant changes. In the case of TNKase, these amino acid substitutions allow for single-bolus administration.

TNKase is administered by weight-adjusted dose, 0.5 mg/kg to 0.6 mg/kg (30 mg in patients weighing less than 60 kg, 50 mg for patients weighing more than 90 kg).

- If signs of cardiogenic shock or contraindications to fibrinolytics, PCI is treatment of choice (Class I) if available
- If PCI is not available, use fibrinolytics (if no contraindications)

Box 11: If Signs of Cardiogenic Shock or Contraindications to Fibrinolytics Are Present

Consideration of fibrinolytic therapy requires a thorough review for contraindications. At this point in decision making the clinician faces a patient

- With ST-segment elevation or new or presumably new BBB
- At less than 12 hours after onset of symptoms

If there are signs of cardiogenic shock or if fibrinolytic therapy is contraindicated, then primary PCI is the treatment of choice. In collaboration with the responsible cardiologist, the clinician should arrange for the patient to go quickly to the catheterization suite. Arrangements for transfer should be initiated if these facilities are unavailable at the hospital of initial presentation. MONA and adjunctive therapy should continue to be administered when indicated.

Primary PCI selected
- Door-to-balloon inflation 90 ± 30 minutes
- Experienced operators
- High-volume center
- Cardiac surgical capability

Box 12: Primary PCI Selected

Goal: Door-to-Dilatation Interval or Arrival-in-Catheterization Suite Interval of 90±30 Minutes

Early Primary PCI: An Equivalent Alternative to Early Fibrinolytic Therapy

The Ischemic Chest Pain Algorithm depicts equal status for angioplasty and fibrinolytics as reperfusion strategies. This equivalence exists, however, only if the primary angioplasty can be performed rapidly at a center with a high volume and a low rate of complications. The interval from arrival at the ED ("door time") to arrival in the catheterization suite should be less than 60 minutes. The interval from door time to inflation of the catheter balloon should be less than 90 minutes ("dilatation time").

In addition, the ACC/AHA Practice Guidelines require that other stringent conditions be met before PCI can be considered an equivalent alternative to fibrinolytic therapy:

- The facility must have cardiac surgery capability.
- Operators must be skilled in the procedure ("skilled" is defined as having performed more than 75 PTCA procedures per year).
- The PCI center must be high volume ("high volume" is defined as a center performing more than 200 PTCA procedures per year).
- PCI center and its operators must operate within a specified "corridor of outcomes" defined by flow rates attained and low complication rates (defined in the 1996 ACC/AHA Practice Guidelines, page 1349).

A total of 20% of US hospitals have cardiac catheterization facilities, and only a portion of these centers can perform emergency PCIs. Therefore, fibrinolytic agents will be used much more often than PCIs. In ACLS training the emphasis will continue to be on rapid identification of those patients who qualify for fibrinolytic therapy and rapid initiation of therapy.

Although only a portion of US hospitals can provide PCIs, the procedure is available for 70% of the population within 30 minutes. ACLS providers need to be able to identify patients who should be considered for emergency coronary catheterization with possible angioplasty or stent placement. These are listed below.

Recommended Angioplasty for Patients With ST-Segment Elevation

Angioplasty (with or without stent placement) is recommended for the following patients:

- Patients with signs and symptoms of a large AMI of less than 12 hours' duration who have a contraindication to fibrinolytic therapy because of a risk of bleeding (Class I)
- Patients with possible "stuttering" infarction with ECG changes but without clear indications for fibrinolytic therapy (Class IIa)
- Patients with AMI who develop cardiogenic shock or pump failure within 18 hours (Class IIa)
- Patients with a history of previous CABG surgery in whom a recent occlusion of a vein graft may have occurred (Class IIa)
- Patients with a witnessed possible AMI in-hospital with rapid access to a catheterization facility (Class IIb)
- Patients who receive fibrinolytic therapy for appropriate reasons but fail to reperfuse and who develop or continue having symptoms

Critical Actions: Assessment and Management

Critical Action Checklist for ACS

The checklist below identifies steps in the immediate and subsequent assessment and treatment of a patient with an ACS. Review—do not memorize—the checklist until you understand the order and rationale for all steps. For in-depth information about these topics, consult the *ECC Guidelines 2000* and the *ECC Handbook*. (See the section Read More About It at the end of this case). You will learn the details in the course.

Critical Actions Checklist: ACLS Case 6
Acute Coronary Syndromes

Scene Survey Steps	Assess: Do or Monitor	Manage: Do or Delegate
Recognize emergency and respond	☐ Note signs and symptoms of ACS ***Immediate assessment (<10 min)*** ☐ Check vital signs with automatic or standard BP cuff ☐ Determine oxygen saturation ☐ Obtain IV access ☐ Obtain 12-lead ECG (physician reviews) ☐ Perform brief, targeted history and physical examination; focus on eligibility for fibrinolytic therapy ☐ Obtain blood for electrolyte and coagulation measurements ☐ Measure initial cardiac marker levels ☐ Obtain portable chest x-ray (<30 minutes) ☐ Use the 1-to-10 pain scale to "measure" pain ☐ Note the time pain began	***Immediate general treatment:*** ☐ Learn *oxygen-IV-monitor* as one word that should be memorized for easy recall and fast action in cardiac emergencies — *Oxygen* = provide supplemental oxygen — *IV* = initiate an IV — *Monitor* = attach monitor to patient ☐ Continue to assess status of airway, movement of air, and status of ventilations ☐ Provide rescue breathing and tracheal intubation as indicated ☐ Obtain heart rate and blood pressure ☐ Begin to take history ☐ Perform Primary and Secondary Surveys ☐ Obtain a 12-lead ECG within minutes, particularly if patient complains of chest pain. ☐ Oxygen at 4 L/min ☐ Aspirin 160 to 325 mg ☐ If indicated: — Nitroglycerin SL or spray — Morphine IV (if pain not relieved with nitroglycerin)
Classify patient	***Assess the 12-lead ECG*** (See Figures 1 and 2): ☐ Classify patient into 1 of 3 categories: — ST-segment elevation or — New (presumably new)-onset bundle branch block — ST-segment depression or — Ischemic T-wave inversion — Nondiagnostic or normal ECG	***For ST-segment elevation or depression:*** ☐ Apply indication and exclusion criteria for use of fibrinolytics ☐ Know *why?*, *when?*, *how?*, and *watch out!* for PCI

Scene Survey Steps	Assess: Do or Monitor	Manage: Do or Delegate
Adjunctive therapy	☐ Assess whether other major drugs are indicated or contra-indicated: — Heparin — β-Blockers — Lidocaine — ACE inhibitors	☐ Know actions, dosing, and precautions of listed drugs
Anatomic location of ischemia, injury, or infarct	☐ Know the basics of ECG localization of ischemia, injury, or infarct. Relate changes to cardiac anatomy and coronary vessel: — Anterior myocardium — Inferior myocardium — Septal myocardium — Lateral myocardium — Right ventricle — BBB (to distinguish new from old)	☐ Know which arrhythmias and other complications are most likely to develop according to which cardiac sites are injured

This critical actions checklist is limited to those actions specific to assessment and management of problems related to ACS. To avoid unnecessary repetition, this checklist does not repeat all the assessment and management steps of the *Primary and Secondary ABCD Surveys.* Please understand that *those steps must be performed for all patients.*

This checklist assumes that the following equipment and personnel are available:

Equipment: 12-lead ECG device

Personnel: other ACLS providers available from the time you are involved

Medications:

- Morphine
- Oxygen
- Nitroglycerin
- Aspirin
- Heparin (UFH, LMWH)
- GP IIb/IIIa inhibitors
- β Blockers
- Fibrinolytic agents
- ACE inhibitors

Unacceptable Actions: Perils and Pitfalls

The ACLS provider will not have successfully realized the objectives of Case 6 if he or she

- Fails to provide immediate assessment and general treatment to a patient with chest pain suggestive of ischemia
- Fails to obtain a 12-lead ECG in a timely fashion (less than 10 minutes from ED arrival to ECG) in patients with chest pain suggestive of ischemia
- Fails to initiate oxygen for patients with chest pain suggestive of ischemia
- Fails to aggressively attempt to control a patient's chest pain
- Fails to recognize exclusion criteria for use of fibrinolytic therapy
- Fails to recognize contraindications for medications listed in the Ischemic Chest Pain Algorithm

Read More About It

The most comprehensive and up-to-date material on the acute coronary syndromes is in the *ECC Guidelines 2000,* Section 1: Acute Coronary Syndromes (Acute Myocardial Infarction) of Part 7: The Era of Reperfusion, written by John M. Field, MD, ACLS editor.

Another excellent resource and summary is the acute coronary syndromes section of the *ECC Handbook* and the *ACLS Reference Textbook.*

Workbook Review

1. **You are an EMS paramedic evaluating a 50-year-old man at his home. He complains of crushing substernal chest pain, profuse sweating, and shortness of breath. His vital signs are as follows: temperature = 37°C; HR = 100 bpm; BP = 170/110 mm Hg; resp = 32; oxygen saturation = 90%. Which of the following includes the best immediate treatment for this patient?**

   a. oxygen, morphine, aspirin, followed by sublingual nitroglycerin if morphine fails to relieve pain

   b. oxygen, sublingual nitroglycerin, morphine, but withhold aspirin unless the ST segment is elevated more than 3 mm

   c. oxygen, sublingual nitroglycerin, followed by morphine if the nitroglycerin fails to relieve the pain, aspirin

   d. oxygen, sublingual nitroglycerin, no morphine because of the high blood pressure, no aspirin until admitted to the hospital

   Read more about it in the ECC Guidelines 2000, *page 25: "Out-of-Hospital Care for ACS" and the algorithm on page 26; and pages 176-180: "Initial General Measures"*

2. **You are an ED physician evaluating the recently arrived 50-year-old man in question 1. The 12-lead ECG shows 3-mm ST-segment elevation in leads V_2 through V_4. Despite prehospital administration of oxygen, aspirin, nitroglycerin, and morphine, the man continues to have severe chest pain, which is now of more than 20 minutes' duration. His blood pressure is 170/110 mm Hg; his heart rate is 120 bpm. Which of the following treatments would be most appropriate for this patient at this time?**

   a. calcium channel blocker PO plus bolus of heparin

   b. ACE inhibitor IV plus lidocaine infusion

   c. magnesium sulfate plus aspirin

   d. IV β-blocker, tPA, heparin

   Read more about it in the ECC Guidelines 2000, *pages 182-184: "ST-Segment Elevation MI"; and pages 191-194: "Adjunctive Therapy for A09CS"*

3. **You are a healthcare provider working in a community medical clinic. A 65-year-old man begins to experience "heavy chest pressure" and shortness of breath, and perspiration is trickling down his face. When you tell him you are calling 911 for care and transport to the ED, he protests, *"No lights and sirens! My wife will drive me to the hospital."* Which of the following would be the *best* reasons to give for transporting this patient to the hospital in an ACLS mobile unit?**

   a. EMS personnel can radio ahead to the ED, activate the acute chest pain protocol, and make the ED aware of an incoming patient with a possible acute coronary syndrome

   b. EMS personnel can provide immediate assessment, including use of a 12-lead ECG if available and immediate treatment with prearrival notification of the receiving hospital

   c. EMS personnel can obtain a blood sample for evaluation of cardiac markers to diagnose the cause of the chest pain

   d. EMS personnel can admit the patient directly to the coronary care unit and not waste time in the ED

   Read more about it in the ECC Guidelines 2000, *pages 24-26: "Recognition and Actions for Acute Coronary Syndromes," including the algorithm on page 26; and pages 173-176: "Out-of-Hospital Management"*

4. **A patient presents to the ED complaining of severe, crushing, midsternal chest pain of 30 minutes' duration. He has a history of smoking and diet-controlled diabetes. His blood pressure is 110/70 mm Hg; his heart rate is 90 bpm. The 12-lead ECG shows a regular sinus rhythm of 90 bpm. Aspirin is administered, and oxygen 2 L/min is provided through a nasal cannula. Nitroglycerin provides no relief for the chest pain. Which of the following drugs should be administered next?**

   a. atropine 0.5 mg IV

   b. lidocaine 1 to 1.5 mg/kg

   c. furosemide 20 to 40 mg IV

   d. morphine sulfate 2 to 4 mg IV

   Read more about it in the ECC Guidelines 2000, *pages 24-26: "Recognition and Actions for Acute Coronary Syndromes," including the algorithm on page 26; and pages 173-176: "Out-of-Hospital Management"*

5. **Which of the following adjunctive therapies is a component of management of an uncomplicated ST-segment elevation AMI?**

   a. amiodarone

   b. aspirin

   c. epinephrine

   d. heparin

   Read more about it in the ECC Guidelines 2000, *pages 24-26: "Recognition and Actions for Acute Coronary Syndromes," including the algorithm on page 26; and pages 173-176: "Out-of-Hospital Management"*

6. Which of the following includes the major components of therapy for the 60-year-old patient presenting with ST-segment elevation MI within 30 minutes of the onset of symptoms of acute ischemic chest pain?

a. reperfusion therapy (fibrinolytics or PCI), aspirin, heparin, IV β-blockers

b. antithrombin therapy with heparin, antiplatelet therapy with aspirin, glycoprotein IIb/IIIa inhibitors, IV β-blockers, and nitrates, monitoring for "high-risk" status

c. serial ECGs with ST-segment monitoring, serum cardiac markers, further risk assessment with perfusion radionuclide imaging and stress echocardiography, aspirin

d. administer prophylactic lidocaine, fluid bolus, and vasopressor infusion

Read more about it in the ECC Guidelines 2000, *pages 178-179: Figure 3: Acute Ischemic Chest Pain Protocol and Figure 4: Acute Coronary Syndrome Algorithm; and pages 180-193: "Risk Stratification, Initial Therapy, and Evaluation for Reperfusion in the ED," "ST-Segment Elevation MI," "ST-Segment Depression: Non–Q-Wave MI/High-Risk Unstable Angina," and "Nondiagnostic ECG"*

7. Which of the following includes the major components of *initial* therapy for the patient with acute ischemic chest pain and a nondiagnostic ECG?

a. reperfusion therapy, aspirin, heparin, β-blockers, and nitrates

b. antithrombin therapy with heparin, antiplatelet therapy with aspirin, glycoprotein IIb/IIIa inhibitors, β-blockers, and nitrates, monitoring for "high-risk" status

c. serial ECGs with ST-segment monitoring, serum cardiac markers, and further risk assessment with perfusion radionuclide imaging and stress echocardiography, aspirin

d. prophylactic lidocaine, fluid bolus, and vasopressor infusion

Read more about it in the ECC Guidelines 2000, *pages 178-179: algorithms; and pages 180-193: "Risk Stratification, Initial Therapy, and Evaluation for Reperfusion in the ED," "ST-Segment Elevation MI," "ST-Segment Depression: Non–Q-Wave MI/High-Risk Unstable Angina," and "Nondiagnostic ECG"*

8. Which of the following patients with acute continuing ischemic chest pain is *most likely* to benefit from β-adrenoreceptor blocking agent therapy?

a. the patient with second- or third-degree heart block

b. the patient with severe left ventricular failure

c. the patient with a systolic arterial blood pressure of 90/60 mm Hg and sinus rhythm of 55 bpm

d. the patient with ST-segment elevation infarction and a blood pressure of 180/104 mm Hg.

Read more about it in the ECC Guidelines 2000, *pages 178-179: algorithms; and pages 180-193: "Risk Stratification, Initial Therapy, and Evaluation for Reperfusion in the ED," "ST-Segment Elevation MI," "ST-Segment Depression: Non–Q-Wave MI/High-Risk Unstable Angina," and "Non-diagnostic ECG"*

9. For which of the following patients would PCI, including angioplasty/stent, be a Class I recommendation and a better option than a conservative strategy with initial medical therapy?

a. a patient with non–ST-segment elevation MI but no "high-risk" characteristics

b. a patient less than 75 years of age with acute coronary syndromes and signs of severe left ventricular dysfunction and cardiogenic shock presenting within 16 hours of symptom onset

c. a patient with ST-segment elevation inferior MI, no signs of shock or left ventricular dysfunction, and no contraindications to fibrinolytic therapy, presenting within 2 hours of onset of symptoms

d. a patient with ST-segment depression who responds to initial treatment

Read more about it in the ECC Guidelines 2000, *pages 178-179: algorithms; and pages 180-193: "Risk Stratification, Initial Therapy, and Evaluation for Reperfusion in the ED," "ST-Segment Elevation MI," "ST-Segment Depression: Non–Q-Wave MI/High-Risk Unstable Angina," and "Non-diagnostic ECG"*

10. Which of the following patients presenting with AMI would be most likely to present with atypical, unusual, or vague signs and symptoms?

a. a 65-year-old woman with a past medical history of typical angina and moderate coronary artery disease according to prior angiogram

b. a 56-year-old man with no prior history of heart disease

c. a 45-year-old woman diagnosed with type I diabetes 22 years ago

d. a 48-year-old man in the intensive care unit after coronary bypass surgery

Read more about it in the ECC Guidelines 2000, *page 24: "Recognition and Actions for Acute Coronary Syndromes"; and page 174: "Patient Education and Delays in Therapy"*

(Continued on next page)

Advanced Question: Management of ACS for Experienced Providers

11. Which of the following includes the major components of therapy for the patient with ST-segment depression MI, good left ventricular function, and no prior MI?

a. reperfusion therapy, aspirin, heparin, β-blockers

b. antithrombin therapy with heparin, antiplatelet therapy with aspirin, glycoprotein IIb/IIIa inhibitors, β-blockers, and nitrates, and monitoring for "high-risk" status

c. serial ECGs with ST-segment monitoring, serum cardiac markers, further risk assessment with perfusion radionuclide imaging and stress echocardiography, aspirin

d. prophylactic lidocaine, fluid bolus, and vasopressor infusion

Read more about it in the ECC Guidelines 2000, *pages 178-179: algorithms; and pages 180-193: "Risk Stratification, Initial Therapy, and Evaluation for Reperfusion in the ED," "ST-Segment Elevation MI," "ST-Segment Depression: Non-Q-Wave MI/High-Risk Unstable Angina," and "Nondiagnostic ECG"*

Bradycardias

Description

In these bradycardia cases you manage patients with *symptomatic* **bradycardia.** The cornerstones of managing bradycardia cases are to

- Differentiate between signs and symptoms **caused** by the slow rate versus those **not caused** by the slow rate
- Correctly diagnose the presence and ***type of AV block,*** a critical factor in management, both acutely and after the patient is stabilized
- Select **atropine,** when appropriate, as the intervention of first choice
- Decide (correctly) when to start TCP
- Decide when to start ***catecholamines*** *(epinephrine, dopamine, and isoproterenol)* to maintain heart rate and blood pressure

What's New in the Guidelines... Bradycardias

The *ECC Guidelines 2000* contain no revisions in the recommended treatments for bradycardia. The principles driving the therapy of bradycardias continue to be

- Treat only symptomatic bradycardias
- The bradycardia must cause the symptoms
- Recognize the red flag bradycardias that are likely to deteriorate (even if asymptomatic):
  — Second-degree AV block type II
  — Third-degree AV heart block (complete heart block)
- The overall treatment approach remains the same as that used in 1994 to 1997:
  — Atropine
  — Transcutaneous pacing (TCP)
  — Dopamine
  — Epinephrine (see the Bradycardia algorithm)

Settings and Scenarios

Setting: Prehospital, Unmonitored Patient

You are a paramedic. You and your partner arrive at the home of a 67-year-old woman who is short of breath. Her husband says she collapsed when she rushed to answer an earlier knock at the door, but she never became unconscious. She is lying on the floor, awake and alert, but pale and sweaty. You begin to manage this patient now.

Setting: Emergency Dept, Unmonitored Patient

You are on duty as a nurse in the Emergency Department (ED). A 67-year-old woman who has experienced chest pain for 2 hours walks into the ED. She is changing slowly into a gown when she slumps onto the bed. She is drowsy, pale, and sweaty.

Setting: In-Hospital, Unmonitored Patient

A 67-year-old woman with unstable angina is being admitted by her general practitioner. She slumps onto the bed. She is drowsy, pale, and sweaty. Describe your initial management.

Setting: Critical Care Unit, Monitored Patient

A 67-year-old woman who has had chest pain for 2 hours has just been admitted from the ED. She presses the call button because she feels nauseated. She is pale and sweaty.

Learning and Skills Objectives

At the end of Case 7 you should be able to describe and discuss

1. Distinctions between **bradycardia** and ***symptomatic* bradycardia**
2. Specific signs and symptoms to look for to determine whether a *bradycardia is symptomatic*
3. *Interventions* to use *in symptomatic bradycardias* and the sequence to follow (see the algorithm)
4. Recognition of *first-degree, second-degree type I and II, and third-degree heart blocks*
5. The coronary artery and cardiac conduction system pathology most likely to cause the 4 types of heart block listed in item 4
6. The significance of bradycardia in a person having an AMI and the particular significance of a right ventricular (RV) infarction combined with bradycardia
7. The pharmacology of *atropine* and how and why atropine is effective in some heart blocks and not others
8. How to prepare the patient, set up the equipment, and start and troubleshoot *TCP*
9. What actions to take when bradycardia of 45 bpm changes to *broad QRS-complex bradycardia* (either rate-related **ventricular escape beats** *or rate-related ischemia with ventricular irritability*)
10. Whether to advise the use of ***lidocaine*** in the situation described in item 9: treatment of ventricular complexes occurring in a slow heart rate

Major Learning Points: Overview of the Bradycardias

Symptomatic bradycardia exists clinically when 3 criteria are present:

1. The heart rate is slow.
2. The patient has symptoms.
3. The symptoms are due to the bradycardia.

You must perform a focused history and physical examination to identify symptomatic bradycardia.

> **The key clinical question is whether the bradycardia is making the patient ill or some other illness is "making" the bradycardia.**

Key Learning Points

1. **Treatment of bradycardias**

   The treatment of bradycardias, like the treatment of tachycardias, challenges the clinician to remember the admonition ***"treat the patient, not the monitor."*** Both autonomic influences and the intrinsic pathology of the conducting system can lead to bradycardia. In particular, AMI can lead to ischemic damage to the conducting system of the heart, producing bradycardias that range from sinus bradycardia to complete third-degree heart block.

   The initial steps of treatment for bradycardia can be organized into the following "quadrads" for easy recall:

   - Secondary ABCD Survey
   - Oxygen–IV–monitor–fluids
   - Vital signs: Temperature, blood pressure, heart rate, respirations

   These quadrads are used to assess and treat symptomatic bradycardia. This approach helps ensure that the *patient*—not the patient's ECG—is treated. The initial steps should always include the third (oxygen–IV–monitor–fluids) and fourth quadrads (vital signs).

2. **Bradycardia caused by AMI**

   If AMI is the cause of bradycardia and the bradycardia is *symptomatic*, you must treat either the AMI or the bradycardia. A cardinal rule in ECC is that you should *treat the original pathology* (the AMI) *rather than the sequelae of the pathology.* This generally means that "MONA" (morphine-oxygen-nitroglycerin-aspirin) is given for the AMI before atropine is given for the bradycardia.

3. **Clinical effects of bradycardia**

   The clinical effects of *significant* or *symptomatic bradycardia* include the following:

   Symptoms: chest pain, shortness of breath, and decreased level of consciousness, weakness, fatigue, exercise intolerance, lightheadedness, dizziness, and "spells"

   Signs: hypotension, drop in blood pressure upon standing, diaphoresis, pulmonary congestion on physical examination or chest x-ray, frank congestive heart failure or pulmonary edema, chest pain, acute coronary syndrome (unstable angina, angina, or other symptoms of AMI), and premature ventricular complexes (PVCs)

4. **The treatment sequence for symptomatic bradycardia is**

   - ***Atropine***
   - ***TCP***
   - ***Dopamine***

Bradycardia Algorithm.

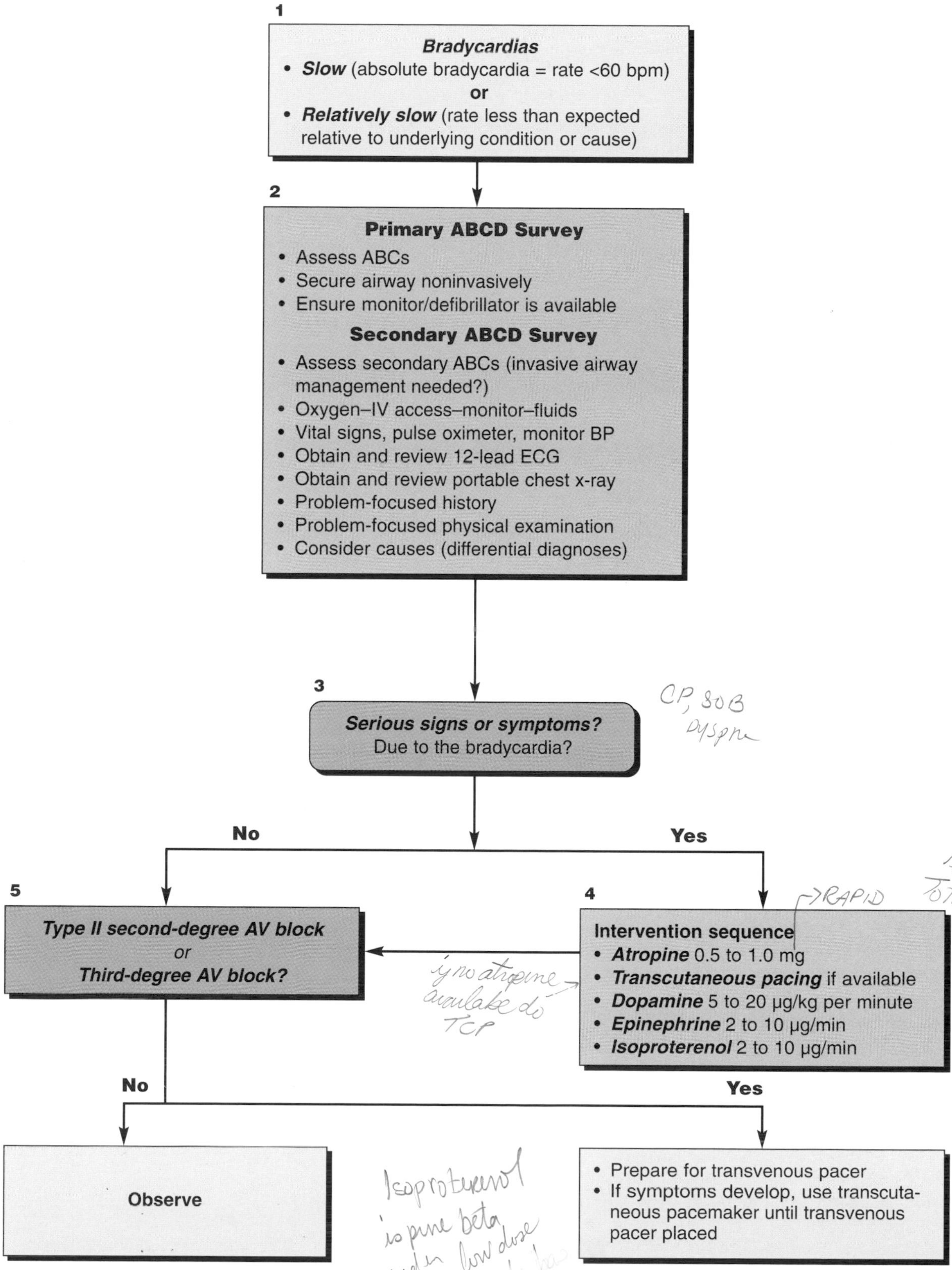
1
Bradycardias
• Slow (absolute bradycardia = rate <60 bpm)
or
• Relatively slow (rate less than expected relative to underlying condition or cause)
2
Primary ABCD Survey
• Assess ABCs
• Secure airway noninvasively
• Ensure monitor/defibrillator is available
Secondary ABCD Survey
• Assess secondary ABCs (invasive airway management needed?)
• Oxygen–IV access–monitor–fluids
• Vital signs, pulse oximeter, monitor BP
• Obtain and review 12-lead ECG
• Obtain and review portable chest x-ray
• Problem-focused history
• Problem-focused physical examination
• Consider causes (differential diagnoses)
3
Serious signs or symptoms?
Due to the bradycardia?
No
Yes
4
Intervention sequence
• Atropine 0.5 to 1.0 mg
• Transcutaneous pacing if available
• Dopamine 5 to 20 µg/kg per minute
• Epinephrine 2 to 10 µg/min
• Isoproterenol 2 to 10 µg/min
5
Type II second-degree AV block
or
Third-degree AV block?
No
Yes
Observe
• Prepare for transvenous pacer
• If symptoms develop, use transcutaneous pacemaker until transvenous pacer placed

- *Epinephrine (see the Bradycardia Algorithm)*
- *Isoproterenol*

The more severe the clinical situation, the more quickly you must carry out this sequence. In more compromised patients you may sometimes run through this sequence without waiting to see whether an earlier treatment has had an effect. If the victim does not appear to respond to the first 4 treatments, you may give isoproterenol, but with extreme caution.

5. Rate-related (escape) PVCs associated with third-degree heart block

If bradycardia drops below the intrinsic rate of the ventricles (30 to 40 bpm), *escape PVCs* (rate-related) may occur. Carefully determine whether these PVCs are effective, ie, does each PVC produce a ventricular contraction that produces a pulse? Consider the following:

- Should you try to eliminate the PVCs by speeding up the rate with atropine? (The likelihood of response is small.)
- Should you instead try TCP or both atropine and TCP?
- *Forbidden:* Do *not* try to treat (eliminate) such PVCs with lidocaine.

6. Profoundly symptomatic bradycardia?

There are interesting *overlaps* among several cardiac syndromes:

- ***Profoundly symptomatic bradycardia:*** what could be more symptomatic than cardiac arrest from a slow heart rate?
- ***Asystole:*** what could be more bradycardic than no beats at all?
- ***Pulseless electrical activity (PEA):*** slow PEA is certainly "symptomatic bradycardia"
- ***Severe hypotension:*** what could be more hypotensive than no blood pressure at all (cardiac arrest)?

Decisions about which algorithm to apply become complicated because of these overlaps. Questions about which treatments to use, however, are simple to answer because the top agents recommended for each of these conditions are the same: ***atropine*** and ***epinephrine.***

New Skills to Master: Transcutaneous Pacing

TCP is appropriate for most cases of symptomatic bradycardia. Operation of a transcutaneous pacemaker is a core skill required of all ACLS providers. Details about indications, technique, and hazards of TCP are presented in an appendix at the end of this case.

New Rhythms to Learn

Heart Blocks

ACLS providers should be able to recognize the major heart blocks:

- First-degree
- Second-degree type I
- Second-degree type II
- Third-degree

Major treatment decisions are based on the type of block present. See the ACLS textbook.

New Drugs to Learn

ACLS providers should know the *what?, how?, when?, why?,* and *watch out!* for the following drugs and therapies:

- Atropine
- Dopamine
- Epinephrine
- TCP
- Isoproterenol for those patients with bradycardias that meet the indications for isoproterenol

See the *2000 Handbook of Emergency Cardiovascular Care for Healthcare Providers,* "Advanced Cardiovascular Life Support Drugs and Electrical Therapy."

A Walk Through the Bradycardia Algorithm

Box 1: Bradycardias

Bradycardias

- ***Slow*** (absolute bradycardia = rate <60 bpm)

or

- ***Relatively slow*** (rate less than expected relative to underlying condition or cause)

Box 2: ABCD Surveys

Primary ABCD Survey

- Assess ABCs
- Secure airway noninvasively
- Ensure monitor/defibrillator is available

Secondary ABCD Survey

- Assess secondary ABCs (invasive airway management needed?)
- Oxygen–IV access–monitor–fluids
- Vital signs, pulse oximeter, monitor BP
- Obtain and review 12-lead ECG
- Obtain and review portable chest x-ray
- Problem-focused history
- Problem-focused physical examination
- Consider causes (differential diagnoses)

Comments for Boxes 1 and 2

Although cardiology usually defines bradycardia as a heart rate less than 60 bpm, the hearts of many people, particularly trained athletes, may normally beat at much slower rates and produce effective systemic perfusion. Clinicians must be aware of the concepts of *absolute bradycardia* (heart rate less than 60 bpm) and *relative bradycardia.* A person with a heart rate of 65 bpm and a systolic blood pressure measurement of 80 mm Hg may be experiencing a "relative" bradycardia: the pulse rate relative to the blood pressure is too low.

Box 3

Serious signs or symptoms?
Due to the bradycardia?

Comments for Box 3

The key clinical questions are

- *Does the slow rate make the patient ill?*
- *Are there "serious" signs or symptoms?*
- *Are the signs and symptoms related to the slow heart rate?*

Look for adverse results of the bradycardia:

- *Symptoms* (chest pain, shortness of breath, decreased level of consciousness)
- *Signs* (hypotension, congestive heart failure, PVCs in the setting of AMI)

Sometimes the *"symptom"* the clinician treats when reacting to *symptomatic bradycardia* is not due to the bradycardia. For example, hypotension associated with bradycardia may be due to myocardial dysfunction or hypovolemia rather than to autonomic problems or problems of the conduction system.

The Intervention Sequence for Symptomatic Bradycardia

Box 4

Intervention sequence
- ***Atropine*** 0.5 to 1.0 mg ***(Note 1)***
- ***Transcutaneous pacing*** if available ***(Note 2)***
- ***Dopamine*** 5 to 20 μg/kg per minute
- ***Epinephrine*** 2 to 10 μg/min
- ***Isoproterenol*** 2 to 10 μg/min

Note 1: Denervated transplanted hearts will not respond to ***atropine.*** Go at once to pacing, ***catecholamine*** infusion, or both.

Overview

The treatment sequence in the Bradycardia algorithm is listed in order of increasing clinical severity, from therapies for the least severe bradycardias to therapies for the most severe bradycardias. You should not, however, move slowly through this intervention sequence with symptomatic bradycardic patients. Patients may be "pre–cardiac arrest" and may merit multiple interventions simultaneously, such as attaching a transcutaneous pacemaker, alerting a cardiologist of the possible need for a transvenous pacemaker, giving IV atropine, and starting an infusion of dopamine, epinephrine, or isoproterenol. All recommendations must be followed intelligently—by thinking clinicians—with regard to individual patients.

1. Atropine

Think carefully before starting treatment for symptomatic bradycardias. Atropine is the agent of choice for an initial intervention.

- Atropine works by blocking the effects of vagal nerve discharges. Areas of the heart not served by the vagus nerve will not respond to atropine. Therefore, atropine is ***not*** indicated for third-degree heart block and wide-complex ventricular escape beats or for Mobitz type II second-degree heart block. Atropine may accelerate the atrial rate and produce increased AV nodal block.
- Atropine should be used with caution, particularly if you suspect that the patient has AMI. Atropine may exacerbate ischemia or induce VT or VF or both when used to treat bradycardia associated with AMI. The acceleration in heart rate caused by atropine may induce rate-related ischemia in a person with AMI or ischemia.
- Atropine is ineffective in many patients with a higher-level block or serious conduction system failure.
- Dose:
  - — For mildly symptomatic bradycardia, give *atropine 0.5 to 1 mg IV, repeated every 3 to 5 minutes, to a total of 0.03 mg/kg.* This results in a 2-mg total dose for a person weighing 70 kg. Use shorter dosing intervals (3 minutes) and higher doses (1 mg) in more urgent clinical conditions.
  - — For more urgent clinical conditions such as asystole and PEA arrest, give atropine 1 mg IV every 3 to 5 minutes. This yields the maximum vagolytic dose of 0.04 mg/kg. Select the shorter interval of 3 minutes for patients in greater distress.

2. Transcutaneous Pacing

Note 2: If patient is symptomatic, do not delay TCP while awaiting IV access or atropine to take effect. Go quickly to TCP.

- Details of how to provide TCP are presented in the appendix to this case.
- TCP is a Class I intervention for all symptomatic bradycardias. If you are concerned about the use of atropine in higher-level blocks, remember that TCP is always appropriate, though not as readily available as atropine.
- If the bradycardia is very slow with urgent symptoms and the patient's clinical condition is unstable, perform TCP immediately.
- Start TCP for patients who do not respond to atropine or who are severely symptomatic, especially when the block is at or below the His-Purkinje level.
- TCP technology has advanced rapidly over the past decade. Now many defibrillator/monitors contain a TCP module and are capable of performing pacing. Unlike transvenous pacing, TCP is available to and can be performed by nearly all ECC providers. Skill in operation of transcutaneous pacemakers is required for ACLS competency.
- ***Comparison of TCP with transvenous pacing:***
  - — TCP can be started quickly and conveniently at the bedside
  - — TCP requires no special equipment such as fluoroscopy
  - — Common clinical impression: TCP fails more often to produce mechanical contractions

— Many patients cannot tolerate the TCP stimulus to the skin. In these patients IV analgesics or sedatives (short-acting benzodiazepines) or both may afford relief and allow the patient to tolerate the stimulus.

3. Catecholamine Infusions: Dopamine, Epinephrine, Isoproterenol

Dopamine

- After the maximum dose of **atropine** is reached (0.04 mg/kg), add a **dopamine infusion** (start at 5 μg/kg per minute) and increase the infusion dose quickly (up to 20 μg/kg per minute) if low blood pressure is associated with the bradycardia.
- It is now widely recognized that the concept of "renal doses" of dopamine (1 to 5 μg/kg per minute) is invalid. It was previously thought that at low doses dopamine has a dopaminergic effect that causes renal, mesenteric, and cerebrovascular dilation, which was thought to produce an increase in renal output. Low-dose dopamine was therefore considered a specific treatment for oliguric renal failure. Once it was learned that these effects did not really occur, the starting dose of dopamine was increased to 5 μg/kg per minute.
- ***Moderate-dose dopamine: 5 to 10 μg/kg per minute ("cardiac doses").*** At moderate doses dopamine has a β_1- and an α-adrenergic effect, causing enhanced myocardial contractility, increased cardiac output, increased heart rate, and increased blood pressure. Note that the Bradycardia Algorithm recommends starting dopamine at 5 μg/kg per minute for *symptomatic* bradycardias. If the dopamine is to effectively increase heart rate for the patient with bradycardia, it should do so in the range of 5 to 10 μg/kg per minute.
- ***High-dose dopamine: 10 to 20 μg/kg per minute ("vasopressor doses").*** At high doses dopamine has a predominantly α-adrenergic effect, producing peripheral arterial and venous constriction. These doses are used to treat low blood pressure with signs and symptoms of shock.

Epinephrine

- If the patient has severe bradycardia with hypotension, the drug of choice is epinephrine. For hypotensive bradycardic patients, start an epinephrine infusion.
- Epinephrine infusion is also indicated when higher doses of dopamine appear ineffective.
- Symptomatic bradycardic patients are often close to PEA or even asystole, and epinephrine is the agent of choice for these 2 arrhythmias. Epinephrine is the catecholamine common to the PEA and Asystole algorithms.
- Epinephrine infusions are prepared in the same manner as isoproterenol infusions: mix a 1-mg ampule of either agent in 500 mL normal saline to produce a concentration of 2 μg/mL. This can then be infused at 1 to 5 mL/min.

Isoproterenol Hydrochloride

- Since 1986 experts have considered isoproterenol to be contraindicated for patients in cardiac arrest and useful only for severe bradycardia. Isoproterenol can also stimulate the denervated heart of cardiac transplant patients.
- For patients with severe symptomatic bradycardia, isoproterenol is generally acceptable only as a temporizing measure until TCP or transvenous pacing becomes available. Negative effects of isoproterenol include an increase in myocardial oxygen consumption and peripheral vasodilatation.
- Isoproterenol provides chronotropic support, thus increasing heart rate.
- As a vasodilator, isoproterenol is relatively contraindicated in patients who are hypotensive, which is usually the case in patients with severe, symptomatic bradycardia.
- Although isoproterenol has been used to speed up the heart rate of asymptomatic patients, isoproterenol is indicated only for *symptomatic* patients, and its use otherwise is inappropriate.
- The use of isoproterenol requires an understanding of the risk-benefit balance: *patients who are ill enough to need isoproterenol are probably too ill to tolerate it.* Some experts, however, argue that at *low* doses isoproterenol causes little vasodilatation but can still speed up the heart rate, which increases blood pressure.
- Use isoproterenol, if at all, with extreme caution. At low doses it is a *Class IIb (possibly helpful)* intervention; at all other doses it is a *Class III (harmful)* intervention.

Box 5

Type II second-degree AV block
or
Third-degree AV block? (Note 3)

Note 3: Never treat the combination of *third-degree heart block* and *ventricular escape beats* with **lidocaine** (or any agent that suppresses ventricular escape rhythms).

Acute Type II Second-Degree AV Block and New Third-Degree AV Heart Block

These arrhythmias are serious even when a patient is asymptomatic.

- These heart blocks are most often caused by occlusion of the septal branch of the left anterior descending artery.
- Like other infranodal blocks, type II second-degree blocks can convert to complete third-degree AV block without warning.
- If bradycardia develops acutely in association with either anterior or anterior-septal infarction, prepare urgently for insertion of a transvenous pacer.
- Arrange for insertion of a transvenous pacemaker as soon as type II second-degree heart block and third-degree AV heart block are identified.
- TCP can be used as a bridge intervention for third-degree AV heart block until a transvenous pacer becomes available. Place the adhesive pads of the TCP even if the patient is asymptomatic.

Critical Actions: Assessment and Management

This critical actions checklist reviews the assessment and treatment of a patient with symptomatic bradycardia. You are not required or expected to memorize the checklist, but you should review it until you understand the order and rationale for all steps. This critical actions checklist is limited to those actions specific to symptomatic bradycardia. To avoid unnecessary repetition, this checklist *does not* repeat all the assessment and management steps of the Primary and Secondary ABCD Surveys. Please understand that *the steps of the Primary and Secondary ABCD Surveys are always performed on all patients.*

Unacceptable Actions: Perils and Pitfalls

- Not preparing for TCP (attach anterior-posterior pacing electrodes) or transvenous pacing (alerting invasive cardiology team, etc) while trying atropine initially
- Not recognizing the clinical importance of distinguishing type II second-degree AV block from type I second-degree AV block (need for more permanent pacing)
- Not limiting isoproterenol to the fourth drug of choice for symptomatic bradycardia; not recognizing the dangers of isoproterenol
- Inappropriately giving lidocaine for lifesaving escape rhythms
- Attempting to increase the heart rate in asymptomatic bradycardic patients
- Inappropriately treating an asymptomatic patient with bradycardia

Read More About It

For more information about the new topics covered in Case 7, see the *ECC Guidelines 2000.*

Also see the following sections of the *ACLS Reference Textbook:*

Chapter 14: Bradycardias: Atrioventricular Blocks and Emergency Pacing

Importance of Heart Block and Infarct Location

RV Infarction

Patients with inferior or RV infarction often present with excessive parasympathetic tone. The parasympathetic effects will cause bradycardia, but hypotension, if present, is probably due to hypovolemia rather than bradycardia.

- ***Give a careful fluid challenge with normal saline (250 to 500 mL over 15 to 30 minutes). For these patients this action may be lifesaving.***

The slow rate is in effect a relative bradycardia—the heart should be beating faster given the low blood pressure. The fluid bolus increases RV filling pressures, which causes an increase in the strength of the RV contractions *(Starling mechanism).*

Acute inferior MIs (right coronary artery events) often produce second- or third-degree heart block with a junctional, narrow-complex escape rhythm. If the patient remains hemodynamically stable, you may not need a transvenous pacemaker.

- Use ***atropine*** to increase the heart rate and blood pressure if these patients become symptomatic.
- If there is no response to atropine, give ***dopamine*** or ***epinephrine.*** The conduction defect is often transient. Standby TCP should be used (and tested) for these patients while awaiting transvenous pacing or resolution of the block.

Third-Degree Heart Block With Anterior AMI

- *Begin preparations to insert a* ***transvenous pacemaker*** (call cardiology and the fluoroscopy suite, alert the CCU).
- *Avoid causing increased ischemia through unnecessary use of* ***atropine.***
- *Use* ***TCP (or catecholamines)*** *if severe symptoms develop; continue pacemaker preparations.*

Third-Degree Heart Block With Inferior AMI

- *Use standby* ***TCP*** *(verify patient tolerance and mechanical capture).*
- *Use* ***atropine*** *if symptoms require it.*

Critical Actions Checklist: ACLS Case 7
Bradycardia

Scene Survey Steps	Assess: Do or Monitor	Manage: Do or Delegate
Recognize emergency and respond	☐ Assess the **Primary and Secondary ABCDs** ***Bradycardia observed:*** ☐ Assess vital signs ☐ Take focused history ☐ Conduct focused physical examination	☐ Secure the airway ☐ Initiate oxygen–IV–monitor–fluids: ☐ Administer oxygen ☐ Start IV; hang NS ☐ Attach monitor, pulse oximeter, and automatic blood pressure cuff ☐ Order a 12-lead ECG ☐ Order a portable chest x-ray
Bradycardia	☐ Assess heart rate and clinical signs and symptoms ☐ Specifically consider signs and symptoms of AMI	☐ Determine if symptoms are severe enough to merit treatment
Symptomatic bradycardia	☐ Assess ECG to identify specific type of bradycardia: — Sinus bradycardia — First-degree heart block — Second-degree heart block, type I or type II — Third-degree heart block ***Bradycardia causing serious signs and symptoms:*** ☐ Identify type of block — Sinus bradycardia — First-degree heart block — Type I second-degree AV block — Type II second-degree AV block — Third-degree heart block	***If second-degree type II block or third-degree block:*** ☐ Avoid atropine ☐ Attach transcutaneous pacer ☐ Conduct trial of TCP to see if pacing captures and how patient tolerates stimulus ☐ Prepare for transvenous pacing ☐ If no block, continue to monitor patient (ABCDs) ☐ ***Start intervention sequence:*** — Atropine: acceptable, all types of heart block except second degree type II or third degree — TCP: recommended for all types of heart block — Dopamine: contraindicated in hypovolemia — Epinephrine: profoundly symptomatic bradycardia refractory to earlier interventions — (Isoproterenol: only when earlier interventions fail)

Read More About It

(Continued from page 151)

Chapter 13: The Basics of Rhythm Interpretation
Chapter 11: Pharmacology 1: Drugs for Cardiac Output and Peripheral Vascular Resistance
Chapter 12: Pharmacology 2: Agents to Control Rate and Rhythm

Appendix: How to Safely and Effectively Use Transcutaneous Pacing

A variety of devices can pace the heart by delivering an electrical stimulus through electrodes. This causes electrical depolarization and subsequent cardiac contraction. A TCP system delivers pacing impulses to the heart through the skin by cutaneous electrodes. Most defibrillator manufacturers have added a pacing mode to their conventional defibrillators. Because the ability to perform TCP is now as close as the nearest defibrillator, ACLS providers need to know the indications for TCP, the techniques, and the hazards.

Recommendations for the Use of Transcutaneous Pacing

Class I

Hemodynamically significant (symptomatic, compromising) bradycardias (too slow), unresponsive to atropine (Class I)

These specific types of bradycardia are the most frequent indication for TCP (see Table: Indications for Emergency Pacing and Pacing Readiness). The precise heart rate is less important than the clinical signs and symptoms produced by the bradycardia. Signs of hemodynamic significance (too slow) include hypotension (systolic blood pressure <80 mm Hg), change in mental status, angina, and pulmonary edema. Use atropine or catecholamines first, before pacing. These agents may increase the heart rate, improve hemodynamics, and eliminate the need for pacing. Start pacing at once if drug therapy is not immediately available. If both pharmacologic therapy and pacing are available, start them simultaneously.

Class IIa

Bradycardia with escape rhythms (Class IIa)

The bradycardia is so slow that it leads to pause-dependent or bradycardia-dependent ventricular rhythms. These ventricular rhythms often fail to respond to pharmacologic therapy. With severe bradycardia some patients will develop wide-complex ventricular beats that precipitate VT or VF. Pacing may increase the intrinsic heart rhythm and eliminate pause- or bradycardia-dependent ventricular rhythms.

Pacing for patients in cardiac arrest with profound bradycardia or PEA due to drug overdose, acidosis, or electrolyte abnormalities (Class IIa)

These patients may have a normal myocardium with a disturbed conduction system. After correction of electrolyte abnormalities or acidosis, rapid pacing can stimulate effective myocardial contractions until the conduction system can recover.

Standby pacing (pacing readiness) (Class IIa)

Several bradycardic rhythms in AMI are due to acute ischemia of conduction tissue and pacing centers. Persons who are clinically stable may decompensate or become unstable over minutes to hours from worsening heart block. These bradycardias may deteriorate to complete heart block and cardiovascular collapse. Therefore, TCP electrodes should be placed in anticipation of clinical deterioration for these rhythms:

- Symptomatic sinus node dysfunction
- Mobitz type II second-degree heart block
- Third-degree heart block
- Newly acquired left, right, or alternating bundle branch block (BBB) or bifascicular block

Workbook Review

1. Which of the following bradycardias is most likely to be associated with clinical symptoms?

a. a heart rate of 53 bpm in an athlete

b. a heart rate of 53 bpm in a patient with cardiovascular disease, presenting with shortness of breath and decreased level of consciousness

c. a heart rate of 53 bpm in a patient who has just vomited after insertion of a nasogastric tube

d. a heart rate of 53 bpm in a patient with first-degree heart block receiving digoxin

Read more about it in the ECC Guidelines 2000, *pages 155-157: Figure 6: Bradycardia Algorithm and Notes*

2. Which of the following would be an appropriate indication for transcutaneous pacing?

a. asymptomatic sinus bradycardia

b. normal sinus rhythm with hypotension and shock

c. complete heart block with pulmonary edema

d. prolonged asystole

Read more about it in the ECC Guidelines 2000, *page 155: paragraph beginning "Transcutaneous pacing ..."*

3. You are evaluating a patient with a heart rate of 45 bpm; a complaint of dizziness; cool, clammy extremities; and prolonged capillary refill. What is the *first* drug of choice you would administer to this patient?

a. atropine 0.5 to 1 mg

b. epinephrine 1 mg IV push

c. isoproterenol infusion 1 to 10 μg/kg per minute

d. adenosine 6 mg rapid IV push

Read more about it in the ECC Guidelines 2000, *pages 155-156: Figure 6: Bradycardia Algorithm and notes*

4. Which of the following signs and symptoms are most likely to result from symptomatic bradycardia?

a. headache, pain or pressure in the center of the chest, palpitations

b. nausea, diaphoresis, pain radiating to the back and between the shoulder blades

c. chest pain, shortness of breath, hypotension, dizziness or altered level of consciousness, congestive heart failure, premature ventricular contractions

d. difficulty with speech, unilateral limb weakness, severe headache, facial droop

Read more about it in the ECC Guidelines 2000, *pages 155-156: Figure 6: Bradycardia Algorithm and notes; and Part 3: "Adult Basic Life Support"*

5. You are treating a patient with a slow heartbeat. For which of the following patients would *atropine* be effective?

a. a 55-year-old man with severe, crushing chest pain and sinus bradycardia at 35 bpm

b. a 55-year-old man with weakness and fatigue on walking short distances and a third-degree AV block at 35 bpm

c. a 55-year-old man with weakness and fatigue on walking short distances and with a history of a heart transplant 6 months ago.

d. a 55-year-old man with weakness and fatigue following acute symptoms of nausea and vomiting and with a slow sinus rhythm at 35 bpm.

Read more about it in the ECC Guidelines 2000, *page 121: "Atropine"; and pages 155-157: Figure 6: Bradycardia Algorithm and notes*

Class IIb

Overdrive pacing of refractory tachycardias (Class IIb)

This technique can terminate malignant supraventricular and ventricular tachycardias. Overdrive pacing is indicated only after pharmacologic treatment or electrical cardioversion has failed. Perform overdrive pacing by pacing the heart for a few seconds at a rate faster than the tachycardia rate. Stop the pacemaker and allow the intrinsic rhythm of the heart to return. Overdrive pacing is limited by the maximum pacing rate of the device, which is usually 170 to 180 bpm.

Bradyasystolic cardiac arrest (Class IIb)

Pacing is not routinely used in these patients. Although it has been studied extensively, only a few studies have shown encouraging results and then only when pacing was initiated within 10 minutes of cardiac arrest. Prehospital studies of TCP for asystolic arrest have shown no benefit from pacing.

TABLE. Indications for Emergency Pacing and Pacing Readiness

Class I

Hemodynamically symptomatic, compromising bradycardias that are too slow and unresponsive to atropine.* Symptoms can include systolic blood pressure less than 80 mm Hg, change in mental status, angina, pulmonary edema.

Class IIa

- Bradycardia with escape rhythms unresponsive to pharmacologic therapy
- Pacing for patients in cardiac arrest with profound bradycardia or PEA due to drug overdose, acidosis, or electrolyte abnormalities
- Standby pacing: prepare for pacing for specific AMI-associated rhythms:
  — Symptomatic sinus node dysfunction
  — Mobitz type II second-degree heart block
  — Third-degree heart block†
  — New left, right, or alternating BBB or bifascicular block

Class IIb

- Overdrive pacing of either supraventricular or ventricular tachycardia refractory to pharmacologic therapy or electrical cardioversion
- Bradyasystolic cardiac arrest

*Includes complete heart block, symptomatic second-degree heart block, symptomatic sick sinus syndrome, drug-induced bradycardias (ie, digoxin, β-blockers, calcium channel blockers, procainamide), permanent pacemaker failure, idioventricular bradycardias, symptomatic atrial fibrillation with slow ventricular response, refractory bradycardia during resuscitation of hypovolemic shock, and bradyarrhythmias with malignant ventricular escape mechanisms.

Class III (relative and absolute contraindications)

Severe hypothermia (Class III)

Bradycardia may be physiological in these patients, caused by the decreased metabolic rate associated with hypothermia. Cold ventricles are more prone to fibrillation and more resistant to defibrillation.

Bradyasystolic cardiac arrest of more than 20 minutes' duration

Pacing is relatively contraindicated in patients with this condition because of the well-documented poor resuscitation rate for these patients and the high probability that those who do survive will have profound brain damage.

Bradycardia in children

Most bradycardia in children results from hypoxia or hypoventilation and will respond to adequate airway intervention with or without drug therapy. Thus, pacing is rarely required in pediatric arrests. Consider pacing for children with bradycardia secondary to drug toxicity or electrolyte abnormalities. Also consider pacing for children with primary bradycardia from congenital defects or bradycardia after open-heart surgery.

Details on Standby or Prophylactic Pacing

Many responsive patients with stable bradycardias may not need TCP if the bradycardia and cardiovascular system remain stable. Clinicians, however, cannot accurately predict which patients will improve steadily versus those who will deteriorate clinically. The practice of standby or prophylactic pacing has therefore developed: attach pacing electrodes to at-risk patients and leave the pacemaker in the standby mode to respond at once to hemodynamic deterioration if it occurs.

Continue efforts to treat the patient's underlying disorder. Use this approach in patients with new type II second-degree and third-degree heart block, especially in the setting of cardiac ischemia and infarction. Try a preliminary trial of pacing with the transcutaneous device to ensure that the pacer can achieve capture and can be tolerated by the patient. If the patient cannot tolerate the pain from the pacing, give diazepam (for treatment of anxiety and muscle contractions) or morphine (for analgesia), or both.

Equipment for TCP

A single pair of anterior-posterior or sternal-apex electrodes allows hands-off defibrillation, pacing, and ECG monitoring. Pediatric electrodes are also available and are useful in pediatric patients with bradycardia of nonrespiratory origin.

Most transcutaneous pacemakers allow operation in either a fixed-rate (nondemand or asynchronous mode) or a demand mode. Most allow rate selection in a range from

30 to 180 bpm. Current output is usually adjustable from 0 to 200 mA. Pulse durations on available units vary from 20 to 40 milliseconds.

An ECG monitor should be an integral part of the unit, configured to blank out the large electrical spike from the pacemaker impulse. This allows interpretation of the much smaller ECG complex. Without blanking, the standard monitor is overwhelmed by the pacemaker spike, and the rhythm appears uninterpretable. This could be disastrous because large pacing artifacts can mask treatable VF.

Technique of TCP

1. Place the anterior electrode to the left of the sternum, centered as close as possible to the point of maximum cardiac impulse.

2. Place the posterior electrode on the back, directly behind the anterior electrode and to the left of the thoracic spinal column.

3. Shave the hair to ensure good skin contact or use alternative pacing electrode positions in patients with excessive body hair. Clip rather than shave excessive hair to avoid tiny nicks in the skin that can increase pain and skin irritation in conscious patients.

4. Activate the device (usually at a rate of 80 bpm).

   — With bradyasystolic arrest, turn the stimulating current to maximum output, then decrease output if capture is achieved.

   — In patients with a hemodynamically compromising bradycardia (but not in cardiac arrest), slowly increase output from the minimum setting until capture is achieved.

   Electrical capture is usually characterized by a widening of the QRS complex (looks like a PVC) by a broad T wave, with the T wave opposite the polarity of the QRS complex. Sometimes only a change in the intrinsic morphology indicates pacing.

5. Assess the hemodynamic response to pacing by pulse, blood pressure cuff, or arterial catheter.

   — Take pulse at the right carotid or right femoral artery to avoid confusion between the jerking muscle contractions caused by the pacer and a pulse.

   — Continue pacing at an output level slightly (10%) higher than the threshold of initial electrical capture.

6. Give analgesia with incremental doses of a narcotic, sedation with a benzodiazepine, or both, to make the pain of chest wall muscle contractions tolerable until transvenous pacing can be instituted.

7. For standby pacing, document that capture is possible by test pacing at a rate slightly faster than the patient's intrinsic rate, then return the device to the standby mode.

Hazards of TCP

The 2 major hazards of transcutaneous pacing are

- Failure to recognize the presence of underlying treatable VF
- Failure to recognize that the pacemaker is not capturing

These complications are due to the large pacing artifact on the monitor. Clinicians formerly feared that TCP might induce arrhythmias or VF. Few if any such cases have been reported. The current required to induce fibrillation through cutaneous electrodes is probably greater than the output of external pacers.

One third of patients rate the pacing stimulus pain as severe or intolerable. Tissue damage can occur with prolonged TCP, but following the manufacturer's recommendations can markedly reduce these problems. Third-degree burns have been reported in pediatric patients with improper or prolonged pacing. With prolonged use, pacing thresholds can change, leading to capture failure. Frequent skin inspection and repositioning of the electrodes can remedy this problem.

Unstable Tachycardia

Description

Case 8 focuses on initial assessment and management of the patient with a rapid, ***unstable*** heart rate. For satisfactory completion of this case, it is critical for ACLS providers to understand the meaning of the term *unstable:*

- The patient displays serious *symptoms* (shortness of breath, chest pain, dyspnea on exertion, altered mental status) *or*
- *Signs* (pulmonary edema, rales, rhonchi, hypotension, orthostasis, jugular vein distention, peripheral edema, ischemic ECG changes), *plus*
- The tachycardia is the immediate cause of the signs and symptoms
- The tachycardia requires immediate treatment with synchronized cardioversion to prevent further hemodynamic deterioration

Settings and Scenarios

Setting: Prehospital

EMTs are dispatched to a 911 call concerning a 52-year-old man who is complaining of shortness of breath, palpitations, and severe chest pain. He is pale and sweaty. *(The rhythm is paroxysmal supraventricular tachycardia.)*

What's New in the Guidelines...

Unstable Tachycardia

The recommendations for treatment of *unstable* tachycardia in the *ECC Guidelines 2000* remain the same as those in the previous guidelines. ACLS providers should be aware of new concepts that will affect the management of both *stable* and *unstable* tachyarrhythmias:

- Significant new developments in the management of *stable* tachycardias will result in a much greater use of electrical cardioversion to treat *stable* tachycardias than previously existed.
- The major new development in the treatment of arrhythmias is the recognition that *antiarrhythmics can actually act as proarrhythmics* much more often than previously suspected. Consequently, after administration of 1 and occasionally 2 antiarrhythmic agents, clinicians should turn to cardioversion as the next treatment modality.
- Patients with compromised cardiac function or an impaired myocardium should seldom—if ever—receive multiple different antiarrhythmics. This recommendation represents a revision of past guidelines. The net effect is that after use of 1 or perhaps 2 agents to control a stable tachycardia in a patient with impaired cardiovascular function, the ACLS provider should select cardioversion as the next treatment.
- Biphasic waveforms are used in many defibrillators available today and will likely be used in most future defibrillators. Most conventional, stand-alone defibrillators will soon incorporate an option for biphasic waveform cardioversion as well as biphasic waveform defibrillation. We all rely on defibrillator manufacturers to provide clinical evidence of safety and effectiveness of their particular biphasic waveform for defibrillation or cardioversion.

  Manufacturers can obtain market approval for new devices by simply supplying clinical data to the Food and Drug Administration. This approval process does not require publication of articles in peer-reviewed scientific journals. At present the AHA can make no recommendations, pro or con, on biphasic cardioversion other than a strong admonition to examine peer-reviewed evidence as it becomes available.

Setting: Emergency Department

A 45-year-old woman presents to the Emergency Department complaining of palpitations, difficulty breathing, and severe pressure in her chest. She complains of extreme weakness and says she feels like she is going to faint. *(The rhythm is VT.)*

Setting: In-Hospital, Unmonitored Patient

A 58-year-old man returns to the surgical floor after an operation for a bowel obstruction. He is known to have angina and takes β-blockers daily. He complains of severe chest pain, shortness of breath, and a feeling of apprehension. *(The rhythm is VT.)*

Setting: Critical Care Unit, Monitored Patient

A 60-year-old man is admitted to the critical care unit for unstable angina. The monitor alarm is activated. The patient states that he is having palpitations, chest pain, and shortness of breath. He says that he feels very light-headed. *(The rhythm is torsades de pointes.)*

Stable Versus Unstable Congestive Heart Failure

Note that it is possible for people to experience a rapid heart rate and impaired cardiac function, such as reduced ejection fraction or signs of congestive heart failure, and yet remain clinically stable. These patients are discussed in Case 9: Stable Tachycardia. Usually these patients are chronically ill with heart disease and have stabilized at a reduced level of function. Immediate cardioversion is not warranted in these cases. ACLS providers should be able to distinguish between acute congestive heart failure due to sudden, sustained tachycardia and "chronic" or "stable" congestive heart failure associated with a chronic tachycardia.

Learning and Skills Objectives

New Skills to Learn

At the end of Case 8 you should be able to describe or demonstrate the following:

1. Initial assessment and management of a patient with unstable tachycardia using the Primary and Secondary ABCD Surveys
2. Rapid application of the tachycardia algorithms and tables
3. Identification of tachycardic patients who are "unstable" from tachycardia
4. Identification of the specific tachycardia, with particular attention to the following tachycardias, which are also emphasized in Case 9: Stable Tachycardia:
   - Atrial fibrillation/flutter
   - Narrow-complex tachycardias, including
     - — Junctional tachycardia
     - — PSVT
     - — Multifocal or ectopic atrial tachycardia
   - Stable wide-complex tachycardias, including
     - — SVT with aberrant conduction
     - — Stable monomorphic VT
     - — Stable polymorphic VT (with and without normal baseline QT interval)
     - — Torsades de pointes
5. Operation of a defibrillator/monitor to perform both defibrillation and cardioversion, including
   - The difference between defibrillation and cardioversion
   - How to switch from the defibrillator/monitor mode to cardioverter mode
   - How to rapidly attach rhythm monitor leads in a modified lead II configuration to a patient
   - How to recognize when the device is in active *synchronization* mode
   - How to switch from synchronized cardioversion to unsynchronized defibrillation and vice versa
6. How to monitor the rhythm through monitor cables and defibrillator paddles
7. How to safely and effectively perform synchronized electrical cardioversion
8. Major elements of postresuscitation and postcardioversion care, including supplemental oxygen, IV access, continuous rhythm monitoring, and postconversion antiarrhythmic therapy if necessary

Key Learning Points: Overview

1. ***Unstable tachycardia*** exists when the heart beats too fast for the patient's cardiovascular condition. The word *too* conveys the concept that the rapid heart rate is directly responsible for a variety of symptoms. The heart is doing 1 of 2 things:
   - Beating so fast that the diastolic period between beats is too short to allow sufficient blood to flow into the heart (reduced diastolic filling time). A reduced blood volume in the ventricles means that stroke volume is reduced (lower amounts of blood are pumped on subsequent beats). Common examples of tachycardias producing a fall in stroke volume include atrial fibrillation or PSVT.
   - Beating fast but beating ineffectively: the strength and coordination of ventricular contractions is

insufficient to maintain stroke volume (pump out satisfactory blood volumes). Stroke volume may be particularly compromised if atrial depolarization and atrial systole do not precede ventricular depolarization and systole (eg, junctional or ventricular tachycardia), because atrial systole normally contributes the final 25% of ventricular filling.

2. This unstable tachycardia leads to serious signs and symptoms. Review the 4 examples of unstable, symptomatic tachycardia in the Settings and Scenarios above. These scenarios capture the broad range of "symptoms" demonstrated by patients in tachycardia.

3. The 2 keys to management of patients with unstable tachycardia are (1) rapid recognition that the patient is *significantly symptomatic* or even *unstable* and (2) rapid recognition that the *signs and symptoms are caused by the tachycardia.* The clinician must quickly determine whether the patient's tachycardia is producing hemodynamic instability and serious signs and symptoms or whether the *signs* and *symptoms* (eg, the pain and distress of an AMI) are producing the tachycardia.

- The concept of "unstable tachycardia" is something of a misnomer—is it the tachycardia that is unstable or the patient's condition?
- *The answer:* ***both.*** The most important concern is the likelihood that a rapid tachycardia could rapidly deteriorate to VF. This is a particular concern when the tachycardia is VT, either monomorphic, polymorphic, or—most unstable—torsades de pointes. VF is a lethal complication, and death follows if VF is not recognized within minutes.

4. Like rhythms that are "too slow" or bradycardic, tachycardia leads to other hemodynamic problems: *hypotension, signs and symptoms of congestive heart failure, weakness, fatigue, shortness of breath on exercise, decreased level of consciousness, persistent chest pain, or continued PVCs in the setting of a possible AMI.* Learn to assess not just for the presence or absence of these symptoms and signs but also for their *severity.*

5. ACLS providers often make the mistake of thinking that any symptomatic tachycardia needs to be immediately cardioverted even if the symptoms are only minor. Chest pain from an acute coronary syndrome can cause tachycardia, which provides an excellent example of this problem. New-onset or unstable angina, for example, will cause pain, anxiety, and discomfort. A tachycardia soon develops as a reaction to the pain and anxiety. It would be a serious error to decide that this tachycardia represents "unstable, symptomatic tachycardia" requiring countershock therapy. In this case the symptoms of chest pain and shortness of breath are due to the cardiac ischemia, not the tachycardia. The best therapeutic approach would be to manage the pain and shortness of breath, not the tachycardia. Once those signs are under control, the tachycardia will disappear.

6. The Tachycardia Algorithms: For further information, refer to the following sections of the *ECC Handbook:*

- Figure 7: The Tachycardias: Overview Algorithm. The branch point for unstable tachycardias is depicted in Figure 7.
- Tachycardias: Atrial Fibrillation and Flutter
- Figure 8: Narrow-Complex Tachycardia
- Figure 9: Stable Ventricular Tachycardia gives a broad overview of multiple related arrhythmias and their recommended treatments.
- If serious signs and symptoms are associated with the tachycardia, the ACLS provider should go immediately to Figure 10: Electrical Cardioversion Algorithm.

7. The treatment of tachycardias, like the treatment of bradycardias, challenges the clinician to remember the admonition *"treat the patient, not the monitor."* Initial assessment with the *ACLS Approach,* using the *Primary and Secondary ABCD Surveys,* helps ensure that ACLS providers assess critical systems and obtain essential information before making treatment decisions.

8. The patient should receive supplemental oxygen, ECG monitoring, and an IV line as soon as possible (oxygen–IV–monitor–fluids).

9. In cases of symptomatic tachycardia, rapid identification of the specific tachycardia will help you decide whether to prepare for immediate cardioversion. For example:

- Sinus tachycardia is not a form of symptomatic tachycardia. It is not an arrhythmia and will not respond to cardioversion.
- Atrial flutter typically produces a heart rate of approximately 150 bpm (lower rates may be present in patients who have received antiarrhythmic therapy). At rates this high symptoms are often present and cardioversion is often required.
- Cardioversion of atrial flutter can often be accomplished with lower energy levels (50 J) than might be required for cardioversion of other tachyarrhythmias.

10. ACLS providers must know when cardioversion is indicated, how to prepare the patient for it (including appropriate medication), and how to switch the defibrillator/monitor to operate as a cardioverter.

11. ACLS providers must know how to use the monitor/defibrillator for synchronized electrical cardioversion. Be familiar with

- Use of the synchronized mode
- Identification of synchronization on the monitor/defibrillator
- Different energy levels required for different tachyarrhythmias
- The need to resynchronize on some defibrillators after each cardioversion attempt
- Establishing when to proceed to unsynchronized shock (ventricular defibrillation) if necessary. The Electrical Cardioversion Algorithm identifies the steps to follow once the decision for cardioversion is made.

12. If cardioversion or clinical deterioration produces VF, treat with immediate defibrillation. Follow the VF/Pulseless VT Algorithm (see Case 3).

13. Postresuscitation/postcardioversion care includes monitoring the ECG, the pulse, and blood pressure, reviewing the ABCs, considering antiarrhythmic therapy, and establishing the level of consciousness and neurologic status.

Specific Skills to Learn

1. How to operate a defibrillator/monitor for cardioversion

2. How to attach patient monitor leads in a modified lead II configuration to a patient

3. How to switch a defibrillator/monitor from defibrillator mode to cardioverter mode

4. How to turn on the synchronization mode and recognize when that mode is active

5. How to move back and forth between synchronized cardioversion and unsynchronized defibrillation

6. How to display the patient's rhythm through either monitoring cables or defibrillator paddles

New Drugs to Learn

It is acceptable to use antiarrhythmics before you have determined that the tachycardia is unstable and needs cardioversion. These antiarrhythmic agents are often the same agents used to treat the stable tachycardias discussed in Case 9: Stable Tachycardias and displayed in the Tachycardia Algorithms (see the *ECC Handbook*). An alphabetical list of these agents is shown here:

Adenosine	Isoproterenol
Amiodarone	Lidocaine
β-Blockers	Phenytoin
Ca^{2+} channel blockers	Procainamide
Digoxin	Propafenone
Flecainide	Sotalol

Several agents are used to provide analgesia and sedation during electrical cardioversion. They include

- ***Sedatives,*** such as diazepam, midazolam, barbiturates, etomidate, ketamine, or methohexital
- ***Analgesics,*** such as fentanyl, morphine, or meperidine

A Walk Through the Unstable Tachycardia Algorithm: Electrical Cardioversion

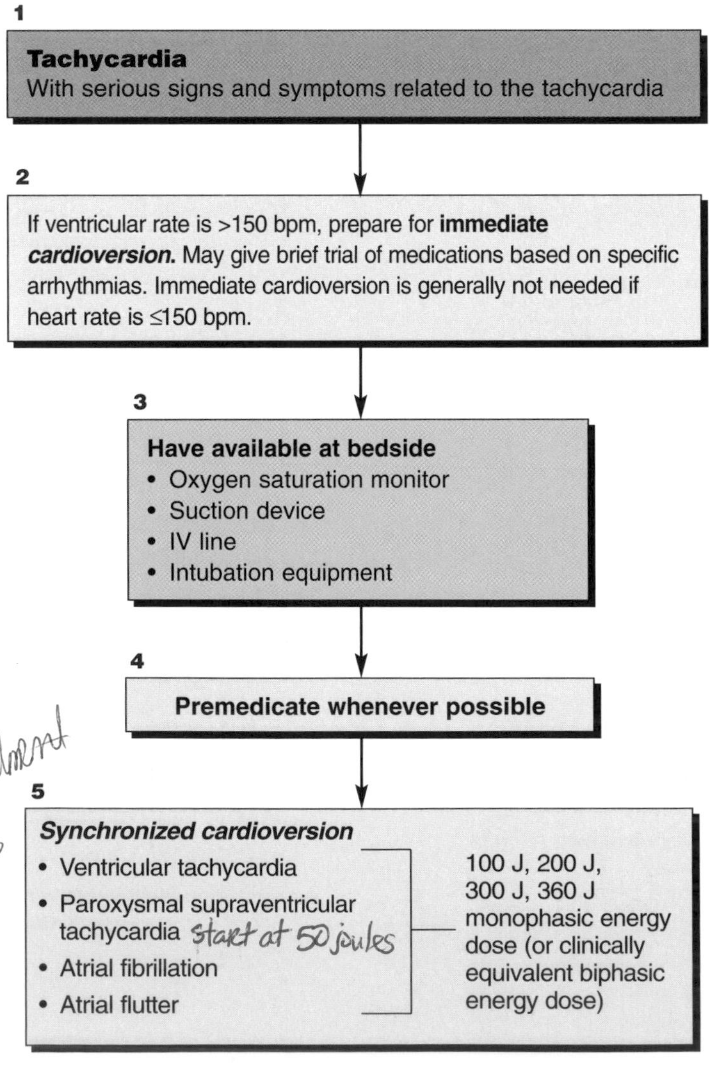
1
Tachycardia
With serious signs and symptoms related to the tachycardia
2
If ventricular rate is >150 bpm, prepare for immediate cardioversion. May give brief trial of medications based on specific arrhythmias. Immediate cardioversion is generally not needed if heart rate is ≤150 bpm.
3
Have available at bedside
• Oxygen saturation monitor
• Suction device
• IV line
• Intubation equipment
4
Premedicate whenever possible
5
Synchronized cardioversion
• Ventricular tachycardia
• Paroxysmal supraventricular tachycardia
• Atrial fibrillation
• Atrial flutter
100 J, 200 J, 300 J, 360 J monophasic energy dose (or clinically equivalent biphasic energy dose)

Box 1

Tachycardia
With serious signs and symptoms related to the tachycardia

Box 1 Comments

The unstable condition must be related to the tachycardia. Signs and symptoms may include chest pain, shortness of breath, decreased level of consciousness, low blood pressure, shock, pulmonary congestion, congestive heart failure, and AMI.

Box 2

If ventricular rate is >150 bpm, prepare for **immediate cardioversion.** May give brief trial of medications based on specific arrhythmias. Immediate cardioversion is generally not needed if heart rate is ≤150 bpm.

Box 2 Comments

For the hemodynamically unstable patient, use cardioversion before antiarrhythmic therapy.

- Inexperienced ACLS providers sometimes misinterpret this approach and think that they should completely forego giving antiarrhythmics in unstable patients with a pulse. Delay is the issue.
- When patients with symptomatic tachycardia are able to maintain a pulse and measurable blood pressure, the clinician can perform the cardioversion in a controlled manner.
- Clinicians should perform cardioversion as first-line therapy if it takes several minutes to locate, prepare, and administer medications.
- Once the clinician has made the decision to perform cardioversion, however, he or she may still administer medications if they are immediately available. One member of the resuscitation team can, for example, administer adenosine while another prepares the defibrillator for cardioversion so that it will be available if the antiarrhythmic therapy is ineffective.

Box 3

Have available at bedside
- Oxygen saturation monitor
- Suction device
- IV line
- Intubation equipment

Box 3 Comments

If ACLS providers have followed the ACLS Approach, the patient will already be attached to a monitor and an oxygen source, with an IV catheter inserted or IV access in progress.

- If available, attach an oxygen saturation monitor and a noninvasive blood pressure device to the patient and verify access to an operational suction device.
- If care is being provided in-hospital, have qualified personnel assist with airway and anesthesia.

Box 4

Premedicate whenever possible

Box 4 Comments

If time and the patient's clinical condition permit, give conscious sedation or some effective combination of analgesia and sedation.

Some experts recommend near-general anesthesia before cardioversion. Effective regimens have included sedatives with or without an analgesic agent. Use such medications carefully, safely, and judiciously. The clinical goal is to alleviate pain caused by the procedure without causing adverse effects.

Box 5

Synchronized cardioversion
- Ventricular tachycardia
- Paroxysmal supraventricular tachycardia 50J
- Atrial fibrillation
- Atrial flutter

100 J, 200 J, 300 J, 360 J monophasic energy dose (or clinically equivalent biphasic energy dose)

Box 5 Comments

- For ease of recall the Electrical Cardioversion Algorithm recommends a standard sequence of energy levels for synchronized cardioversion: 100 J → 200 J → 300 J → 360 J.
- The 2 exceptions to this are atrial flutter, which often responds to lower energy levels (such as 50 J), and polymorphic VT (irregular morphology and rate), which often requires higher energy levels.
- These doses are for defibrillators that use monophasic waveforms. Biphasic waveform shocks are acceptable if documented as clinically equivalent to reports of monophasic shock success. For polymorphic VT, start with 200 J.

Steps for Synchronized Cardioversion

1. Consider "conscious sedation" with analgesic and sedative agents.
2. Turn on monitor/defibrillator (models have either one power switch controlling ON-OFF for both monitor and defibrillator or separate POWER controls for monitor and defibrillator).
   - Select lead II on *lead select switch.* Make sure the lead select switch is not placed in *paddles* mode.
3. Attach monitor leads to the patient *("white to right, red to ribs, what's left over to the left shoulder").* Make sure the monitor displays the patient's rhythm clearly without artifact.
4. Engage the synchronization mode by pressing the "SYNC" control button.
5. Look for markers on R waves indicating sync mode.
6. If necessary adjust R-wave gain until sync markers occur with each R wave.
7. Select appropriate energy level.
8. Position conductor pads on the patient (or apply gel to paddles).
9. Position paddles on patient (sternum-apex).
10. Announce to team members: *"Charging defibrillator—stand clear!"*
    - Make one more quick check of the monitor to confirm that tachycardia continues.
11. Press the CHARGE button on the apex paddle (right hand).
12. When the defibrillator is charged, begin the final clearing chant. State firmly in a forceful voice the following chant before each shock:
    - *"I'm going to shock on three. One, I'm clear."* (Check to make sure you are clear of contact with the patient, stretcher, and equipment.)
    - *"Two, you're clear."* (Make a visual check to ensure that no one continues to touch the patient or stretcher. In particular, don't forget about the person providing ventilations. That person's hands should not be touching the ventilatory adjuncts, including the tracheal tube! Turn off the oxygen supply or divert the flow away from the patient's chest.)
    - *"Three, everybody's clear."* (Check yourself one more time before pressing the SHOCK button.)
13. Apply 25 lb pressure on both paddles (should deform the shape of the chest).
14. Press the DISCHARGE buttons simultaneously, and hold them down until the device discharges. (There can be a delay of several seconds while the device attempts a proper synchronization between the last part of the R wave and the discharge of current.)
15. Check the monitor. If tachycardia persists, increase the joules according to the Electrical Cardioversion Algorithm.
    - Reset the sync mode after each discharge of current, because most defibrillators default to unsynchronized mode. This default allows immediate defibrillation if cardioversion produces VF.

Critical Actions: Assessment and Management

Critical Actions Checklist for Unstable Tachycardia

The checklist identifies steps in the assessment and treatment of a patient with ***unstable tachycardia.*** Do not try to memorize the checklist. Review the checklist until you understand the order and rationale for all the steps.

For in-depth information about the new topics covered in Case 8, consult the *ECC Guidelines 2000* (see Read More About It at the end of this case).

Equipment and Personnel

Completion of the checklist requires that the following equipment and personnel be available:

Equipment

- Conventional defibrillator/monitor capable of synchronized cardioversion
- *Optional for course:* 12-lead ECG
- Equipment for noninvasive airway management
  - — Oxygen source (simulated in course)
  - — Nasal cannula
  - — Oropharyngeal airways
  - — Bag mask
  - — Venturi mask
  - — Pocket face mask
  - — Equipment for IV access
  - — Over-the-needle cannula
  - — IV fluids
  - — ACLS drugs

Personnel

- The ACLS learner
- One healthcare professional who knows CPR
- One healthcare professional who has successfully completed the ACLS provider course

Critical Actions Checklist: ACLS Case 8
Unstable Tachycardia

This critical actions checklist is limited to those actions specific for unstable tachycardia. To avoid unnecessary repetition, this checklist does not repeat all of the assessment and management steps of the Primary and Secondary ABCD Surveys. Remember that *those steps are always performed on all patients.*

Scene Survey Steps	Assess: Do or Monitor	Manage: Do or Delegate
Recognize emergency and respond	☐ Assess using the Primary and Secondary ABCD Surveys *Not in cardiac arrest or VF; tachycardia observed:* ☐ Assess vital signs: HR >150 bpm ☐ Take focused history ☐ Conduct focused physical examination	☐ Secure airway. ☐ Start oxygen–IV–monitor–fluids: ☐ Administer oxygen ☐ Start IV ☐ Attach monitor, pulse oximeter, and automatic blood pressure cuff ☐ Order 12-lead ECG ☐ Order portable chest x-ray
Symptomatic tachycardia?	☐ Look for serious cardiovascular signs and symptoms ☐ Is tachycardia causing serious signs and symptoms? *Check:* ☐ Oxygen saturation ☐ Suction device: available/working ☐ IV line ☐ Intubation equipment: available	*Tachycardia >150 bpm plus serious signs and symptoms* *Tachycardia causing signs and symptoms* *Prepare for immediate cardioversion:* ☐ Premedicate with sedative plus analgesic agent or consult anesthesiologist as needed ☐ Safely perform synchronized cardioversion (see Steps for Synchronized Cardioversion) ☐ Verify in sync mode ☐ Select appropriate current level (see algorithm) ☐ Follow all safety guidelines ☐ Deliver cardioversion shock ☐ Resynchronize defibrillator after each synchronized shock ☐ Recognize change in rhythm
Postconversion care	☐ Closely monitor vital signs ☐ Continue oxygen–IV–monitor–fluids ☐ Search for causes of tachycardia ☐ If VF occurs, recognize need to defibrillate	☐ Give bolus of lidocaine if not already given ☐ Start lidocaine infusion if bolus given earlier

Unacceptable Actions: Perils and Pitfalls

The following actions contribute to complications or poor patient outcome and should be immediately identified by the instructor and corrected. Unacceptable actions include

1. Inability to recognize cardiovascular instability in a timely fashion
2. Treating the monitor instead of the patient
3. Failure to resynchronize the defibrillator after the initial synchronized shock if further synchronized shocks are necessary
4. Failure to turn off synchronizing circuit if unsynchronized shocks are needed for VF
5. Failure to provide antiarrhythmic therapy after electrical cardioversion for the patient with VT
6. Failure to follow up with a history, physical examination, and identification of the possible cause of the arrhythmia

Read More About It

For details about the topics covered in Case 8 see the *ECC Guidelines 2000:*

- Part 6: Advanced Cardiovascular Life Support: Section 7: The Tachycardia Algorithms, pages 158-165
- Part 6: Advanced Cardiovascular Life Support: Section 2: Defibrillation, pages 90-94

Additional information may be obtained from the *ACLS Reference Textbook:*

- Chapter 11: Pharmacology 1
- Chapter 12: Pharmacology 2
- Chapter 13: The Basics of Rhythm Interpretation
- Chapter 15: Narrow-Complex Supraventricular Tachycardias
- Chapter 16: Stable Wide-Complex Tachycardias

Workbook Review

1. You are working in the ED when a 34-year-old woman arrives with a complaint of palpitations. She has a history of mitral valve prolapse and a heart rate of 165 bpm, a respiratory rate of 14 breaths/min, and blood pressure of 118/82 mm Hg. Her lungs are clear to auscultation, and she has no hepatomegaly. She denies having any shortness of breath. She is placed on an ECG monitor, which indicates that a narrow-complex, regular tachycardia is present. Which of the following phrases best characterizes this patient's condition?

a. stable tachycardia

b. unstable tachycardia

c. heart rate appropriate for clinical condition

d. tachycardia with poor cardiovascular function

Read more about it in the ECC Guidelines 2000, *page 117: "Paroxysmal Supraventricular Tachycardia"; and page 118: "Atrial Tachycardia and Atrial Fibrillation/Flutter"*

2. You are working in a clinic when a 58-year-old man walks in complaining of chest pain. He is diaphoretic and complains of dizziness. He sits in a chair at the triage desk while you check his pulse, which is rapid. As you prepare to attach a cardiac monitor to the patient, the man suddenly slumps over unresponsive. Which of the following best describes his condition?

a. stable tachycardia

b. unstable tachycardia, possible cardiac arrest

c. heart rate appropriate for clinical condition

d. tachycardia with adequate cardiovascular function

Read more about it in the ECC Guidelines 2000, *page 115: "New Concerns From the International Guidelines 2000 Conference: Impaired Hearts and 'Proarrhythmic Antiarrhythmics,'" "Summary: Treatment of Hemodynamically Stable, Wide-Complex Tachycardias," and "Hemodynamically Stable (Monomorphic) VT"; page 116: "Polymorphic VT and VF/Pulseless VT"; and pages 117-120: "Paroxysmal Supraventricular Tachycardia, Atrial Tachycardia, Atrial Fibrillation/Flutter, and Junctional Tachycardia"*

3. **For which of the following patients would immediate cardioversion be indicated?**

   a. a 62-year-old man with rheumatic mitral and aortic valve disease, an irregularly irregular heart rate of 153 bpm, and a blood pressure of 88/70 mm Hg

   b. a 78-year-old woman with fever, pneumonia, mild chronic congestive heart failure, and sinus tachycardia of 133 bpm

   c. a 55-year-old man with multifocal atrial tachycardia, a respiratory rate of 12 breaths/min, and a blood pressure of 134/86 mm Hg

   d. a 69-year-old with a history of coronary artery disease who presents with chest pain, a heart rate of 118 bpm, and ST-segment elevation

   Read more about it in the ECC Guidelines 2000, *page 117: "Paroxysmal Supraventricular Tachycardia"; page 118: "Atrial Tachycardia and Atrial Fibrillation/Flutter"; and page 91: "Cardioversion"*

4. **Which of the following groups of signs would *not* be consistent with evidence of *unstable* tachycardia?**

   a. heart rate of 140 bpm, tachypnea, wheezing, and pneumonia in a patient receiving albuterol

   b. heart rate of 140 bpm with rapid atrial flutter in a patient with aortic stenosis and AMI, blood pressure of 90/55 mm Hg, faint peripheral pulses, diaphoresis, tachypnea, and rales

   c. VT in a man complaining of chest pain, shortness of breath, and palpitations

   d. heart rate of 155 bpm in a 55-year-old woman with severe chest pain, difficulty breathing, extreme weakness and dizziness, and blood pressure of 88/54 mm Hg

   Read more about it in the ECC Guidelines 2000, *page 115: "New Concerns From the International Guidelines 2000 Conference: Impaired Hearts" and 'Proarrhythmic Antiarrhythmics,'" "Summary: Treatment of Hemodynamically Stable, Wide-Complex Tachycardias," and "Hemodynamically Stable (Monomorphic) VT"; page 116: "Polymorphic VT and VF/Pulseless VT"; and pages 117-120: "Paroxysmal Supraventricular Tachycardia, Atrial Tachycardia, Atrial Fibrillation/Flutter, and Junctional Tachycardia"*

5. **You decide to convert an unstable, symptomatic tachycardia. You place the cardioverter/defibrillator in synchronization mode and administer a sedative and an analgesic to the patient. Suddenly the patient becomes unresponsive and pulseless, and the ECG rhythm becomes highly irregular, resembling VF. When you attempt to deliver the shock, nothing happens: no shock is delivered and there is no energy transfer. What is the explanation for the failure to deliver a shock?**

   a. the defibrillator/cardioverter battery has failed

   b. the SYNC switch is not functioning properly

   c. the patient has developed VF and the defibrillator will not deliver a charge because it is attempting to synchronize shock delivery with an R wave

   d. the monitor cannot synchronize the cardioversion shock because a lead has come loose

   Read more about it in the ECC Guidelines 2000, *page 92: "Synchronized Cardioversion"; and page 164: Synchronized Cardioversion Algorithm*

Stable Tachycardia

Description

Case 9 focuses on the recognition and management of the following tachycardias:

- Paroxysmal (reentrant) SVT and automatic tachycardias, including junctional tachycardia, ectopic tachycardia, and multifocal atrial tachycardia
- Atrial fibrillation/atrial flutter
- Stable VTs: monomorphic and polymorphic VT, including polymorphic VT in the context of QT prolongation during sinus rhythm (torsades de pointes)
- Wide-complex tachycardia, type undetermined

Remember that Case 9 presents *stable* tachycardias. The treatment of patients with *unstable* tachycardias is presented in Case 8.

Settings and Scenarios

Setting: Prehospital, Unmonitored Patient

A paramedic has evaluated a 47-year-old woman with sudden onset of palpitations but no chest pain or shortness of breath. Physical examination reveals that her blood pressure is 150/90 mm Hg, her pulse is 160 bpm and regular, and she is alert and oriented. Her respiratory rate is 20 breaths/min, and her lungs are clear. There are no carotid bruits. ECG monitoring shows PSVT. The paramedic calls medical control and requests permission to treat.

What's New in the Guidelines...

Stable Tachycardia

From 1 Algorithm to 3 Algorithms and a Table

Many ACLS providers consider the single tachycardia algorithm from the 1994 *ACLS Textbook* complex and difficult to learn. In an attempt to clarify the principles of management of patients with tachycardia, the *ECC Guidelines 2000* provide recommendations for management of tachycardia in 3 algorithms and a table spread over 2 pages. Although this expanded format does not simplify the recommendations and expands them rather than making them more concise, the goal of this expanded information is to clarify important aspects of patient management. In the *ECC Handbook* the new materials are

Figure 7: The Tachycardias: Overview Algorithm (including wide-complex tachycardias)

Table: Tachycardias: Atrial Fibrillation and Flutter

Figure 8: Narrow-Complex Tachycardia

Figure 9: Stable Ventricular Tachycardia: Monomorphic and Polymorphic

Important New Management Principles

As in the past, decisions about the treatment of clinically significant tachycardias require clinicians to ask and answer 2 key questions:

1. **The clinical question: Is the patient *stable* or *unstable?* with serious signs and symptoms that are due to the tachycardia?**

   In general, stable tachycardias are treated with drugs (at least initially) whereas unstable tachycardias require immediate electrical cardioversion.

2. **The ECG question: Is the QRS complex wide or narrow?**

   This is important primarily because it guides the choice of drug therapy.

Although these classic questions are still fundamental and should be answered in all cases, the new guidelines for tachycardias also present several new management principles. Cardiologists who specialize in arrhythmia management helped to develop the new guidelines. Although

(Continued on next page)

Setting: Prehospital, Unmonitored Patient

A 62-year-old man calls 911 complaining of palpitations. Paramedics find him alert, friendly, and complaining of palpitations but not dyspnea or chest pain. Physical examination reveals a heart rate of 167 bpm and blood pressure of 130/80 mm Hg. His lungs are clear. There are no carotid bruits. The ECG monitor shows PSVT. The paramedic calls medical control for permission to treat.

Setting: Emergency Dept, Unmonitored Patient

A 35-year-old man enters the ED complaining of being awakened by a rapid heart rate and a pounding headache that won't go away. He has no chest pain or shortness of breath. Physical examination shows a blood pressure of 130/80 mm Hg, a heart rate of 160 bpm, a clear chest, and no carotid bruits. The ECG monitor shows PSVT.

Setting: Unmonitored Patient, In-Hospital Medical Unit

While working on the medical floor, you are asked to see a 49-year-old woman with pneumonia who complains that her heart is beating rapidly. She is alert and oriented and has no chest pain or dyspnea. Her heart rate is 160 bpm and irregular. Her blood pressure is 150/90 mm Hg. Her lungs are clear. There are no carotid bruits. A 12-lead ECG shows no ischemia. A monitor tracing shows an irregular rhythm that you identify as rapid atrial fibrillation.

Setting: Intensive Care Unit, Monitored Patient

A 58-year-old man is on mechanical ventilation after surgery. The rapid heart rate alarm sounds. The patient is sedated. His blood pressure is 150/80 mm Hg, and his pulse is 160. His lungs are clear. There are no carotid bruits. A 12-lead ECG shows no ischemia. The monitor shows a *wide-complex tachycardia of uncertain type.*

this led to a more complicated set of algorithms—and, unavoidably, to more complicated decision trees—the new approach is important because it should improve clinical outcomes. Thus, in addition to considering the 2 key questions above, ACLS providers can better serve their patients by understanding and applying 5 new principles as well:

1. ***Antiarrhythmics are also proarrhythmic.*** All antiarrhythmic agents are now recognized to possess some degree of proarrhythmic activity. This new insight has profoundly altered the use of antiarrhythmics, especially for management of tachycardia.
2. ***One antiarrhythmic may help; more than one may harm.*** The use of 2 or more antiarrhythmics to treat tachycardia is undesirable because it increases the risk of complications to heart function and rhythm. The use of more than 1 agent is not routinely recommended.
3. ***Antiarrhythmics can make an impaired heart worse.*** If the patient with a symptomatic rapid heart rate has impaired myocardial function, most antiarrhythmics will make cardiac function worse.
4. ***Electrical cardioversion can be the intervention of choice or a "second antiarrhythmic."*** In the modern era DC electrical cardioversion is either the intervention of choice or the second "antiarrhythmic." The threshold to perform electrical cardioversion should be much lower than recommended in previous guidelines. In the *"stable vs unstable"* decision, consider this rule of thumb: an antiarrhythmic administered to a patient with persistent tachycardia may itself render that patient *"unstable."*
5. ***First diagnose—then treat.*** In the acute setting the new *ECC Guidelines 2000* place a much higher priority on identification of the arrhythmia if time and clinical status permit. Several new agents have been approved for use for the stable tachycardias, most notably amiodarone, as well as flecainide, propafenone, sotalol, and ibutilide.

Summary of New Recommendations in the Tachycardia Algorithms

New agents and approaches have been recommended to make treatment of the tachycardias accurate, safe, and effective. These include the following:

Control of Rate and Rhythm in Atrial Fibrillation and Flutter

- A new table summarizes the major treatment considerations for atrial fibrillation and atrial flutter:
  - — Is the patient clinically unstable? (If so, consider cardioversion.)
  - — Is cardiac function impaired? (If so, consider cardioversion.)
  - — Is an accessory conduction pathway and/or pre-excitation syndrome present, such as Wolff-Parkinson-White syndrome? (If so, avoid drugs that selectively block the atrioventricular node, such as adenosine, calcium channel blockers, b-blockers, and digoxin.)
  - — Has the duration of atrial fibrillation been longer than 48 hours? (If so, avoid cardioversion—either electrical or chemical—if at all possible. When AF persists for several hours, stasis of blood in the atrium can lead to clot formation. Abrupt termination of AF and return of atrial contractions can cause a mural thrombus to break

(Continued on next page)

off and become an embolus, which in turn can cause a stroke or other embolic complications.

- Treat atrial fibrillation/atrial flutter in a "staged" fashion depending on several factors:
  - — If unstable, cardiovert at once.
  - — If stable, first control the rate, then convert the rhythm if necessary and/or appropriate.

Stable Ventricular Tachycardias

- Treatment of hemodynamically stable ventricular VT depends on whether the VT is *monomorphic* or *polymorphic and whether left ventricular function is normal or impaired.*
- Polymorphic VT is typically self-terminating but recurrent. Treatment is usually initiated after the rhythm has spontaneously terminated and is directed at preventing its recurrence. Ongoing polymorphic VT is usually hemodynamically unstable and should be treated according to the pulseless VT/VF algorithm.
- Treatment of polymorphic VT depends on whether *QT intervals* are normal or prolonged (as in torsades de pointes) when VT is not present (ie, during normal sinus rhythm). When polymorphic VT develops in patients who have prolonged QT during sinus rhythm, treatment with magnesium is recommended. Polymorphic VT in the *absence* of QT prolongation is treated the same as monomorphic VT as described below.
- *IV procainamide, sotalol (not available in the United States), amiodarone, and lidocaine are acceptable choices for treatment of hemodynamically stable monomorphic VT in patients with normal left ventricular function; use of amiodarone or lidocaine is preferred in patients with impaired left ventricular function.*

Narrow-Complex Supraventricular Tachycardia

- First, consider carotid sinus massage or other vagal maneuvers.
- *Adenosine* is the typical drug of choice for treatment of narrow-complex SVTs.
- If the tachycardia persists after use of adenosine, consider whether the rhythm is one of the following:
  - — A *paroxysmal supraventricular tachycardia (PSVT) due to reentry,* or
  - — *An automatic rhythm such as ectopic atrial tachycardia, multifocal atrial tachycardia, or junctional tachycardia.*

This distinction is important because PSVT is usually caused and sustained by a reentry circuit and therefore usually responds to DC cardioversion. In contrast, junctional tachycardia and ectopic and multifocal atrial tachycardia are usually caused by an automatic or "irritable" focus rather than a reentry phenomenon and therefore do not respond to cardioversion.

For each patient with narrow-complex SVT, consider whether cardiac function is preserved or impaired, because treatment may differ if there is significant ventricular dysfunction or congestive heart failure. Specifically you should avoid drugs that have significant potential to impair cardiac function if cardiac function is already impaired.

Setting: Unmonitored Patient, ED or In-Hospital Medical Unit

A 35-year-old man has just reported palpitations. He mentions a similar sensation followed by a syncopal episode 6 months ago. He denies having chest pain, chest discomfort, shortness of breath, dizziness, or abnormal sweating. He is alert and his mental status is normal. His blood pressure is 130/80 mm Hg, and his pulse is 160. The lungs are clear. There are no carotid bruits.

Setting: Telemetry or Coronary Care Unit, Monitored Patient

A 58-year-old man is on telemetry 4 days after an acute inferior MI. The rapid heart rate alarm sounds. He denies having chest pain, chest discomfort, and shortness of breath, dizziness, or abnormal sweating. He is alert, and his mental status is normal. His blood pressure is 125/75 mm Hg, and his pulse is 160, firm and regular. The lungs are clear. There are no carotid bruits.

Learning and Skills Objectives

By the end of Case 9 you should be able to describe and discuss

1. The ECG and monitor strip criteria that distinguish
   - Atrial fibrillation and atrial flutter
   - PSVT
   - Tachycardias with narrow or wide QRS complexes
   - VT
2. At least 3 signs and symptoms that suggest a tachycardia is *stable*
3. At least 3 signs and symptoms that suggest that a tachycardia is *unstable*
4. The sequence of treatments for atrial fibrillation and atrial flutter
5. The sequence of treatments for PSVT
6. The sequence of treatments for stable VT

7. The sequence of treatments for wide-complex tachycardia of uncertain cause

8. Why it is important to determine the onset of atrial fibrillation and atrial flutter and how this knowledge can assist with diagnosis and treatment

9. The clinical issues surrounding use of anticoagulants for atrial fibrillation

10. How to perform vagal maneuvers safely and effectively

11. How to perform DC electrical cardioversion safely and effectively

12. The management of patients with PSVT who remain in rapid ventricular response after vagal maneuvers, 2 doses of adenosine, and 2 doses of verapamil (or other appropriate drug)

13. The distinction between reentry and automatic tachycardias and why the latter generally do not respond to electrical cardioversion

14. Why it is important to have or attempt to obtain information about cardiac function or impairment when treating either supraventricular or ventricular tachycardia

15. Drugs to use and drugs to avoid in patients with accessory conduction pathways and pre-excitation syndromes such as Wolff-Parkinson-White syndrome, particularly when the rhythm is atrial fibrillation or atrial flutter

Major Learning Points: Understanding the Tachycardias

1. Stable tachycardia refers to a condition in which the patient has
   - Heart rate more than 100 bpm
   - No significant signs or symptoms caused by increased rate
   - An underlying *cardiac* abnormality that generates the rhythm (eg, fever and exercise are systemic conditions, *not* cardiac conditions).

2. Initial assessment of the patient according to the ACLS Primary and Secondary ABCD Surveys often provides the information needed to make a working diagnosis or to identify underlying conditions that could be causing the tachycardia.

3. The terms *stable* and *unstable* are widely used but can be ambiguous and potentially misleading. ACLS providers must understand a critical concept: *clinical stability* is a *continuum,* not a *yes/no* or *present/absent* state.

4. The 1-page Tachycardia Algorithm used from 1992 to 1999 offered 4 *classes* or *triage boxes* for stable tachycardia:

   a. *Atrial fibrillation/flutter*

   b. *Narrow-complex tachycardias*

   c. *Wide-complex tachycardias of unknown type*

   d. *VT (either monomorphic or polymorphic-normal QT versus polymorphic-prolonged QT tachycardia.)*

The *ECC Guidelines 2000* preserve these same 4 boxes. The ACLS experts and consultants working with the *ECC Guidelines 2000,* however, argued persuasively for expansion of the recommendations for tachycardia management.

- The major reason to expand the tachycardia recommendations was the growing awareness that several subgroups of tachycardic patients required special assessment and treatment. The tachycardia algorithms had to provide more precision and detail to provide the best care for all patients. Although this requires ACLS providers to learn and apply elements of advanced rhythm diagnosis and treatment, there is widespread conviction that both ACLS instructors and providers can meet the challenge. The 2000 edition of the algorithms provided each of the 4 tachycardia boxes with notes and comments that gives greater details and sharper perspective.

5. Classification of the tachycardias depends on the careful clinical response to 4 questions:
   - Is the QRS complex narrow or wide?
   - Is the rhythm supraventricular or ventricular?
   - Is the patient stable or unstable?
   - Does the patient have a significant degree of ventricular dysfunction, such as a reduced ejection fraction (EF) or congestive heart failure?

   The answers guide subsequent diagnosis and treatment.

6. If at any point the patient starts to become hemodynamically unstable, the ACLS provider must move to the unstable tachycardia branch of the Tachycardia Algorithm:
   - Begin preparations for synchronized conversion.
   - Know the indications, procedures (including conscious sedation), and complications of synchronized cardioversion.
   - Know the basics of postconversion care (including monitoring the patient's neurologic status and distinguishing respiratory depression or hypotension from sedation).

7. When ***atrial fibrillation*** or ***flutter*** produces a rapid ventricular response, your first priority is to *slow* the ventricular response:
   - Do not attempt immediate cardioversion (unless serious signs and symptoms due to the tachycardia are present).
   - Spontaneous conversion to normal sinus rhythm often occurs once the rate is controlled by medication, eg, calcium channel blockers or β-blockers.
   - If the stable tachycardia begins to cause rate-related angina, shortness of breath, dizziness, diaphoresis, weakness, or other signs or

symptoms of hemodynamic or clinical deterioration, then the patient is becoming *unstable,* and prompt cardioversion becomes an urgent priority.

- Conversion to a normal sinus rhythm can be accomplished either *electrically* (ie, by DC cardioversion, which is generally preferred) or *chemically* (eg, with procainamide, ibutilide, or amiodarone).
- Patients who have been in atrial fibrillation for longer than 48 hours should receive anticoagulation therapy before conversion to sinus rhythm is attempted.
- An increasing number of cardiologists and emergency physicians are performing urgent echocardiography to look for blood clots (thrombus formation) inside the heart (best assessed with transesophageal echocardiography [TEE]). Echocardiography is also used to look for areas of the ventricular wall that are not moving *(akinetic)* or that are moving in an uncoordinated pattern *(dyskinetic).*

8. Vagal maneuvers increase vagal nerve stimulation and can slow an SVT and even convert it to a normal sinus rhythm:

- In addition to a therapeutic value, vagal maneuvers have diagnostic value. If vagal maneuvers appear to change the heart rate, then the tachycardia is much more likely to be of supraventricular origin. Typically vagal maneuvers will either "break" PSVT or have no effect on PSVT. Conversely, vagal maneuvers will usually not convert atrial flutter to sinus rhythm but will unmask any hidden flutter waves, thus clarifying the diagnosis.
- The old practice of pressing on the eyeballs to achieve a strong vagal effect has been discredited. Eliminate this practice from your list of acceptable vagal maneuvers.
- Carotid sinus massage (CSM) is contraindicated in those who are known to have—or who are at significant risk for—carotid atherosclerosis. Because older patients often have undiagnosed carotid atherosclerosis and because carotid bruits are not always present even with significant atherosclerosis, most experts avoid CSM in patients who are elderly or even in late middle age. In such cases consider other vagal techniques such as the Valsalva maneuver.
- Occult diseases or pathologies often cause wide–QRS complex tachycardias. Evaluate the patient's vital signs and use a problem-focused history to gather clues to possible causes. Common etiologies include ischemic heart disease, hypoxia, hypovolemia, hypoglycemia, electrolyte abnormalities, and drug toxicities. The D of the Secondary ABCD Survey is an admonition to search for underlying conditions and correct any that are identified.

9. Stable wide-complex tachycardias can be of either ventricular or supraventricular origin. Identification of the specific type and origin of the arrhythmia may be either *(a) impossible* from a surface ECG or *(b) unnecessary* for initial treatment. Two rules for managing stable patients with wide-complex tachycardia are

- Rule 1. Wide-complex tachycardia should be considered VT until proven otherwise.
- Rule 2. Always remember Rule 1.

This aphorism is not meant to encourage simplistic thinking about VT but rather represents an extreme caution about possibly giving medications that can be harmful to patients with this precarious arrhythmia.

10. The 2 drugs to consider for treatment of stable wide-complex tachycardia thought to be *monomorphic VT* are *procainamide or amiodarone.* If patients have impaired ventricular function such as clinical signs of congestive heart failure or poor EF, the drugs to consider are *amiodarone* or *lidocaine*.

11. The usual drugs of choice for wide-complex tachycardia *of uncertain type* are either *procainamide* or *amiodarone*. Those with impaired ventricular function should receive amiodarone rather than procainamide. Each of these drugs is effective for both narrow- and wide-complex tachycardia and both supraventricular and ventricular tachycardia. Each is considered safe and effective for treating tachycardia associated with an accessory conduction pathway or pre-excitation syndrome, such as Wolff-Parkinson-White syndrome.

12. Note that in general *verapamil and adenosine are contraindicated for treatment of wide-complex tachycardia.* Use of verapamil in this setting can produce catastrophic, even fatal results. This caution holds true for VT, in which the vasodilatory and negative inotropic effects of verapamil can cause severe hemodynamic compromise. This caution also applies to certain types of SVT. When used for SVT, verapamil selectively blocks the AV node. If an accessory conduction pathway or pre-excitation syndrome is present, verapamil can increase conduction through the accessory pathway and paradoxically increase the heart rate. For patients with atrial fibrillation or atrial flutter, this poses severe risks and is associated with a very high incidence of clinical deterioration. Thus, no patient with wide-complex tachycardia should receive verapamil (or another calcium channel blocker, β-blocker, or digoxin) unless the patient has had electrophysiological studies that identified the specific type of tachycardia involved and ruled out a pre-excitation syndrome. Since few patients present with such documentation, providers of emergency cardiovascular care should rarely if ever use calcium channel blockers, β-blockers, or digoxin for the treatment of wide-complex tachycardia.

13. Similarly, in general *adenosine is no longer recommended for routine use in treatment of patients with a wide-complex tachycardia.* First, adenosine is ineffective for VT, which is the underlying rhythm in nearly 70% of wide-complex tachycardias of unknown type. Adenosine, like verapamil, blocks the AV node but not accessory pathways. Therefore, adenosine carries a verapamil-like risk for paradoxical and dangerous acceleration of heart rate in patients with a pre-excitation syndrome. Because of its short half-life (about 10 seconds), risks of adenosine administration are lower than risks of verapamil administration. Nevertheless, other agents are available. Procainamide and amiodarone block both the AV node *and* any accessory pathway. A large accumulation of data demonstrates a higher incidence of serious side effects with adenosine than previously recognized. Because of these factors and the availability of amiodarone and procainamide, adenosine for wide-complex tachycardia has fallen into disfavor.

14. Finally this case reinforces the need to

- Continually assess the ABCs
- Promptly take a problem-focused history
- Perform a focused but adequate physical examination
- Within a code setting, consider "oxygen–IV–monitor" 1 word and order it as soon as possible
- Continuously monitor and reassess the patient
- Treat not only the obvious clinical problems but also search for and treat any underlying causes and conditions

Specific Skills to Learn

At the end of this case you should be able to demonstrate

1. How to perform an initial patient assessment that can identify stable tachycardia caused by an underlying cardiac condition versus tachycardia caused by a systemic condition
2. How to identify tachycardias with narrow or wide QRS complexes
3. How to treat stable tachycardias according to the Tachycardia Algorithm
4. How to perform vagal maneuvers safely and effectively
5. How to perform synchronized cardioversion safely and with appropriate initial energy levels

New Drugs to Learn

ACLS providers should know the actions, indications, administration, and precautions for the pharmacologic agents recommended for treatment of tachycardias. The table below lists all agents mentioned in the new tachycardia algorithms and table, divided into the most commonly used drugs and the less commonly used drugs, including one drug recommended but not yet approved for use in the United States.

New Rhythms to Learn

1. Atrial fibrillation
2. Atrial flutter
3. Paroxysmal (reentrant) SVT
4. Automatic SVT (junctional tachycardia, ectopic atrial tachycardia, multifocal atrial tachycardia)
5. VT, monomorphic
6. VT, polymorphic; normal baseline QT interval
7. VT, polymorphic; prolonged baseline QT interval (torsades de pointes)
8. Wide-complex tachycardia of uncertain type

A Walk Through the Tachycardia Algorithms

Overview

The *ECC Guidelines 2000* recommendations for tachycardias have expanded to 3 algorithms and a 2-page table. In the *ECC Handbook* the new materials are:

Figure 7: The Tachycardias: Overview Algorithm (including wide-complex tachycardias)

Table: *Tachycardias: Atrial Fibrillation and Flutter*

Most Commonly Used Drugs or Classes of Drugs*	Less Commonly Used Drugs
Adenosine	Flecainide
β-blockers (esmolol, atenolol, metoprolol)	Propafenone
Calcium channel blockers (diltiazem,verapamil)	Sotalol (not approved for use in the United States)
Digoxin	
Procainamide	
Amiodarone	
Lidocaine	
Ibutilide	
Magnesium sulfate	

*Drugs in parentheses are the most frequently used drugs within a class of agents.

The Tachycardias: Overview Algorithm.

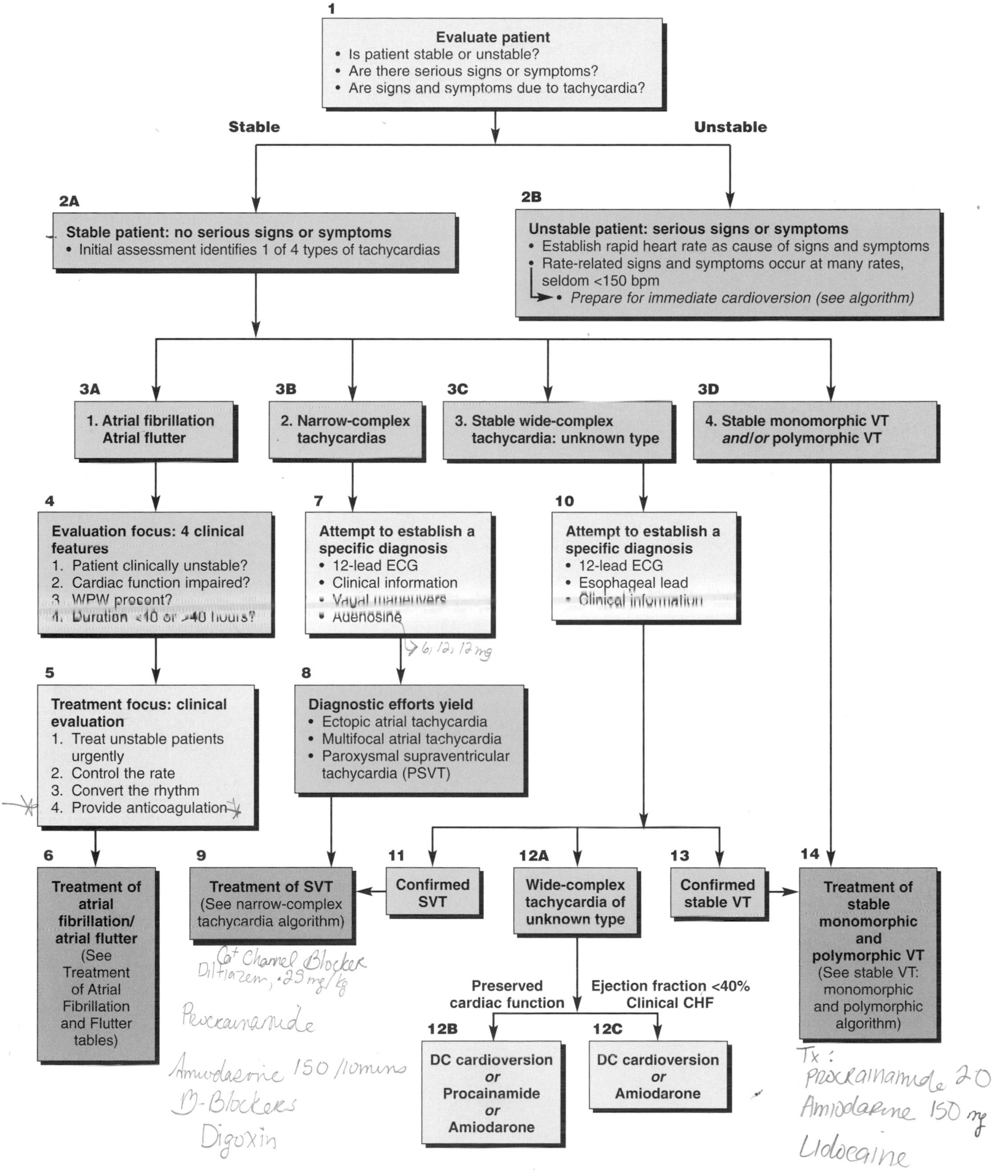

1
Evaluate patient
• Is patient stable or unstable?
• Are there serious signs or symptoms?
• Are signs and symptoms due to tachycardia?
Stable
Unstable
2A
Stable patient: no serious signs or symptoms
• Initial assessment identifies 1 of 4 types of tachycardias
2B
Unstable patient: serious signs or symptoms
• Establish rapid heart rate as cause of signs and symptoms
• Rate-related signs and symptoms occur at many rates, seldom <150 bpm
• Prepare for immediate cardioversion (see algorithm)
3A
1. Atrial fibrillation Atrial flutter
3B
2. Narrow-complex tachycardias
3C
3. Stable wide-complex tachycardia: unknown type
3D
4. Stable monomorphic VT and/or polymorphic VT
4
Evaluation focus: 4 clinical features
1. Patient clinically unstable?
2. Cardiac function impaired?
3. WPW present?
4. Duration <48 or >48 hours?
7
Attempt to establish a specific diagnosis
• 12-lead ECG
• Clinical information
• Vagal maneuvers
• Adenosine
6, 12, 12 mg
10
Attempt to establish a specific diagnosis
• 12-lead ECG
• Esophageal lead
• Clinical information
5
Treatment focus: clinical evaluation
1. Treat unstable patients urgently
2. Control the rate
3. Convert the rhythm
4. Provide anticoagulation
8
Diagnostic efforts yield
• Ectopic atrial tachycardia
• Multifocal atrial tachycardia
• Paroxysmal supraventricular tachycardia (PSVT)
6
Treatment of atrial fibrillation/ atrial flutter (See Treatment of Atrial Fibrillation and Flutter tables)
9
Treatment of SVT (See narrow-complex tachycardia algorithm)
11
Confirmed SVT
12A
Wide-complex tachycardia of unknown type
13
Confirmed stable VT
14
Treatment of stable monomorphic and polymorphic VT (See stable VT: monomorphic and polymorphic algorithm)
Preserved cardiac function
Ejection fraction <40% Clinical CHF
12B
DC cardioversion or Procainamide or Amiodarone
12C
DC cardioversion or Amiodarone
Ca+ Channel Blocker
Diltiazem, .25 mg/kg
Procainamide
Amiodarone 150/10mins
B-Blockers
Digoxin
Tx:
Procainamide 20
Amiodarone 150 mg
Lidocaine

Figure 8: Narrow-Complex Tachycardia

Figure 9: Stable Ventricular Tachycardia: Monomorphic and Polymorphic

The tachycardia algorithms were conceived as useful *educational groupings* to give a broad overview of all the tachycardias and link them to the recommended treatments. Underlying the new algorithms and table are 3 simple questions of stratification:

- Is the patient stable or unstable?
- Is the QRS complex wide or narrow?
- Is the baseline cardiac function normal or impaired?

The answers will yield the following broad stable tachycardia categories:

- Stable *narrow* QRS complex with *normal* heart
- Stable *narrow* QRS complex with *impaired* heart
- Stable *wide* QRS complex with *normal* heart
- Stable *wide* QRS complex with *impaired* heart

Evaluate patient
- Is patient stable or unstable?
- Are there serious signs or symptoms?
- Are signs and symptoms due to tachycardia?

Box 1: Initial Evaluation of the Tachycardic Patient

This box poses the critical clinical questions that must be asked—and asked repeatedly—during the evaluation and treatment of every patient with a rapid heart beat:

1. *Is the patient stable or unstable?*
2. *Are there serious signs or symptoms?*
3. *Are the signs and symptoms due to the tachycardia?*

In general, stable tachycardias are treated with drugs (at least initially), and unstable tachycardias are treated with immediate electrical DC cardioversion. Before treatment is initiated, however, the ACLS provider should determine whether the *tachycardia* is actually causing the clinical symptoms or whether some underlying medical *condition* is causing a secondary tachycardia.

For example, a patient with signs and symptoms of an acute MI might have a rapid heart rate—eg, a sinus tachycardia at a rate of 150 bpm—as well as chest pain due to myocardial ischemia and hypotension due to pump failure. It would be an error to assume that the tachycardia is the *primary* cause of this patient's clinical and hemodynamic instability. Another example is an elderly patient with a history of both chronic atrial fibrillation and congestive heart failure who presents with acute pulmonary edema and a heart rate of 150 bpm. This patient does display rapid atrial fibrillation, but the rapid rate is more likely to be a *response* to the pulmonary edema than the *cause* of the pulmonary edema.

It would be a serious mistake to treat these 2 patients with electrical cardioversion because the tachycardia is not the *primary* problem. The general rule is that *any* tachycardia that is *causing* clinical or hemodynamic instability should be shocked promptly. That is why the final step in the first box is to ask whether the signs or symptoms are *due* to the tachycardia.

Finally, it must be acknowledged that the "stable vs unstable" decision in emergency cardiovascular care is an example of a ubiquitous challenge throughout all clinical medicine—the need to render a dichotomous, sharply defined, black or white, yes or no judgment on a question that is intrinsically *fuzzy* or *gray*. These important dilemmas in clinical care are further elaborated on in the sidebar "Fuzzy Logic in Clinical Medicine."

Stable patient: no serious signs or symptoms
- Initial assessment identifies 1 of 4 types of tachycardias

Box 2A: Initial Assessment: Stable Patient: No Serious Signs or Symptoms

In the *ECC Guidelines 2000,* stable patients are classified into 4 general groups. Separate algorithms and tables provide recommendations for management of each of these conditions.

Unstable patient: serious signs or symptoms
- Establish rapid heart rate as cause of signs and symptoms
- Rate related signs and symptoms occur at many rates, seldom <150 bpm
  - *Prepare for immediate cardioversion (see algorithm)*

Box 2B: Unstable Patient: Serious Signs or Symptoms

Promptly shock any tachycardia causing clinical or hemodynamic instability. This is a fundamental principle of emergency cardiovascular care. The more unstable the patient, the more urgent the need for electrical cardioversion. Note, however, that the determination as to whether a given patient is stable or unstable is a clinical judgment call. In making such a decision the ACLS provider should consider the *total clinical picture,* not just a single parameter such as blood pressure or heart rate, and recognize that there is a *continuum* of clinical stability. The sidebar "Fuzzy Logic in Clinical Medicine" elaborates on these points for the interested provider.

**1. Atrial fibrillation
Atrial flutter**

Box 3A: 1. Atrial Fibrillation and Atrial Flutter

(Box numbers refer to boxes in the Tachycardia Overview Algorithm)

Box 4: Evaluation Focus, 4 Clinical Features

Evaluation focus: 4 clinical features
1. Patient clinically unstable?
2. Cardiac function impaired?
3. WPW present?
4. Duration <48 or >48 hours?

Box 5: Treatment Focus: Clinical Evaluation

Treatment focus: clinical evaluation
1. Treat unstable patients urgently
2. Control the rate
3. Convert the rhythm
4. Provide anticoagulation

Fuzzy Logic in Clinical Medicine: "Gray Zones" and Other Types of Uncertainty

Fuzzy logic, more properly known as multivalent logic, is a conceptual tool for dealing with vagueness, ambiguity, imprecision, and other types of uncertainty. Rather than seeing things as "black and white"—that is, dichotomizing the world—fuzzy logic recognizes that in the real world many situations are "gray." Fuzzy logic "grades the gray," that is, recognizes that there may be multiple shades of gray. It also requires practitioners to consider multiple variables in making decisions. Originally developed by mathematicians, computer scientists, and engineers, the concepts are very relevant to clinical medicine.

These concepts can be applied to assessment of clinical stability. The determination as to whether a given patient is stable or unstable is a clinical judgment call. To make such decisions, clinicians must consider the *total clinical picture,* not just 1 or 2 parameters such as blood pressure or heart rate.

Most healthcare professionals intuitively recognize that clinical stability exists as a *continuum.* Patients who are "more good than bad" can be treated as "stable": there is time for drug or other nonelectrical therapy.

"More good than bad" does not necessarily mean good! On the other hand, tachycardic patients who are "more bad than good"—with serious signs or symptom—should be considered unstable and given shocks promptly. In reality, *most* patients are in a gray zone between stable and unstable, and even experts may disagree as to the best therapeutic strategy in such cases.

Patients who are *very stable* and patients who are *very unstable* represent the opposite ends of the stable-unstable continuum. The clinical reality is that a specific tachycardic patient may exist at any point along the spectrum.

For patients in the fuzzy *gray zone* between "more stable than unstable" and "more unstable than stable," ACLS providers should think in terms of the *total clinical picture.* Consider whether the patient is in *very good condition (clearly stable), more good than bad, more bad than good,* or in *very bad condition (clearly unstable).* Again, keep in mind that *more good than bad* does not mean good!

Patients deemed *more good than bad* can be treated much like a truly stable patient but should be monitored closely because clinical status can change and patients can deteriorate.

Nevertheless, by definition patients who are *more good than bad* are tolerating their condition reasonably well. Time is available to analyze the situation carefully and treat less aggressively. For example, ACLS providers may provide supportive care while observing clinical progress, or they may use several medications early instead of electrical cardioversion when treating a tachycardia.

In emergency cardiovascular care ACLS providers should consider patients who look *more bad than good* as seriously ill. For practical purposes treat these patients as unstable tachycardic patients.

The Tachycardia Overview Algorithm sets the stage for more detailed and sophisticated management of atrial fibrillation and atrial flutter as outlined in the table below.

Some general principles warrant emphasis. First, the ACLS provider should answer 4 key questions:

1. *Is the patient clinically stable?* If so, there is time for pharmacologic therapy. If not and the duration of atrial fibrillation is less than 48 hours, then electrical cardioversion is indicated.
2. *Is cardiac function impaired* as evidenced by congestive heart failure, ventricular dysfunction, or a poor EF (eg, less than 40%; note that a normal EF is about 55% to 60%)? If so, that will affect the choice of drugs, because it is important to avoid drugs that can further impair pump function (eg, those with negative inotropic effects).
3. *Does the patient have Wolff-Parkinson-White syndrome or some other pre-excitation syndrome?* If so, certain drugs are preferred (eg, amiodarone or procainamide), and other drugs are contraindicated. Drugs that selectively block the AV node without also blocking coexisting accessory conduction pathways (eg, adenosine, calcium channel blockers, β-blockers, and digoxin) are relatively contraindicated when pre-excitation syndromes are present.
4. *Has the duration of atrial fibrillation been less than 48 hours or more than 48 hours?* The longer a patient remains in atrial fibrillation, the greater the chance that one or more blood clots (thrombi) will be present within the atria. Once clots form, conversion of the rhythm—by either electrical or chemical therapy—can induce an atrial thrombus to break off and become an arterial embolus. This embolus can be carried "downstream" and cause arterial vascular occlusion with associated organ infarction. The most feared complication is a stroke, but

Treatment of Atrial Fibrillation or Flutter Based on Duration and Ventricular Function

Duration 48 Hours or Less

1. Control the Rate

Ventricular Function Preserved	Ventricular Function Impaired
CLASS I • **Diltiazem** (or another calcium channel blocker) *or* • **Metoprolol** (or another β-blocker) *or*	**CLASS IIb** • **Diltiazem** (only recommended calcium channel blocker) *or* • **Digoxin** *or* • **Amiodarone**
1 (and only 1) of the following:	
CLASS IIb • Flecainide • Propafenone • Procainamide • Amiodarone • Digoxin	

2. Convert the Rhythm

DC Cardioversion
(recommended)
or
Amiodarone (IIb)
or

Ventricular Function Preserved	Ventricular Function Impaired
CLASS IIa • Ibutilide • Flecainide • Propafenone • Procainamide	**CLASS IIa** • No antiarrhythmic other than amiodarone is recommended

Duration Greater Than 48 Hours

1. Control the Rate

Ventricular Function Preserved	Ventricular Function Impaired
CLASS I • **Diltiazem** (or another calcium channel blocker) *or* • **Metoprolol** (or another β-blocker)	**CLASS IIb** • **Diltiazem** (only proven calcium channel blocker) *or* • **Digoxin** *or* • **Amiodarone**
NOTE: Avoid the following antiarrhythmics for rate control if AF duration >48 hours or unknown:	
CLASS III • Flecainide • Propafenone • Procainamide • Amiodarone	

2. Convert the Rhythm

Urgent Cardioversion

- Begin IV heparin at once
- Transesophageal echocardiography to exclude atrial clot

then

- Cardioversion within 24 hours

then

- Anticoagulation for 4 more weeks

Delayed Cardioversion

- Anticoagulation (INR = 2 to 3) for at least 3 weeks

then

- Cardioversion

then

- Anticoagulation for 4 more weeks

Treatment of Atrial Fibrillation or Flutter Associated With Wolff-Parkinson-White (WPW) Syndrome

1. Control the Rate
and
2. Convert the Rhythm

Note: Do not use the following drugs to treat AF associated with WPW (can be harmful):

CLASS III

- **Adenosine**
- **β-Blockers**
- **Calcium channel blockers**
- **Digoxin**

Duration 48 Hours or Less

DC Cardioversion **(Recommended) or**

Ventricular Function Preserved	**Ventricular Function Impaired**
CLASS IIb • Amiodarone • Procainamide • Flecainide* • Propafenone* • Sotalol* *Parenteral form not available in United States	**CLASS IIb** • Amiodarone • No antiarrhythmic other than amiodarone is recommended

Duration Greater Than 48 Hours

Urgent Cardioversion (<24 Hours)	***Delayed Cardioversion (>3 weeks)***
• Begin IV heparin at once • Transesophageal echocardiography to exclude atrial clot ***then*** • Cardioversion within 24 hours ***then*** • Anticoagulation for 4 more weeks	• Anticoagulation (INR = 2 to 3) for at least 3 weeks ***then*** • Cardioversion ***then*** • Anticoagulation for 4 more weeks

an embolus can cause other serious complications, depending on the organ involved.

Note that 48 hours is not a rigid cutoff point. In some patients, particularly those with other risk factors for thromboembolism, such as rheumatic mitral valve disease, an atrial thrombus can form in less than 48 hours. For this reason some clinicians use TEE to rule out an atrial thrombus before attempting cardioversion in high-risk patients with atrial fibrillation even if the duration is somewhat less or more than 48 hours. Such decisions require advice from cardiologists or other critical care specialists with considerable expertise in the treatment of cardiac arrhythmias.

Patients with atrial fibrillation of more than 48 hours' duration or unknown duration are often sufficiently stable to wait several weeks for *elective* cardioversion. A minimum of 3 weeks of therapeutic anticoagulation is recommended before *elective* cardioversion of atrial fibrillation or flutter, with an additional 4 uninterrupted weeks of treatment to be provided after cardioversion.

Another critical issue in the initial management of atrial fibrillation and atrial flutter is whether to merely reduce the ventricular rate (which is often sufficient) or to actually terminate the arrhythmia. Termination may be unnecessary if the patient is tolerating the tachycardia. Termination should be attempted only if the tachycardia is known to be of recent onset (48 hours or less) or an atrial thrombus has been ruled out by TEE and anticoagulation precautions have been taken. Drugs used to slow ventricular rate include calcium channel blockers (verapamil or diltiazem), β-blockers (such as atenolol and propranolol), and digoxin.[1] Drugs used to convert atrial fibrillation or atrial flutter to sinus rhythm include procainamide, ibutilide, and amiodarone among others.

[1]Use digoxin only when the situation is not urgent. Digoxin has a slow onset of action and is used primarily for long-term rate control.

Management of complex cases of atrial fibrillation and atrial flutter can require subtle, sophisticated decision making, a discussion of which is beyond the scope of this manual. Providers are referred to the ACLS *textbook* for additional information.

Box 3B: 2. Narrow-Complex Tachycardias

(Box numbers refer to boxes in the Tachycardia Overview Algorithm)

2. Narrow-complex tachycardias

Box 7: Attempt to Establish a Specific Diagnosis

Attempt to establish a specific diagnosis
- 12-lead ECG
- Clinical information
- Vagal maneuvers
- Adenosine

Box 8: Diagnostic Efforts Yield

Diagnostic efforts yield
- Ectopic atrial tachycardia
- Multifocal atrial tachycardia
- Paroxysmal supraventricular tachycardia (PSVT)

Box 9: Treatment of SVT: Algorithm for Narrow-Complex Tachycardia

Treatment of SVT
(See Narrow-Complex Tachycardia Algorithm)

Narrow-complex tachycardias are nearly always *supraventricular* in origin. The ACLS Narrow-Complex Tachycardia Algorithm (Figure 8 in the *ECC Handbook*) divides SVTs into 3 general groups:

1. *Junctional tachycardia*
2. *Paroxysmal SVT*
3. *Ectopic or multifocal atrial tachycardia*

Electrophysiologists view these 3 groups from the perspective of the mechanism that originates and propagates the tachycardia. Narrow-complex tachycardias have just 2 causal mechanisms: *reentry circuit* or *automatic focus* (possibly more than one).

The *reentry-circuit mechanism* propagates and sustains the tachycardia by a repetitive feedback loop of electrical impulses within the conduction system. Cardiologists refer to this phenomenon as a "circus movement" because the electrical impulses start in one location and travel in a circle. The *reentry-circuit*

Note on Box 7:

Box 7 of the Tachycardia Overview Algorithm lists 2 initial treatments for narrow-complex tachycardia: vagal maneuvers and adenosine therapy. Because the vagal maneuver carotid sinus massage is often poorly understood and performed, a separate sidebar describes the proper technique.

The technique used to administer adenosine is the major determinant of its effectiveness. Proper administration of adenosine is well described in the *ECC Handbook* and is not repeated here. Ironically, after the single appearance of the word "adenosine" in the overview algorithm, a great deal of "box space" is devoted in 2 algorithms to the treatment of persistent narrow-complex tachycardias. In most narrow-complex tachycardias (nearly 90%), however, adenosine converts the tachycardia to normal sinus rhythm. The need for further treatment considerations after adenosine simply disappears in the vast majority of tachycardias.

prototype is PSVT. *Reentry tachycardias,* both supraventricular and ventricular, respond well to certain antiarrhythmic drugs and are very responsive to electrical cardioversion.

The prototype of the *automatic focus* tachycardias is *ectopic* or *multifocal atrial tachycardia* (MAT). One or more "irritable" foci within the atria fire repetitively to generate MAT. Automatic focus tachycardias *do not respond* to electrical cardioversion. Electrical cardioversion disrupts and terminates repetitive reentry loops, but there is no reentry feedback loop in MAT. Treat automatic focus tachycardias with medications that suppress the ectopic foci, such as β-blockers, calcium channel blockers, and amiodarone. Equally important, try to identify and correct underlying causes.

Junctional tachycardia is another automatic focus tachycardia. By definition junctional tachycardias originate within or near the AV node, near the junction of the atria and ventricles. Because junctional tachycardias are automatic tachycardias, treat them exactly the same as MAT, with β-blockers, calcium channel blockers, and amiodarone. Junctional tachycardias seldom respond to electrical cardioversion because there is rarely an associated reentry loop. (In some patients the mechanism of a junctional tachycardia can be a reentry circuit in the vicinity of the junction.)

ACLS providers should base their treatment of narrow-complex tachycardia on 2 considerations.

Cardioversion vs Defibrillation for Tachycardias

The therapeutic effect of electrical cardioversion is profoundly different from the therapeutic effects of electrical defibrillation. *Cardioversion* terminates repetitive reentry loops; *defibrillation*—either atrial or ventricular—terminates fibrillation by depolarizing the entire fibrillating myocardium.

1. *Is the tachycardia due to a reentry circuit mechanism or a focus of automaticity?* Each of these mechanisms dictates a separate treatment approach, including whether to consider DC cardioversion and which drugs to use.

2. *Is the function of the heart preserved or impaired?* If pump function is impaired, carefully select a drug unlikely to have a further adverse effect on the heart. In most narrow-complex tachycardias this agent will

How to Perform Carotid Sinus Massage

Anatomy and Physiology

The carotid sinus is an area in the common carotid artery located at the branch point of the internal and external carotid arteries.

- The carotid sinus contains baroreceptors that respond to pressure changes in the carotid artery.
- The carotid sinus contains nerve endings which, when stimulated, convey impulses to the heart and vasomotor control centers in the brain stem.
- These control centers in turn stimulate the vagus nerve.
- Stimulation of the vagus nerve increases vagal tone, which inhibits the sinus node and upper conducting pathways.
- This in turn typically slows the heart rate.

This classic feedback loop is called the *vaso-vagal reflex* because it starts in the carotid artery *(vaso-)*, loops up to the brain and central nervous system, then moves down the fibers of the vagus nerve *(vagal)* to the sinus node and upper portions of the conducting system.

Preparation

Avoid carotid sinus massage in older patients. Note that the absence of a carotid bruit *does not* rule out carotid atherosclerosis. Assess for the following:

- Working IV line in place
- Availability of atropine
- Availability of transcutaneous pacing if clinically indicated
- Working ECG monitor, rhythm displayed

Possible Hazards

Numerous complications/hazards of carotid sinus massage have been reported, including

- Stroke (embolic and occlusive)
- Syncope
- Sinus arrest
- AV block
- Asystole

Technique

1. Turn the patient's head to the left.
2. Locate the right carotid sinus by finding the maximum impulse in the carotid artery at the level of the top of the thyroid cartilage.
3. Using 2 fingers of the right hand, press down with some force and begin a firm up-and-down massage for 5 to 10 seconds.
4. Repeat this massage 2 to 3 times, pausing 5 to 10 seconds between each attempt.
5. If this is not successful, try the same technique using the left carotid artery.
6. Never attempt simultaneous bilateral massage.
7. If carotid sinus massage is not effective, consider combining it with another vagal maneuver such as the Valsalva maneuver or placement of a cold ice pack on the skin.

Synchronized Cardioversion

Modern defibrillator/cardioverters can deliver either *unsynchronized* or *synchronized* shocks. An unsynchronized shock simply means that the electrical shock will be delivered whenever the operator pushes the control button to discharge the machine. Thus the shock may fall anywhere within the cardiac cycle, essentially at random. In contrast, the defibrillator/cardioverter delivers a synchronized shock in *synchrony* with the peak of the QRS complex (highest point of the R wave).

This is done via a sophisticated sensor in the defibrillator/cardioverter. When the SYNC option is engaged, the operator presses the discharge buttons to deliver the shock. The defibrillator/cardioverter may seem to pause before it shocks because it is awaiting the next QRS complex. The shock is delivered a few milliseconds after the R wave so that it appears to land on the QRS complex. This avoids delivery of a shock during cardiac repolarization (represented on the surface ECG as the T wave), a period of particular vulnerability during which a shock can precipitate VF.

In theory synchronization is simple; the operator merely pushes the "SYNC" control on the face of the defibrillator/cardioverter. In practice, however, there are potential problems. For example, if the R-wave peaks of a tachycardia are undifferentiated or of low amplitude, the monitor sensors may be unable to identify an R-wave peak and therefore will not deliver the shock.

In addition, cardioverters synchronize only to the signal from the monitor electrodes and never through the hand-held quick-look paddles. An unwary practitioner may try to synchronize—unsuccessfully in that the machine will not discharge—and may not recognize the problem.

Yet another problem is that synchronization can take extra time (eg, if it is necessary to attach electrodes or if the operator is unfamiliar with the equipment).

The ACLS recommendation is to synchronize for patients with stable tachycardias and patients with unstable tachycardias who are not *so* unstable that even a few moments' delay might lead to further clinical deterioration. (Obviously this is a clinical judgment call.)

Otherwise, to avoid dangerous delays, very unstable patients, such as those in severe shock or pulseless VT, should receive an unsynchronized shock. Should the unsynchronized shock cause VF (which, despite the theoretical risk, occurs in only a very small minority of patients), immediately attempt defibrillation.

be amiodarone. In PSVT and impaired pump function, place the priority on early DC cardioversion, which is safe and effective.

The algorithm cites an EF of less than 40% as indicative of impaired cardiac function. Despite use of an imprecise upper limit, the "less than 40%" cutoff is somewhat arbitrary. Accurate assessment of EF is impossible without sophisticated equipment and imaging techniques. Most ACLS providers will need to use patient history, reported symptoms, and physical signs to assess cardiac function. Relevant physical signs of impaired myocardial function include rales, jugular venous distention, an S_3 gallop, and other findings of congestive heart failure. With the clinical examination providing only limited sensitivity and specificity for assessment of EF, most practitioners will need to accept a degree of uncertainly, particularly in borderline cases. The main point is to avoid drugs that may further impair contractility in patients with *suspected* pump failure. Precise knowledge of the EF or extent of heart failure is not required.

Last, remember that this section addresses the diagnosis and treatment of *stable* narrow-complex tachycardias. Should a given patient become *unstable*, this algorithm no longer applies, and defibrillation or cardioversion should be attempted promptly as described in Case 8.

Box 3C: 3. Stable Wide-Complex Tachycardia: Unknown Type

3. Stable wide-complex tachycardia: unknown type

Box 10: Attempt to Establish a Specific Diagnosis

Attempt to establish a specific diagnosis
- 12-lead ECG
- Esophageal lead
- Clinical information

Box 12A: Wide-Complex Tachycardia of Unknown Type

Wide-complex tachycardia of unknown type

Box 12B: Preserved Cardiac Function; DC Cardioversion

DC cardioversion
or
Procainamide
or
Amiodarone

Box 12C: Ejection Fraction <40% Clinical CHF

DC cardioversion *or* Amiodarone

Ideally clinicians should attempt to identify the specific type of wide-complex tachycardia present and treat accordingly. The challenge, however, is to distinguish between VT and SVT with aberrant conduction. AV dissociation is nearly always diagnostic of VT, and a very wide QRS interval (more than 0.14 seconds) also suggests VT. Nevertheless, making a precise diagnosis from a surface ECG can be difficult or even impossible. *The wise ACLS provider should assume that any wide-complex tachycardia is VT until proven otherwise.* This is a good strategy for 2 reasons. First, about 90% of wide-complex tachycardias actually are VT, so from a statistical perspective the *always-VT assumption* is correct 90% of the time. Second, the *always-VT assumption* fits better with the need to avoid harm to patients.

There is little danger in treating a wide-complex SVT as if it were VT. Wide-complex SVT is stable and unlikely to degenerate with the agents used to treat VT. There is considerable risk, however, if VT is treated with calcium channel blockers and β-blockers often used to treat wide-complex SVT. If treated with calcium channel blockers, particularly verapamil, wide-complex VT can degenerate rapidly into cardiovascular collapse and an unstable, life-threatening arrhythmia.

Amiodarone and procainamide are good choices for wide-complex tachycardias of uncertain type because they are effective for treating both supraventricular and ventricular tachycardias. Another option is to consider synchronized electrical DC cardioversion—even as an alternative to drug therapy—particularly if an experienced specialist is available to advise about the procedure.

As with other tachycardias, the ACLS provider should also stratify patients based on cardiac function. Treat stable patients with *preserved* cardiac function with either procainamide or amiodarone. Treat stable patients with *impaired* cardiac function (such as clinical signs of heart failure or a previously documented low EF) with amiodarone. Avoid procainamide in patients with impaired function because procainamide has negative inotropic effects.

Finally, remember the general rule that it is better to use just one antiarrhythmic agent in a given patient to avoid proarrhythmic effects. If one agent has not converted a tachycardia after an appropriate dose, the next step usually should be DC cardioversion.

Box 3D: 4. Stable Monomorphic VT or Polymorphic VT

4. Stable monomorphic VT *and/or* polymorphic VT

Box 14: Treatment of Stable Monomorphic and Polymorphic VT

Treatment of stable monomorphic and polymorphic VT (See stable VT: monomorphic and polymorphic algorithm)

The final section of the Tachycardia Overview Algorithm ends by referring the ACLS provider to the Stable Ventricular Tachycardia: Monomorphic and Polymorphic Algorithm (*ECC Handbook*, Figure 9).

The *ECC Guidelines 2000* experts recommended that clinicians should attempt to distinguish *monomorphic VT* from *polymorphic VT*. The 2 types of VT have different causes and require different treatments. In *monomorphic VT* the QRS complexes appear almost identical in shape (morphology). In *polymorphic* VT the morphology of the QRS complexes varies significantly. In addition, polymorphic VT can be subdivided into 2 types, those with a *normal baseline QT interval* and those with a *prolonged baseline QT interval.* Note that the references to the baseline QT interval for a specific patient are to a measurement that cannot be obtained from an acute, sustained VT. The baseline QT interval can be obtained only from a patient's 12-lead ECG recorded *before* the onset of acute VT.

Most ACLS providers think of *monomorphic VT* when they think of VT. If cardiac function is normal, the monomorphic form responds well to any of 4 drugs: IV procainamide, amiodarone, lidocaine, or sotalol. Based on the evidence available in 2000, most experts would select either procainamide or amiodarone. Sotalol is not yet available in the United States, and as the *ECC Guidelines 2000* indicate, lidocaine has been determined to be much less effective than previously believed. If cardiac function is impaired, then either amiodarone or lidocaine is acceptable. Patients who do not respond to 1-drug therapy should be considered for DC cardioversion.

Polymorphic VT is often associated with metabolic derangements such as electrolyte abnormalities or drug toxicities. The initial approach should include a search for and correction of such a condition. Acceptable drugs include all of the agents listed for monomorphic VT as well as β-blockers. As with monomorphic VT, consider using DC cardioversion for patients with polymorphic VT who do not respond to the initial drug.

Torsades de pointes is an example of a *wide-complex, polymorphic prolonged baseline QT interval. Torsades* is a form of VT in which the initial deflection of the QRS complexes repeatedly changes from an up (positive) direction to a down (negative) direction. This produces a unique pattern on the rhythm strip. The QRS complexes display a periodic "peak-to-trough" distance that produces a wide-to-narrow-to-wide-to-narrow rise and fall pattern. This pattern has been termed the "spindle-node" pattern or "twisting of the points" pattern—a phrase that is the literal translation of the French *torsades de pointes*.

Torsades de pointes requires special treatment. A metabolic derangement (such as hypokalemia, hypomagnesemia, or hypocalcemia) or a drug toxicity (particularly medications that prolong the QT interval, eg, procainamide, quinidine, or the tricyclics) frequently precipitates *torsades*. Always consider such underlying causes and correct them quickly when torsades occurs. Although the *drug* of choice for treatment of torsades associated with hypomagnesemia is magnesium sulfate, some experts believe the *treatment* of choice should be *overdrive pacing*. The evidence for the efficacy of magnesium sulfate appears only fair. The algorithm lists 3 other acceptable agents: isoproterenol, phenytoin, and lidocaine. Though not common, torsades is not rare. Without early recognition and appropriate treatment, torsades has a high mortality rate. ACLS providers should be familiar with this rhythm and know that it requires special management.

Critical Actions: Assessment and Management

The following table presents critical actions that every ACLS provider should master. This is provided only as a general overview and is not intended to be comprehensive.

Critical Actions Checklist: ACLS Case 9
Stable Tachycardia

Scene Survey Steps	Assess: Do or Monitor	Manage: Do or Delegate
Recognize emergency and respond	☐ Assess the Primary and Secondary ABCD Surveys ***Tachycardia observed:*** ☐ Obtain and assess vital signs ☐ Take problem-focused history ☐ Perform focused physical examination	☐ Secure airway ☐ Order oxygen–IV–monitor? ☐ Order 12-lead ECG ☐ Order portable chest x-ray ☐ Order appropriate laboratory studies
Tachycardia Overview Algorithm for stable tachycardias	☐ Look for serious signs and symptoms of hemodynamic instability ☐ Assess cardiac rhythm and classify it as one of the following: — Atrial fibrillation or flutter — Narrow-complex tachycardia — Wide-complex tachycardia of uncertain type — VT ☐ Continually reassess ABCDs ☐ Remain alert for signs and symptoms of clinical or hemodynamic deterioration	☐ Make diagnosis of stable tachycardia with no serious signs and symptoms due to tachycardia ☐ Follow the algorithm and treatment protocol for the specific tachycardia ☐ If patient's condition deteriorates, prepare for and administer immediate cardioversion

Unacceptable Actions: Perils and Pitfalls

The following actions related to Case 9 are unacceptable and should be immediately identified by the instructor and corrected:

1. Failure to perform initial Primary and Secondary ABCD Surveys
2. Failure to recognize and diagnose a clinically significant tachycardia
3. Failure to promptly order oxygen–IV–monitor
4. Failure to assess patient for clinical and hemodynamic instability
5. Failure to assess patient for cardiac failure or ventricular dysfunction
6. Failure to consider QRS morphology in VT
7. Failure to treat properly in accordance with the appropriate ACLS algorithm—especially failure to promptly cardiovert an unstable tachycardia
8. Failure to search for and treat an underlying cause of the tachycardia
9. Failure to search for and treat other underlying conditions
10. Failure to try vagal maneuvers before drugs in treating stable SVT
11. Failure to use proper technique in electrical cardioversion, including failure to clear the area for safety and failure to synchronize when appropriate
12. Failure to reassess the patient after a change in rhythm or clinical status
13. Failure to clear the area for purposes of safety before attempting electrical cardioversion
14. Attempting to electrically cardiovert an *automatic-focus* SVT

Workbook Review

Questions 1 to 5 are basic. Questions 6 to 10 require a bit more sophistication than the others and are included primarily for more experienced providers.

1. A 75-year-old man presents to the ED complaining of having lightheadedness and palpitations for 1 week. His heart rate is 160 bpm and irregular; his blood pressure is 100/70 mm Hg. The physical examination is normal, with no evidence of cardiac or circulatory failure. The 12-lead ECG shows rapid atrial fibrillation but is otherwise normal. Which of the following should be included in your initial orders for this patient?

- **a.** oxygen–IV–monitor
- **b.** immediate defibrillation
- **c.** no therapy is indicated
- **d.** epinephrine 1 mg IV every 3 to 5 minutes

Read more about it in the ECC Guidelines 2000, *page 118: "Atrial Fibrillation/Flutter"; pages 120-124: "Antiarrhythmic Drugs and the Arrhythmias They Treat"; and pages 158-165: "The Tachycardia Algorithms"*

2. You continue to manage the same patient described in question 1. You conclude that he has been in atrial fibrillation for at least 1 week. His vital signs remain unchanged. Which of the following would be the most appropriate treatment for atrial fibrillation?

- **a.** IV digoxin to slow ventricular response
- **b.** IV diltiazem to slow ventricular response
- **c.** IV amiodarone in an attempt to convert atrial fibrillation to a sinus rhythm
- **d.** synchronized cardioversion

Read more about it in the ECC Guidelines 2000, *page 118: "Atrial Fibrillation/Flutter"; pages 120-124: "Antiarrhythmic Drugs and the Arrhythmias They Treat"; and pages 158-165: "The Tachycardia Algorithms"*

3. A 55-year-old man with known heart failure develops sustained wide-complex tachycardia after an episode of chest pain relieved by nitroglycerin. Currently HR = 150 bpm, BP = 100/60 mm Hg; ECG before the tachycardia = old left bundle branch block, which prevents determination of the wide-complex tachycardia as ventricular or supraventricular in origin. Which of the following is the *most* appropriate initial medication?

a. IV lidocaine

b. IV adenosine

c. IV amiodarone

d. IV verapamil

Read more about it in the ECC Guidelines 2000, *page 118: "Atrial Fibrillation/Flutter"; pages 120-124: "Antiarrhythmic Drugs and the Arrhythmias They Treat"; and pages 158-165: "The Tachycardia Algorithms"*

4. A 25-year-old woman presents to the ED saying "I'm having another episode of *PSVT!*" Her prior medical history includes an electrophysiologic stimulation study that confirmed a reentry tachycardia, no WPW, and no pre-excitation. Her heart rate is 180 bpm; she reports palpitations and mild shortness of breath. Vagal maneuvers with carotid sinus massage have no effect on heart rate or rhythm. Which would be the most appropriate *next* intervention?

a. DC cardioversion

b. IV diltiazem

c. IV propranolol

d. IV adenosine

Read more about it in the ECC Guidelines 2000, *page 118: "Atrial Fibrillation/Flutter"; pages 120-124: "Antiarrhythmic Drugs and the Arrhythmias They Treat"; and pages 158-165: "The Tachycardia Algorithms"*

5. Your patient is an 80-year-old woman who complains of palpitations and lightheadedness. Her physical exam is unremarkable. The initial ECG shows a regular, narrow-complex tachycardia with HR of 150 bpm. The Valsalva maneuver does not produce conversion, but the ventricular rate slows to reveal classic atrial flutter waves. Which of the following would be an acceptable next intervention?

a. IV diltiazem to slow ventricular rate

b. IV metoprolol to slow ventricular rate

c. DC cardioversion

d. any of the above

Read more about it in the ECC Guidelines 2000, *page 118: "Atrial Fibrillation/Flutter"; pages 120-124: "Antiarrhythmic Drugs and the Arrhythmias They Treat"; and pages 158-165: "The Tachycardia Algorithms"*

6. An elderly male patient complains of chest tightness, palpitations, and dizziness. His heart rate is 170 bpm; his blood pressure is 90/60 mm Hg. The ECG shows multifocal atrial tachycardia. Which of the following treatments would be *inappropriate*?

a. DC cardioversion

b. IV metoprolol

c. IV diltiazem

d. IV amiodarone

Read more about it in the ECC Guidelines 2000, *page 118: "Atrial Fibrillation/Flutter"; pages 120-124: "Antiarrhythmic Drugs and the Arrhythmias They Treat"; and pages 158-165: "The Tachycardia Algorithms"*

7. A 66-year-old homeless man with a history of chronic alcoholism presents with polymorphic tachycardia. He is tolerating the tachycardia well. You correctly diagnose torsades de pointes; HR = 160 bpm; BP = 90/60 mm Hg. On physical examination you find a malnourished man with no evidence of heart failure. Which of the following treatments would be *most appropriate* at this time?

a. amiodarone

b. IV magnesium

c. IV lidocaine

d. IV procainamide

Read more about it in the ECC Guidelines 2000, *page 118: "Atrial Fibrillation/Flutter"; pages 120-124: "Antiarrhythmic Drugs and the Arrhythmias They Treat"; and pages 158-165: "The Tachycardia Algorithms"*

8. You have just evaluated a 60-year-old woman with known Wolff-Parkinson-White syndrome. Her chief complaint is palpitations and mild chest discomfort that started 1 hour ago. Her ECG shows rapid atrial fibrillation at a rate of 175 bpm. Which of the following drugs is *contraindicated?*

a. IV diltiazem

b. IV propranolol

c. IV digoxin

d. all of the above

Read more about it in the ECC Guidelines 2000, *page 118: "Atrial Fibrillation/Flutter"; pages 120-124: "Antiarrhythmic Drugs and the Arrhythmias They Treat"; and pages 158-165: "The Tachycardia Algorithms"*

9. Which of the following treatments would also be *contraindicated* in the patient in question 8?

a. IV adenosine

b. IV procainamide

c. IV amiodarone

d. synchronized electrical cardioversion

Read more about it in the ECC Guidelines 2000, *page 118: "Atrial Fibrillation/ Flutter"; pages 120-124: "Antiarrhythmic Drugs and the Arrhythmias They Treat"; and pages 158-165: "The Tachycardia Algorithms"*

10. A 50-year-old man presents to the ED. His chief complaint is that he is "feeling weak and dizzy" since getting up this morning. His previous medical history includes an extensive AMI 1 year ago, known left ventricular dysfunction, and an ejection fraction less than 40%. He is doing well clinically, with only mild exercise intolerance. On physical examination you note fine bibasilar rales that have been documented on every physical exam the patient has had since the AMI. The ECG shows monomorphic VT; his heart rate is 150 bpm; and his blood pressure is 90/60 mm Hg. Which of the following would be the most appropriate treatment sequence for this patient?

a. IV amiodarone, then synchronized cardioversion if the rhythm does not convert

b. IV procainamide, then synchronized cardioversion if the rhythm does not convert

c. IV magnesium, then synchronized cardioversion if the rhythm does not convert

d. immediate synchronized DC cardioversion

Read more about it in the ECC Guidelines 2000, *page 118: "Atrial Fibrillation/ Flutter"; pages 120-124: "Antiarrhythmic Drugs and the Arrhythmias They Treat"; and pages 158-165: "The Tachycardia Algorithms"*

Read More About It

The ECC Guidelines 2000

Pharmacologic agents for arrhythmias are presented in detail in Part 6: Advanced Cardiovascular Life Support, Section 5: Pharmacology I: Agents for Arrhythmias.

The tachycardia algorithms are presented in more detail in Part 6: Advanced Cardiovascular Life Support, Section 7: Algorithm Approach to ACLS Emergencies.

The ECC Handbook

The *ECC Handbook* provides an excellent and readily available source for details of the 3 tachycardia algorithms and the atrial fibrillation/flutter table as well as the recommended pharmacologic agents and electrical cardioversion.

Acute Ischemic Stroke

> **What's New in the Guidelines...**
>
> **Acute Ischemic Stroke**
>
> The Stroke Expert Panels from the Guidelines 2000 Conference made no changes to the Stroke Algorithm. Research has continued to accumulate in support of the effect of fibrinolytic therapy when given to carefully selected patients within 3 hours of the onset of symptoms of acute ischemic stroke. This is a Class I recommendation, with the important caveat that it *must* be given according to the NINDS protocol, which requires a careful search for indications and contraindications.
>
> - Intra-arterial fibrinolytic therapy may be beneficial for patients with middle cerebral artery occlusion 3 to 6 hours after the onset of symptoms (Class IIb recommendation).
> - Intravenous fibrinolytic therapy within 3 to 6 hours of onset of symptoms (this recommendation received an Indeterminate rating because of insufficient evidence to support its efficacy).

Description

A Different ACLS Case

The learning objectives for Case 10 are presented differently from the way they were presented in Cases 1 through 9. The management of patients with acute ischemic stroke is a specialty topic, much of which is beyond the scope of an ACLS provider. Prehospital care should focus on rapid identification and assessment of patients with stroke and rapid transport (with prearrival notification) to a facility capable of providing acute ischemic stroke care. In-hospital acute stroke care includes the ability to rapidly evaluate patients for fibrinolytic therapy and administer therapy to appropriate candidates, with availability of neurologic medical supervision within the target times recommended by the NINDS (later in this chapter).

First-time ACLS providers are already required to master a great deal of resuscitation knowledge and skills. The average ACLS provider is not expected to also master acute management of stroke in its entirety within the short time allotted in the ACLS Provider Course. However, the principles of prehospital management and fundamental aspects of initial acute stroke care should be learned.

The Promise of Fibrinolytic Therapy for Acute Ischemic Stroke

In 1996 the AHA recommended the use of fibrinolytic therapy *within 3 hours of symptom onset for selected patients* with **ischemic stroke.** After an in-depth review of the available evidence, the AHA Stroke Task Force concluded that fibrinolytic therapy was supported by sufficient evidence to receive a Class IIb recommendation. The scientific panel discussions leading to the *ECC Guidelines 2000* concluded that fibrinolytic therapy for eligible patients with acute ischemic stroke within 3 hours of symptom onset should receive a Class I recommendation. The class of recommendation was increased (strengthened) as the result of accumulating scientific evidence. This evidence included additional analysis of the 2-part NINDS study (the 2 key studies documenting positive results of fibrinolytic therapy in carefully selected patients), a published Cochran analysis of 17 studies containing more than 5000 patients, and additional published studies of intra-arterial therapy. These published reports documented no increase in mortality rates and improved functional outcome associated with fibrinolytic therapy administered within 3 hours of symptom onset. It is important to note that fibrinolytic therapy must be carefully administered according to the guidelines, including indications, contraindications, and time requirements.

The major obstacle to optimal care of the acute stroke victim is initial delay in seeking care. Most stroke victims fail to seek care quickly enough to benefit from the newest therapies. *Fibrinolytic therapy must be instituted within 3 hours of symptom onset.* Most strokes occur at home.

Many stroke victims deny the presence of stroke symptoms, and most delay access to care for several hours after the onset of symptoms. This time delay often eliminates any possibility of fibrinolytic or other innovative therapy.

The full potential for fibrinolytic therapy will not be realized until stroke victims, their relatives and friends, prehospital healthcare professionals, and physicians and nurses from the clinic to the ICU recognize and respond to signs and symptoms of stroke. The narrow window of time in which fibrinolytic therapy can be given safely and effectively requires early recognition of stroke signs in the prehospital setting and rapid transport (with prearrival notification) to the ED. In the ED triage, assessment and treatment must be streamlined to ensure rapid evaluation of suitability for fibrinolytics and other new therapies.

All ACLS providers must have a basic awareness of the emergency assessment and treatment of patients with signs and symptoms of stroke. In Case 10 the Stroke Algorithm provides the best expression of the learning objectives. Although this case deviates from the case management format to a more didactic approach, management of stroke is too important a topic not to be included in even the most introductory ACLS course.

The Acute Ischemic Stroke Video*

The *Acute Ischemic Stroke* videotape was developed specifically to give life to the Stroke Algorithm. In the ACLS Provider Course instructors frequently use this video as *"the stroke case."* ACLS course participants can view the videotape while simultaneously following the Stroke Algorithm in the *ECC Guidelines 2000* (page 205), the *ECC Handbook,* or the algorithm in this case. The instructor will stop the video periodically to discuss the content that was just presented. Active participation in the discussions and case presentations provides the most effective learning.

*22:00 minutes; product code 70-2521

Case Content

This case provides an opportunity to review the following information:

- The clinical algorithm for stroke
- The signs and symptoms of stroke
- The pivotal new role of fibrinolytic agents in the care of selected patients with acute ischemic stroke: these agents can reduce the impact and sometimes actually "cure" an acute thrombotic stroke by reopening an occluded cerebral artery. In addition, through unknown mechanisms fibrinolytic agents can reduce the amount of "downstream-threatened" brain tissue that becomes infarcted and dead and decrease the amount that is ischemic and "threatened."
- Early recognition and early interventions, especially actions that can be taken by prehospital providers and ED personnel
- The critical role of urgent CT, with urgent review and interpretation by a skilled physician. These physicians should be specifically trained to review CT scans in the context of eligibility/ineligibility for fibrinolytic therapy.
- Complications of acute stroke

Settings and Scenarios

Case 10 focuses on the stroke victim in the *Acute Ischemic Stroke* video. The instructor can use information from any step in this patient's care to emphasize prehospital screening and prearrival notification, ED triage and diagnostic studies, or in-hospital therapy.

Learning and Skills Objectives

At the end of Case 10 you should be able to

1. Describe why timely action by the patient, friends or family members, EMS providers, and ED personnel plays a crucial role in the care of stroke patients
2. Describe the major signs and symptoms of stroke that serve as red flags signaling the beginning of a stroke
3. State 3 ways in which emergency medical dispatchers (EMDs) can recognize potential stroke patients during 911 calls and can shorten the time from onset of stroke to the beginning of fibrinolytic therapy
4. Describe several of the elements assessed in one of the validated prehospital stroke scales that are now available (either the Cincinnati Prehospital Stroke Scale or the Los Angeles Prehospital Stroke Screen). Describe how to administer the scale and normal versus abnormal findings. *Note:* Both of these stroke scales are described in the *ACLS Reference Textbook,* in the *ECC Guidelines 2000,* pages 206-207, in the *ECC Handbook,* and later in this case.
5. List 4 actions prehospital personnel should take at the bedside of a patient being evaluated for possible ischemic stroke
6. List 4 major protocols that EDs should put in place to ensure the shortest possible "door-to-drug" interval (from arrival at the ED to first infusion of tPA)
7. Describe a quick "walkthrough" of the algorithm for suspected stroke victims, focusing on the 7 potential points of delay in the care of the stroke patient (the 7 "D's" of stroke care). Potential delay can occur at any of the following points:
   - **D**etection of the onset of signs of stroke
   - **D**ispatch of EMS
   - **D**elivery to a hospital capable of providing acute stroke care
   - **D**oor of ED, including triage
   - **D**ata, including CT scan and its interpretation

- Decision about fibrinolytics
- Drug administration and postdrug monitoring

8. Describe the positive benefits of fibrinolytic therapy for ischemic stroke, the potential complications, and how to discuss these with the patient and family

Specific Skills to Master

ACLS care providers must be able to perform a rapid neurologic exam. They should be able to perform either the Cincinnati Prehospital Stroke Scale or the Los Angeles Prehospital Stroke Screen and should be able to determine the Glasgow Coma Scale score.

New Rhythms to Learn

No arrhythmias are specific for stroke patients. Many stroke patients, however, develop cardiac arrhythmias during the first 24 to 48 hours after a stroke. Life-threatening arrhythmias are a potential complication of stroke, particularly intracranial hemorrhages. The healthcare provider should be prepared to identify and treat any arrhythmias that occur.

New Drugs to Learn

The ACLS provider should know the indications, doses, precautions, and contraindications for the following:

- Approved fibrinolytic agents (tPA only as of 2000)
- Medications recommended for antihypertensive therapy for acute ischemic stroke
  - Sodium nitroprusside
  - Labetalol
  - Nitroglycerin (transdermal or intravenous)

(See the *ECC Handbook,* the *ECC Guidelines 2000,* pages 209-212, and the *ACLS Reference Textbook.*)

Critical Actions: Assessment and Management

Critical Actions for ACLS Providers in the Prehospital Setting

The following actions must take place to provide the patient with the best possible outcome. At the end of the case the ACLS provider in the prehospital setting should be able to

- Recognize the signs of transient ischemic attack (TIA) and stroke
- Perform a rapid neurologic examination that includes the elements of the Cincinnati Prehospital Stroke Scale and the Los Angeles Prehospital Stroke Screen
- Determine (if possible) the time of symptom onset
- Provide rapid transport to an ED capable of caring for patients with acute ischemic stroke
- Assess and support cardiorespiratory function as necessary during transport
- When proper equipment is available, perform finger-stick determination of serum glucose levels and treat appropriately
- Notify the receiving hospital early that a possible stroke victim is in transport

Critical Actions for ACLS Providers in the ED

The following actions must take place to provide the patient with the best possible outcome. At the end of the case the ACLS provider in the ED should be able to

- Perform a rapid Primary ABCD triage
- Support cardiorespiratory function if needed
- Support fluid status
- Place a high priority on meeting the national target times for evaluating acute stroke patients (based on NINDS recommendations)
- Arrange for urgent review and interpretation of CT scans of the head by a radiologist familiar with NINDS indications for the use of fibrinolytics
- Control hypertension if necessary (see the *ECC Handbook*)

Critical Actions Related to Fibrinolytic Therapy

The following actions must take place to provide the patient with the best possible outcome. At the end of the case the ACLS provider involved in the care of patients eligible for fibrinolytic therapy should be able to

- Understand the potential risks and benefits of fibrinolytic therapy for selected patients with acute ischemic stroke who present within 3 hours of symptom onset
- Understand the inclusion and exclusion criteria for fibrinolytic therapy
- Discuss clinical findings suggestive of clinical deterioration or possible hemorrhage after fibrinolytic therapy

Unacceptable Actions

Unacceptable Actions by ACLS Providers in the Prehospital Setting: Perils and Pitfalls

The following actions by participants are unacceptable and can contribute to poor patient outcome and potential complications and should be corrected by the instructor:

- Failure to recognize signs or symptoms suggestive of TIA or stroke and evaluate the patient appropriately
- Failure to attempt to determine the time of onset of stroke signs
- Delay in transporting the patient to the ED (eg, delay from multiple attempts to achieve IV access)
- Transporting a potential stroke victim to an ED not capable of treating acute ischemic stroke patients with fibrinolytic

therapy (ie, ED without urgent CT capabilities, experienced on-call radiologists, or experienced neurologists)

- Failure to assess and support cardiorespiratory function during transport
- Attempts to treat hypertension in the field
- Failure to notify the receiving hospital ED well in advance of the impending arrival of a possible stroke victim

Unacceptable Actions by ACLS Providers in the ED: Perils and Pitfalls

The following actions by participants are unacceptable and can contribute to poor patient outcome and potential complications and should be corrected by the instructor:

- Failure to recognize and properly evaluate a patient with signs and symptoms suggestive of TIA or stroke
- Excessive delays in obtaining or reading a CT scan
- Failure to treat complications of stroke, including cardiorespiratory deterioration, severe hypertension, or seizures
- Administration of contraindicated therapies (eg, inappropriate antihypertensive therapy)

Unacceptable Actions by the ACLS Provider Related to Fibrinolytic Therapy: Perils and Pitfalls

The following actions by participants are unacceptable and can contribute to poor patient outcome and potential complications and should be corrected by the instructor:

- Recommendation of fibrinolytic therapy for a patient with obvious hemorrhagic stroke on CT
- Recommendation of fibrinolytic therapy for a patient with ischemic stroke but obvious contraindications to fibrinolysis (eg, severe hypertension unresponsive to therapy, presentation more than 3 hours from symptom onset)
- Failure to anticipate or recognize potential complications of fibrinolytic therapy

A Walk Through the Acute Ischemic Stroke Algorithm

The Stroke Chain of Survival

The stroke patient requires a series of actions to link the victim to the best chance of survival. The "stroke chain of survival" described by the AHA and the American Stroke Association is similar to the Chain of Survival for sudden cardiac arrest and contains the following 4 links:

- Rapid recognition and reaction to stroke warning signs
- Rapid start of prehospital care
- Rapid EMS system transport and hospital pre-notification
- Rapid diagnosis and treatment in the hospital

The 7 "D's" of Potential Delay in Assessment and Care of the Stroke Victim

Optimal care of the victim of acute ischemic stroke must minimize delay in recognition of stroke symptoms, activation of the EMS system, transport to and prearrival notification of a hospital capable of acute stroke care, appropriate evaluation and selection of eligible candidates for fibrinolytic therapy, and administration of fibrinolytics. Delays at any of these major points can make the patient ineligible for fibrinolytic therapy.

Borrowing from the nomenclature of the memory aid of the National Heart Attack Alert Program, *"Door-Data-Decision-Drug,"* Hazinski developed a multistep memory aid for the treatment of acute stroke called *the 7 "D's" of Stroke Survival and Recovery*[1]*:*

1. *Detection* of the onset of stroke signs and symptoms
2. *Dispatch* through activation of the EMS system and prompt EMS response
3. *Delivery* of the victim to the appropriate receiving hospital while providing appropriate prehospital assessment, care, and prearrival notification
4. *Door* (ED triage)
5. *Data* (ED evaluation, including CT)
6. *Decision* about potential therapies
7. *Drug* therapy

At each of these 7 steps care must be organized and efficient to avoid needless delays. The Algorithm for Suspected Stroke (Figure 1) follows the ***7 D's of Stroke Survival and Recovery*** and is discussed below.

1. *Detection:* Early Recognition

Early treatment of stroke depends on the victim, family members, or other bystanders detecting the event.

- Fewer than 1 of 10 stroke victims has been educated about the signs and symptoms of stroke before experiencing his or her own event.
- Unlike a heart attack, strokes are painless and may start quietly. The patient may have only mild facial weakness, a minor problem speaking, or slight dizziness. More dramatic signs, including paralysis of a hand or arm, disabling vertigo, and loss of consciousness, may be observed.
- Mild signs or symptoms may go unnoticed or be ignored by the patient, family, and friends.

2. *Dispatch:* Early EMS Activation and Instructions From EMDs

Stroke victims and their families must be taught to activate the EMS system as soon as they detect signs or symptoms of stroke. Currently half of all stroke victims are driven to the ED by family or friends. But the EMS system provides the safest and

[1]Hazinski MF. Demystifying recognition and management of stroke. *Curr Emerg Cardiac Care.* Winter 1996;7:8.

FIGURE 1. Algorithm for Suspected Stroke.

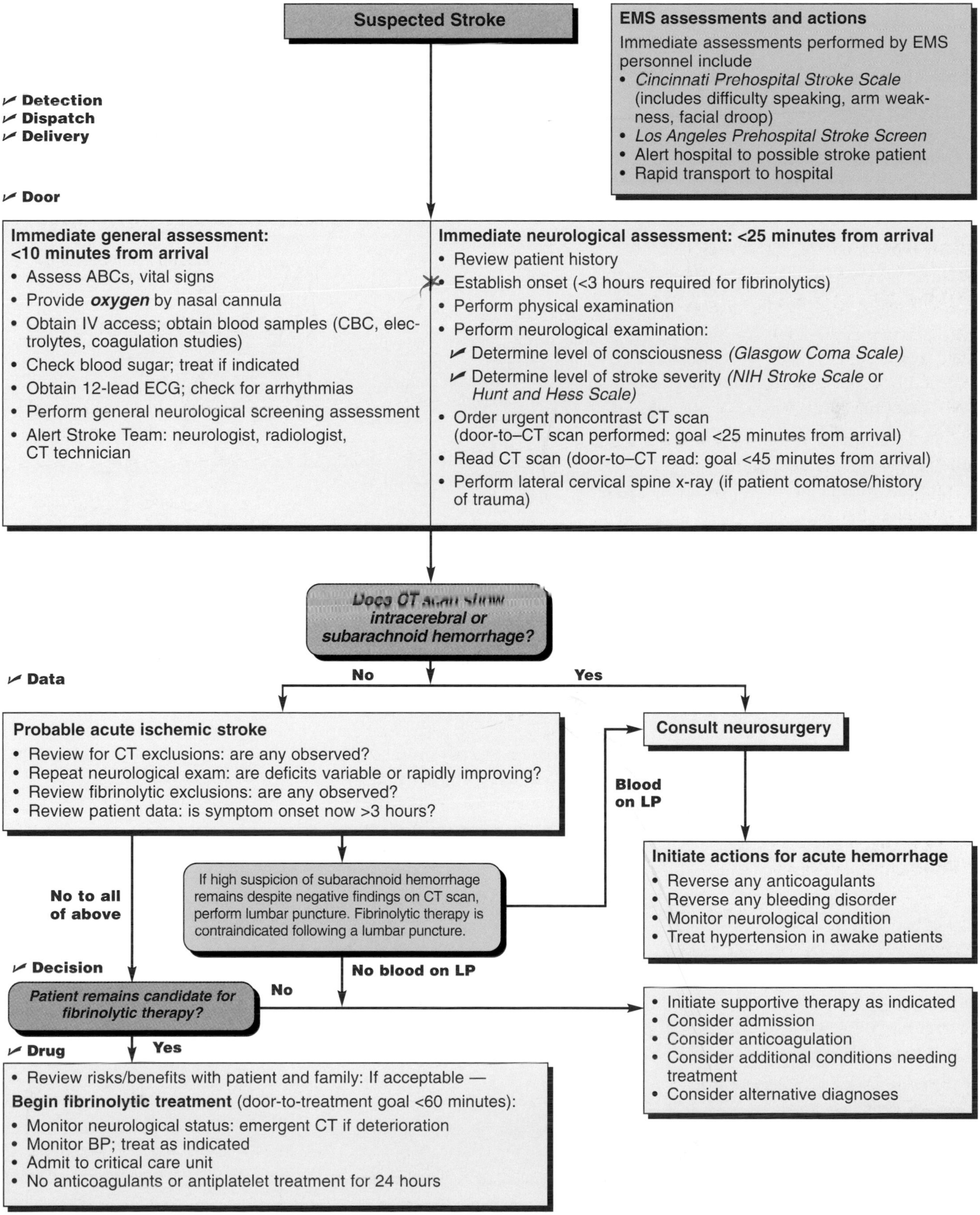

most efficient method for emergency transport to the hospital. In addition, EMS personnel will be able to identify a hospital capable of acute stroke care and provide prearrival notification to the hospital so that it will be prepared to efficiently evaluate and manage the patient.

- Family, friends, or prehospital personnel should not contact primary physicians or specialty providers. This tends to delay arrival in the ED and is not recommended.
- Family transport also delays arrival in the ED and prevents prearrival notification of the ED.
- EMDs play a critical role in the timely treatment of potential stroke victims. Their professional responsibilities include recognition of critical red flag complaints.
- EMDs evaluate patient complaints using specific protocols, which help prioritize the call to ensure a rapid EMS response.
- Highly skilled dispatchers have demonstrated effective skills to triage many cardiovascular emergencies, including possible stroke and acute coronary events. EMDs require additional stroke training, however. In a recent study just over half of EMS dispatchers correctly identified stroke based on complaints and interview responses during the initial EMS call.
- EMDs can also instruct bystanders in lifesaving skills—including airway management, patient positioning, and rescue breathing—while EMS personnel are on their way.

3. *Delivery:* Prehospital Assessment, Transport, and Management

The goals of *delivery* are

- Rapid identification of signs and symptoms indicating a stroke
- Support of vital functions
- Rapid transport of the victim to an appropriate receiving facility
- Prearrival notification of the receiving facility

Importance of Prehospital Care in the Fibrinolytic Era

The advent of new and effective stroke treatments plus the urgent need for rapid administration of these treatments have combined to give a new role to EMS providers. EMS providers must be trained to recognize the signs and symptoms of a possible stroke and to initiate prehospital screening and appropriate supportive therapy. EMS system protocols must assign a high priority to stroke patients. Training programs must incorporate protocols that cover early recognition, early stabilization, early transportation, and early notification of the receiving emergency care facility.

Stroke Identification in the Prehospital Setting

EMTs and paramedics can correctly identify stroke or TIA in 3 of 4 people with either condition. Extensive medical histories and neurologic exams by prehospital personnel are impractical, especially because gathering of this data may delay rapid transport of the patient to the ED.

The Cincinnati Prehospital Stroke Scale

The ***Cincinnati Prehospital Stroke Scale,*** named for the location where it was developed, identifies a high percentage of acute stroke patients by assessing only 3 physical findings:

1. **Facial droop** (have the patient smile or show his or her teeth)
2. **Arm drift** (the patient closes his or her eyes and holds both arms out)
3. **Speech difficulties** (have the patient say "You can't teach an old dog new tricks.")

See Table 1.

Emergency personnel (including emergency medicine physicians and ED nurses) can evaluate the patient with the Cincinnati Prehospital Stroke Scale in less than 1 minute. Patients with 1 of these 3 findings—as a *new* event—have a 72% probability of an ischemic stroke; if all 3 findings are present the probability of an acute stroke is more than 85% (positive predictive value). Immediately contact the medical control providers and the destination ED and provide prearrival notification. These patients require rapid transport to the hospital.

The Los Angeles Prehospital Stroke Screen

The **Los Angeles Prehospital Stroke Screen** (LAPSS) is a much stricter screen for acute stroke; LAPSS adds criteria for age, history of seizures, symptom duration, blood glucose levels, and lack of preexisting ambulation problems to 2 of the 3 physical signs of the Cincinnati scale. Consequently the positive predictive value of the LAPSS is much higher—a person with positive findings on all 8 criteria has a 97% probability of an acute stroke. See Table 1.

"Load and Go"

The interval between the onset of symptoms and arrival at the ED *must be minimized.* This is the responsibility of EMS personnel. The presence of acute stroke is an indication for "load and go." Specific stroke therapy can be provided only in the appropriate receiving hospital ED, so time in the field only delays (and may prevent) definitive therapy. More extensive assessments and initiation of supportive therapies can continue en route to the hospital or in the ED.

Establish the Time of Onset of Stroke Signs

If possible prehospital providers should establish the precise time of the onset of stroke signs and symptoms. The time of onset must be obtained to evaluate the patient for fibrinolytic therapy. If the time of symptom onset is viewed as time "zero," all assessments and therapies can be related to that time.

Early notification of ED personnel enables them to prepare for the imminent arrival

TABLE 1. Prehospital Assessment of Possible Stroke

A. The Cincinnati Prehospital Stroke Scale

(Kothari R, et al. *Acad Emerg Med.* 1997;4:986-990.)

Facial Droop (have patient show teeth or smile):

- Normal—both sides of face move equally
- Abnormal—one side of face does not move as well as the other side

Arm Drift (patient closes eyes and holds both arms straight out for 10 seconds):

- Normal—both arms move the same *or* both arms do not move at all (other findings, such as pronator drift, may be helpful)
- Abnormal—one arm does not move *or* one arm drifts down compared with the other

Abnormal Speech (have the patient say "you can't teach an old dog new tricks"):

- Normal—patient uses correct words with no slurring
- Abnormal—patient slurs words, uses the wrong words, or is unable to speak

Interpretation: If any *1* of these 3 signs is abnormal, the probability of a stroke is 72%.

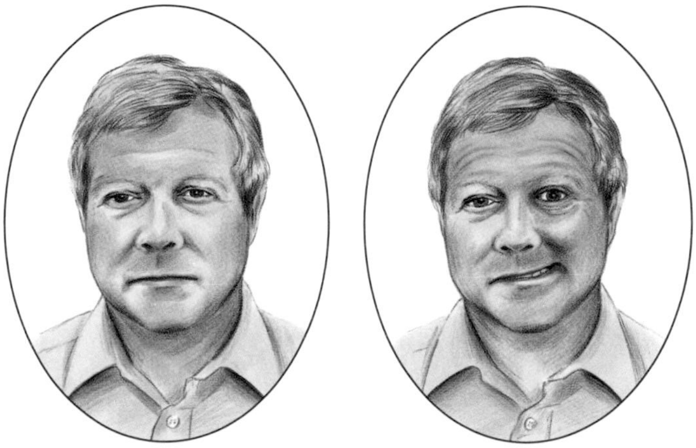

Left: normal. Right: stroke patient with facial droop (right side of face).

B. Los Angeles Prehospital Stroke Screen (LAPSS)

For evaluation of acute, noncomatose, nontraumatic neurologic complaint. If items 1 through 6 are ***all*** **checked "Yes"** (or "Unknown"), provide prearrival notification to hospital of potential stroke patient. If any item is checked "No," return to appropriate treatment protocol. *Interpretation:* 93% of patients with stroke will have a positive LAPSS score (sensitivity = 93%), and 97% of those with a positive LAPSS score will have a stroke (specificity = 97%). Note that the patient may still be experiencing a stroke if LAPSS criteria are not met.

Criteria	**Yes**	**Unknown**	**No**
1. Age >45 years	❑	❑	❑
2. History of seizures or epilepsy **absent**	❑	❑	❑
3. Symptom duration <24 hours	❑	❑	❑
4. At baseline, patient is **not** wheelchair bound or bedridden	❑	❑	❑
5. Blood glucose between 60 and 400	❑	❑	❑

6. ***Obvious asymmetry*** (right vs left) in ***any*** of the following 3 exam categories **(must be unilateral):**

	Equal	**R Weak**	**L Weak**
Facial smile/grimace	❑	❑ Droop	❑ Droop
Grip	❑	❑ Weak grip	❑ Weak grip
	❑	❑ No grip	❑ No grip
Arm strength	❑	❑ Drifts down	❑ Drifts down
	❑	❑ Falls rapidly	❑ Falls rapidly

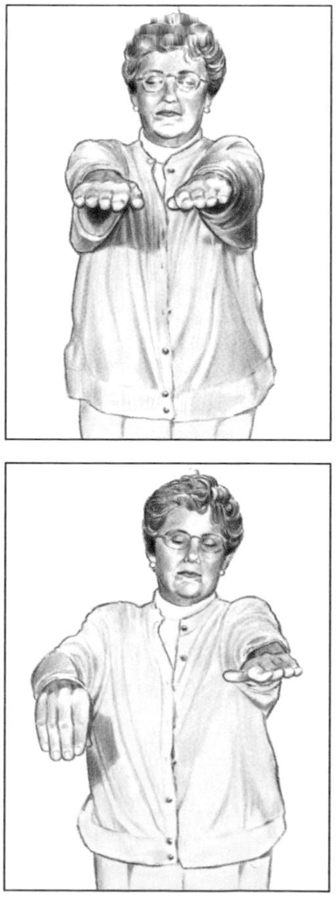

One-sided motor weakness (right arm).

Kidwell CS, Saver JL, Schubert GB, Eckstein M, Starkman S. Design and retrospective analysis of the Los Angeles prehospital stroke screen (LAPSS). *Prehosp Emerg Care.* 1998;2:267-273.

Kidwell CS, Starkman S, Eckstein M, Weems K, Saver JL. Identifying stroke in the field: prospective validation of the Los Angeles Prehospital Stroke Screen (LAPSS). *Stroke.* 2000;31:71-76.

of a stroke patient and shortens the time required to determine whether the patient has indications for acute stroke therapy.

Prehospital Support of Cardiopulmonary Function

Prehospital assessment and management requires evaluation and support of the ABCs of critical care (**A**irway, **B**reathing, and **C**irculation) and close monitoring of vital signs and neurologic function.

Airway

Paralysis of the muscles of the throat, tongue, or mouth can lead to partial or complete upper-airway obstruction. Saliva may pool in the throat and be aspirated. The stroke victim may vomit, and aspiration of vomitus is a concern.

- Suction the oropharynx or nasopharynx as needed. Avoid trauma, which can lead to significant bleeding if the patient is subsequently treated with tPA.
- Turn the patient to a lateral decubitus position or—preferably—the *recovery position* (on the side, with the arm used to sustain neck extension) to facilitate removal of vomitus.
- Support the airway by positioning the head and neck or placing an oropharyngeal or nasopharyngeal airway.
- Administer supplemental oxygen as needed.
- If ventilation is inadequate, provide positive-pressure ventilation.
- Provide advanced airway maneuvers in the field when basic airway management is ineffective. Comatose patients are at particular risk for upper-airway obstruction and often require advanced airway maneuvers (nasotracheal intubation should be avoided because of the increased risk of traumatic bleeding).

Exercise caution in moving the patient's neck if there is a possibility of cervical trauma. A history of cervical trauma will not be known if the patient is comatose.

- Injury to the head or neck may precipitate a stroke.
- The stroke victim may fall with the onset of stroke, producing a secondary cervical injury.
- *If the victim may have sustained trauma to the head or neck, immobilize the head and neck until a firm cervical collar is in place.*

Breathing

Stroke victims may develop breathing abnormalities, and rescue breathing may be needed. Abnormal respirations are common in comatose patients and portend serious brain injury.

- Irregular respiratory rates include prolonged pauses, Cheyne-Stokes respirations, or neurogenic hyperventilation.
- Shallow respirations or inadequate air exchange resulting from paralysis can occur.
- Promptly begin rescue breathing, assisted ventilation, and supplemental oxygen when indicated.
- Severe, coma-producing brain injuries can lead to respiratory arrest, but this is usually preceded by other abnormalities in the respiratory pattern.
- Provide rescue breathing or assisted ventilation immediately if respiratory arrest or inadequate respirations develop.

Circulation

Cardiac arrest is an uncommon complication of stroke. Cardiac abnormalities in stroke patients are usually related to the development of perfusing arrhythmias or respiratory arrest. Very few stroke patients require chest compressions.

- Arrhythmias and changes in blood pressure frequently complicate stroke, and monitoring of both blood pressure and cardiac rhythm is part of the early assessment of a stroke victim.
- Hypotension or shock is rarely caused by stroke, so if these clinical problems develop, seek causes other than the stroke.
- Hypertension is often present in stroke patients, but it typically subsides and does not require treatment. Treatment of hypertension in the field is not recommended. Decisions about this therapy should be made in the ED, where blood pressure can be monitored continuously. Cardiac arrhythmias may point to an underlying cardiac cause of stroke or may be a consequence of the stroke. Bradycardia may indicate hypoxia or elevation of intracranial pressure (ICP).

Other Supportive Measures

Other supportive measures, such as IV access, management of seizures, and diagnosis and treatment of hypoglycemia, can be initiated during transport to the hospital if necessary.

- Isotonic fluids (normal saline or lactated Ringer's solution) are used for IV therapy; hypotonic fluids are contraindicated because they can precipitate an abrupt fall in serum sodium and osmolality and an extravascular fluid shift that can contribute to the development of cerebral edema.
- Glucose-containing solutions should be avoided unless hypoglycemia is documented by rapid glucose test or is strongly suspected from history.
- Bolus administration of fluids is not indicated unless hypovolemia is present.
- Vital signs—pulse, respirations, and blood pressure—should be checked frequently so that changes or abnormalities can be detected. Disturbances in these signs are frequent.

4. *Door:* ED Triage

Even if a potential stroke victim arrives in the ED in a timely fashion, excessive time may elapse before appropriate neurologic consultation and diagnostic studies are performed.

- Hospitals should notify community EMS services whether they have the equipment and personnel to manage patients with acute stroke.
- More and more hospitals have assembled a specific "stroke team" or a designated "stroke unit" to organize personnel and equipment. The purpose of these designated teams or units is to evaluate the patient with acute stroke as efficiently as possible.
- To maximize efficiency, use checklists, standing orders, and written protocols. The NINDS study group has recommended goals that use upper time limits for evaluation of acute stroke patients who are candidates for fibrinolytic therapy (Table 2). These targets define the critical time interval that should be achieved for 80% of patients with acute stroke.

5. *Data:* ED Evaluation and Management

Once the patient arrives in the ED a number of assessment and management activities must occur quickly and without delay. The time clock is blinking the phrase "time is brain."

Assess the ABCs quickly and recheck frequently. The initial neurologic evaluation should be performed as quickly as possible. Confirm the precise time of stroke or onset of symptoms from family or people at the scene: *this is critical.* All the data necessary to make the decision for or against fibrinolytics is gathered at this point. The data assembled in the ED is summarized in the box below and described in the text in more detail.

TABLE 2. NINDS-Recommended Stroke Evaluation Targets for Potential Fibrinolytic Candidates*

Time Targets	
Door to doctor:	10 minutes
Door to CT completion:	25 minutes
Door to CT read:	45 minutes
Door to treatment:	60 minutes
Access to neurologic expertise†:	15 minutes
Access to neurosurgical expertise†:	2 hours
Admit to monitored bed:	3 hours

CT indicates computed tomography.
*Target times will not be achieved in all cases but represent a reasonable goal.
†By phone or in person.

5. *Data:* ED Evaluation and Management

- **A.** Emergency neurologic assessment
  1. Level of consciousness
  2. Type of stroke (hemorrhagic vs nonhemorrhagic)
  3. Location of stroke (carotid vs vertebrobasilar)
  4. Severity of stroke
- **B.** General medical assessment
- **C.** Differential diagnosis
- **D.** Emergency diagnostic studies
  1. CT scan, noncontrast
  2. Lumbar puncture (subarachnoid bleeding suspected)
  3. Electrocardiogram (ECG)
  4. Blood studies, especially all tests related to bleeding: 3 P's: platelets, prothrombin time (PT), partial thromboplastin time (PTT)
  5. Magnetic resonance imaging (MRI)
  6. Cerebral angiography

A. Emergency Neurologic Assessment

Emergency neurologic assessment focuses on 4 key issues:

1. Level of consciousness
2. Type of stroke (hemorrhagic versus nonhemorrhagic)
3. Location of stroke (carotid versus vertebrobasilar)
4. Severity of stroke

Perform focal neurologic examinations frequently so that any change in condition (worsening or improvement) can be detected. Repeat neurologic exams need not be exhaustive.

1. Level of Consciousness and Evaluation of Brain Stem Function

The *level of consciousness* tells you a great deal about what is happening with a patient:

- *Depressed consciousness* within hours of stroke onset indicates a ***severe brain insult,*** with ***increased ICP.*** Most often the cause is an *intracerebral or subarachnoid hemorrhage.*
- *Early stupor or coma* occurs with *massive hemispheric or brain stem infarction.* Stupor and coma are uncommon with ischemic strokes (nonhemorrhagic).
- *Coma,* the lack of any purposeful response to external stimuli, usually indicates damage to *both cerebral hemispheres* or the *brain stem.*
- *Coma* at the *onset* of stroke usually means that a *massive hemorrhage or basilar artery occlusion* has occurred. Coma may also indicate a cardiac arrest with global brain ischemia or metabolic/toxic problems, such as a drug overdose.
- All patients presenting with *depressed consciousness* are at risk of aspiration and death. *Depressed consciousness* may indicate the start of brain herniation occurring in the first few hours after onset of stroke.
- Use the Glasgow Coma Scale (GCS) (Table 3) to appraise neurologic function in patients with altered consciousness. The total score ranges from 3 through 15. It is based on the best responses elicited for eye opening (1 through 4), verbal responses (1 through 5), and movement (1 through 6). A patient with a GCS score of 8 or less has a very poor prognosis.

Examination of the eyes provides an excellent evaluation of brain function, even in comatose patients.

- The size, equality, and reactivity of the **pupils and** the **position** of the eyes should be evaluated at rest and in response to the doll's eyes maneuver (turning of the head from side to side).
- Corneal **reflexes,** gag reflexes, and respiratory pattern should also be evaluated.
- *Unilateral pupil dilation* may be the first sign of brain stem dysfunction due to *uncal herniation (coning).*
- *Fixed, dilated pupil* in an alert patient complaining of intense headache suggests a *ruptured aneurysm.*
- *The doll's eyes test* evaluates brain stem function. In this test the eyes move conjugately in a direction opposite head rotation in a patient with an intact brain stem.
- In an obtunded or comatose patient, if the eyes move fully side to side, the *doll's eyes reflex is positive* (good). This implies that the brain stem is functioning. When the doll's eyes reflex is absent (the eyes do not rotate in their sockets when the head is turned), significant brain stem dysfunction may be present. *Absent corneal response* and *absent gag reflex* imply severe brain stem dysfunction.

TABLE 3. Glasgow Coma Scale

	Score
Eye opening	
■ Spontaneous	4
■ In response to speech	3
■ In response to pain	2
■ None	1
Best verbal response	
■ Oriented conversation	5
■ Confused conversation	4
■ Inappropriate words	3
■ Incomprehensible sounds	2
■ None	1
Best motor response	
■ Obeys	6
■ Localizes	5
■ Withdraws	4
■ Abnormal flexion	3
■ Abnormal extension	2
■ None	1

A variety of irregular respiratory patterns, including Cheyne-Stokes respiration, may also occur with cortical damage, and neurogenic hyperventilation or ataxic respiration may occur with brain stem damage. The absence of any spontaneous respiration is obviously an ominous sign and may imply brain death in the absence of hypothermia or sedating drugs.

2. Type of Stroke: Ischemic or Hemorrhagic

There are *4 classes of stroke,* 2 caused by clots (ischemic stroke) and 2 by hemorrhage (hemorrhagic stroke).

The 4 Classes of Stroke

- *Ischemic stroke:* caused by blood clots
  (85% of all strokes; the only type that can receive fibrinolytics)
  1. Cerebral thrombosis
  2. Cerebral embolism
- *Hemorrhagic stroke:* caused by ruptured blood vessels
  3. Intracerebral hemorrhage
  4. Subarachnoid hemorrhage

The 2 classes of stroke caused by clots are *cerebral thrombosis* and *cerebral embolism.* These are by far the most common types of stroke, accounting for about 85% of all strokes.

The 2 types of stroke caused by hemorrhage and ruptured blood vessels are *intracerebral hemorrhage* and *subarachnoid hemorrhage.* Patients with hemorrhagic stroke are not eligible for fibrinolytic therapy. The histories and physical findings of hemorrhagic and ischemic stroke overlap, and you should not depend solely on the clinical presentation for diagnosis. *In most cases a noncontrast CT scan is the definitive test for differentiating ischemic from hemorrhagic stroke.*

3. Stroke Location (Carotid vs Vertebrobasilar)

In an alert patient with possible stroke, assess the higher cortical functions, including language, visual, cranial nerve, motor, and sensory functions. The neurologic signs help distinguish a stroke involving the anterior circulation from one involving the posterior (vertebrobasilar) circulation.

- **Brain stem location:** suggested by *crossed deficits* (1-sided motor weakness with contralateral sensory deficit) or *bilateral* neurologic signs
- **Subcortical or lacunar infarct** caused by small-vessel disease: suggested by a *pure sensory stroke* or *dysarthria with a clumsy hand*
- Some clinical signs, such as a ***pure motor deficit,*** are rare. In practice it is often difficult to distinguish lacunar from nonlacunar infarcts on the basis of clinical features, especially in the first few hours after stroke onset.

4. Stroke Severity

- The ***National Institutes of Health Stroke Scale*** (NIHSS) (*ECC Guidelines 2000,* pages 212-213: Appendix A) has become the standard, routine in-hospital measure of neurologic function. This scale should routinely be used by all healthcare professionals who care for acute stroke patients in the ED or in-patient setting, especially emergency medicine physicians, nurses, and allied health personnel. Because of the need to use this scale routinely, the AHA ECC Committee and the AHA Stroke Council have included this scale in all ACLS textbooks published since 1997.

- The NIHSS should be performed before administration of fibrinolytic therapy.
- NIHSS scores correlate with stroke severity and long-term outcome and provide a reliable, valid, and easy-to-perform neurologic examination.
- The NIHSS can be performed in less than 7 minutes to enable trending of multiple standardized neurologic evaluations of the patient over time.
- The NIHSS total score ranges from 0 (normal) to 42 points, broken down into 5 major areas:
  - — Level of consciousness
  - — Visual assessment
  - — Motor function
  - — Sensation and neglect
  - — Cerebellar function
- The NIHSS is not a comprehensive neurologic examination (eg, it does not record gait or all cranial nerve deficits), and further neurologic evaluation should be performed on a case-by-case basis.

The NIHSS helps guide decisions about fibrinolytic therapy in ischemic stroke patients:

- Patients with mild (or improving) neurologic deficits (NIHSS less than 4), such as sensory loss or dysarthria with a clumsy hand, are not candidates for fibrinolytic therapy. For these patients with mild deficits, the amount of benefit gained will be minimal and does not justify the risk of intracranial bleeding incurred with fibrinolytic therapy. Exceptions may include isolated severe aphasia (NIHSS 3) or hemianopsia (NIHSS 2 or 3).
- In patients with severe deficits (NIHSS greater than 22), a large area of the brain has probably been infarcted. These patients are at higher risk for developing a symptomatic hemorrhage associated with fibrinolytic therapy. The risk of hemorrhage versus the benefit of treatment must be evaluated on an individual basis.
- The Hunt and Hess Scale (Table 4) for Subarachnoid Hemorrhage is useful for grading severity, probability of survival, and probability of complications. The Hunt and Hess Scale applies only to patients with subarachnoid hemorrhage and is not useful for grading other types of stroke.

TABLE 4. Hunt and Hess Scale for Subarachnoid Hemorrhage

Grade	Neurologic Status
1	Asymptomatic
2	Severe headache or nuchal rigidity; no neurologic deficit
3	Drowsy; minimal neurologic deficit
4	Stuporous; moderate to severe hemiparesis
5	Deep coma; decerebrate posturing

B. General Medical Assessment

The physical examination alone can indicate important causes and complications in a patient with acute stroke. Table 5 provides some examples of signs noted on physical examination and comments on what those signs may indicate.

C. Differential Diagnosis: Sudden Onset of Focal Brain Dysfunction

The ***sudden onset of focal brain dysfunction*** is the ***hallmark of stroke.*** Few nonvascular neurologic diseases cause sudden, focal brain dysfunction. If the patient's neurologic function gradually worsens over several days rather than improves, think more of a nonvascular neurologic disease as the cause of the "stroke."

Hypoglycemia and seizures are 2 problems that merit special comment. **Hypoglycemia** can cause focal neurologic signs, such as aphasia or hemiparesis, with or without an altered mental status. Consider *hypoglycemia* in any patient with a potential stroke. **Seizures** may mimic or complicate stroke. Signs such as paresis or aphasia can persist for several hours after a seizure (Todd's paralysis), often in combination with some clouding of consciousness. A patient found after a seizure may present with only these postictal neurologic signs. With some patients, it will be difficult to distinguish paralysis

Differential Diagnosis of Focal Brain Dysfunction

Cerebrovascular Events

- Hemorrhagic stroke
- Ischemic stroke
- Postcardiac arrest ischemia
- Hypertensive encephalopathy

Trauma: Craniocerebral/cervical trauma

Infection: Meningitis/encephalitis/brain abscess

Intracranial Mass Effects

- Tumor
- Subdural/epidural hematoma

Seizures

- Seizure and persistence of postictal neurologic signs (Todd's paralysis)

Complicated Migraine

- Migraine, hemiplegia: migraine and persistent neurologic signs

Metabolic/Toxic

- Hyperglycemia (nonketotic hyperosmolar coma)
- Hypoglycemia
- Hyponatremia
- Drug overdose

TABLE 5. Physical Examination Findings and Their Potential Significance In Stroke*

Stroke Assessment Finding	Comments/Points to Consider
■ Cardiac arrest associated with onset of stroke	■ Points to an underlying cardiac cause of stroke
■ Bradycardia	■ Classic sign of elevated ICP ■ Response to hypoxia, which may be caused by airway obstruction or hypoventilation
■ Prolonged QT interval ■ Altered P, T, and U waves ■ ST-segment depression or elevation	■ Arrhythmias may complicate stroke, particularly hemorrhagic stroke
■ Atrial fibrillation ■ Atrial flutter and ■ No aspirin or anticoagulant	■ Common causes of embolic stroke—should be ruled out
■ No pulse felt below knees ■ Extremity cool to touch	■ Suggests multiple, recurrent emboli
■ Carotid bruit	■ High-grade carotid stenosis or small emboli from atherosclerotic lesions in carotid artery causing stroke
■ Head or orbit bruits	■ Stroke secondary to large cerebral arteriovenous malformation
■ Petechiae or ecchymoses	■ Hemorrhagic stroke secondary to blood dyscrasia or coagulopathy
■ Preretinal (subhyaloid) hemorrhages	■ Subarachnoid hemorrhage in a comatose patient
■ Papilledema	■ Rarely seen in first hours after stroke ■ When present, consider an intracranial mass such as a tumor or neoplasm
■ Patient with acute stroke and fever	■ Infective endocarditis? Septic emboli from heart through carotid arteries?
■ Irregular rhythm, friction rub, murmur, click, or gallop	■ Might suggest a cardiac cause of emboli
■ Patient with general signs and symptoms of stroke	■ Always check glucose, ethanol, narcotics, other drugs ■ Also check electrolytes, drug overdoses, osmolality problems
■ Altered level of consciousness in general	■ Check for possible head and neck injury ■ Any evidence of cranial or cervical trauma ■ When practical, check blood glucose level before treatment with 50% dextrose

*For the interested reader, see the expanded Table 16 in Chapter 18 of the *ACLS Reference Textbook*.

caused by a stroke from postictal Todd's paralysis. Most stroke patients with paralysis maintain an alert level of consciousness. Be aware that different types of strokes have different associations with seizures in the first 24 hours after the stroke:

- After thrombotic stroke: seizures are rare
- After embolic stroke: seizures occur in 5% to 10% of patients
- After subarachnoid hemorrhage: seizures follow in 15% of patients

The differential diagnosis of a stroke is included in the box on the preceding page.

D. Emergency Diagnostic Studies

Diagnostic studies in the ED establish stroke as the cause of the patient's symptoms, differentiate brain infarction from brain hemorrhage, and determine the most likely cause of the stroke.

CT Scan (Noncontrast)

- A noncontrast CT scan is the single most important diagnostic test for patients with a possible stroke. It is critical to rule out hemorrhagic stroke as soon as possible. Fibrinolytic agents cannot be given until the possibility of a hemorrhagic stroke is eliminated.
- Try to obtain the CT scan within 25 minutes of arrival at the ED door and have it read within the next 20 minutes (total of 45 minutes from arrival at the ED door).
- If CT is not readily available, stabilize the patient and transfer him or her to an appropriate facility. The CT scan is needed even if the patient will not be given fibrinolytics.
- Withhold anticoagulants and fibrinolytics until you exclude a brain hemorrhage with the CT. To avoid confusing blood and contrast, perform CT without contrast enhancement.

What to Look for on a CT Scan (Noncontrast)

- Blood has a density that is about 3% greater than brain tissue. On modern CT scanners this 3% difference in density can be manipulated so that hemorrhage and free blood will appear distinctly white in comparison with surrounding tissues.
- Contrast agents also "light up" on CT scan. Because these agents would obscure the high-contrast areas of free blood, always start with a noncontrast CT. This will prevent any confusion between an acute hemorrhage and the contrast agent.
- With an acute ischemic stroke, however, blood flow is blocked to an area of the brain. Acutely brain structures with or without normal blood flow appear the same on the CT scan. Therefore the CT scan will usually appear "normal" for a few hours after blood flow to an area of the brain that is blocked or reduced. Thus, ischemic brain tissue often cannot be identified on CT scan within hours of a stroke.
- The ischemic brain, however, is damaged and will soon begin to swell and become edematous. After 6 to 12 hours the edema and swelling produce a hypodense area that is usually visible on a CT scan. This well-defined hypodensity, however, rarely develops within the 3-hour limit required for administration of fibrinolytics. *Note:* The time of stroke onset is likely to be more than 3 hours if a hypodensity is present on CT scan. In general a hypodense area on CT scan excludes a patient from fibrinolytic therapy on CT scan. You can certainly say that this hypodense area indicates a recent stroke, but you cannot say exactly how recent the stroke was, and it is probably more than 3 hours old.
- A CT scan may fail to depict small infarctions or ischemic lesions in the cerebellum or brain stem. Large areas of infarction, however, may cause early, subtle CT changes, for example, a blurred or obscure junction of the gray-white matter, effaced sulci, or areas of early hypodensity.
- One helpful comment to remember: *to qualify as a candidate for fibrinolytic treatment, the patient should have an acute CT scan that appears normal—no sign of hemorrhage, no large areas of no flow, and no hypodense areas (which would suggest that the stroke is over 3 hours old).*

Almost all patients with a recent intracerebral hemorrhage will have a CT scan with increased density in the location of the bleeding.

- With subdural bleeding/hematoma, there is a classic display of blood in a fingernail-shaped, crescent moon–shaped, or sickle-shaped hematoma below the dura.
- In epidural bleeding the hemorrhage pattern appears as a lens-shaped, biconvex, football-shaped pattern adhering to the undersurface of the inner table of the skull and the epidural surface of the brain.
- In subarachnoid hemorrhage the hyperdensity of the blood is noted diffusely, spreading along the irregular surface of the brain in the subarachnoid space.
- The CT findings in subarachnoid hemorrhage may also be subtle, showing only a thin white layer adjacent to the brain.
- Specific CT features often indicate the cause of hemorrhage. For example, blood in the basal cisterns occurs commonly with ruptured aneurysms. Acute intracranial complications of stroke, such as hydrocephalus, edema, mass effect, or shift of normal brain structures, can also be seen with CT.

Probable Subarachnoid Hemorrhage + Normal CT Scan = Lumbar Puncture (LP)

The initial CT appears normal in approximately 5% of patients with diagnosed subarachnoid hemorrhage (SAH). Such patients usually have a small SAH and are alert, with no focal neurologic deficits (Hunt and Hess Scale grade 1).

This means, however, that of every 20 patients with confirmed SAH, 1 patient had a normal initial CT scan. The key to diagnosis must be the level of clinical suspicion. With a high clinical suspicion of SAH and a negative CT scan, you must ask "Is this patient really bleeding into his brain with a normal CT scan? Is he one of the 20 SAH victims with a normal CT scan?"

The Current Recommendation:

- If you have a high clinical suspicion that the patient has a SAH despite a normal CT scan, perform an LP to look for acute blood in the cerebrospinal fluid (CSF). *Note:* An LP eliminates any potential use of fibrinolytic therapy. If CT demonstrates blood in a patient with SAH, an LP is not necessary.
- If the spinal tap yields bloody CSF, compare the appearance of the fluid in successive tubes. SAH produces bloody CSF that is the same in all 4 LP tubes. The red blood cell count should not vary from tube to tube.
- Immediately centrifuge the CSF from the LP. Observe whether the supernatant fluid is xanthochromic, ie, an orange-yellow color. This color is from *old* red blood cells and not related to a traumatic tap. It may take several hours—up to 12—after SAH for the fluid to become yellow. Therefore, xanthochromic spinal fluid has a high positive predictive value when symptom onset occurred a number of hours before the emergency evaluation. Repeat CT scans and LPs may be required.

Other Diagnostic Tests: 12-Lead ECG, Chest, and Cervical Spine Radiographs

- Electrocardiography can demonstrate recent MI or arrhythmias such as atrial fibrillation that may be the cause of embolic stroke.
- ECG changes can also be triggered by stroke, especially if intracerebral hemorrhage has occurred.
- Chest x-rays can confirm or rule out cardiomegaly, pulmonary edema, and aspiration.
- In comatose patients or patients unable to give a good history and in whom trauma is suspected, obtain lateral cervical spine x-rays. These radiographs help locate fractures or dislocations.

Important Blood Tests

- A complete blood count, platelet count, International Normalized Ratio (INR)/PT, and PTT are useful screens for hematologic causes of stroke or a blood dyscrasia.
- Coagulation studies are recommended for patients who may receive fibrinolytic therapy or undergo a neurosurgical procedure.
- When a "surgical" lesion is suspected or if the patient with ischemic stroke is a candidate for fibrinolytic therapy, obtain a blood sample for type and screen.
- Specialized studies for hypercoagulative states and hematologic disorders associated with stroke (sickle cell anemia, protein S deficiency) can be performed after admission, especially in young stroke patients.
- Assess the initial oxygen saturation by pulse oximetry (avoid arterial puncture for blood gases if fibrinolytic therapy is being considered).
- Perform a chemistry screen, including electrolytes and glucose.
- Stroke may be a complication of drug or alcohol abuse. Obtain urine or blood specimens if clinically indicated to determine the presence of cocaine, amphetamines, opiates, or alcohol.

Magnetic Resonance Imaging

MRI is not part of the routine evaluation of acute stroke.

- Although MRI is very sensitive and will detect some lesions missed by CT, it is not superior to CT for detecting hemorrhage. Hemorrhage is the most important indication for emergency brain imaging in suspected stroke.
- MRI is time-consuming, not universally available, expensive, and may hamper continuous observation of the acutely ill patient.

Cerebral Angiography

- Most emergency cerebral angiography is performed in patients with SAH.
- This allows neurosurgeons to plan better for aneurysm clipping.
- Neurointerventional procedures such as aneurysm coiling, angioplasty, and intra-arterial fibrinolytic therapy also require emergency angiography in selected patients.
- Many other studies can be performed electively, including echocardiography, carotid artery ultrasound, and transcranial Doppler echocardiography.

6. *Decision:* Specific Stroke Therapies

General Care of the Stroke Patient

The general care of the stroke patient is summarized in Table 6 and discussed in more detail in the section below:

Table 6. General Management of the Patient With Acute Stroke

1. IV fluids	Avoid D_5W and excessive fluid loading.
2. Blood sugar	Determine immediately. Bolus of 50% dextrose if hypoglycemic; insulin if >300 mg%.
3. Thiamine	100 mg if malnourished, alcoholic.
4. Oxygen	Pulse oximetry. Supplement if indicated.
5. Acetaminophen	If febrile.
6. NPO	If at risk for aspiration.

1. Establish IV access and administer either normal saline or lactated Ringer's solution. Avoid hypotonic solutions because they may contribute to brain edema. Unless the patient is hypotensive, rapid infusion of fluids is not required.
2. Administer a bolus of 50% dextrose and water if *hypoglycemia* is shown by rapid blood glucose determinations. Mild *hyperglycemia* is typically not corrected because such attempts often produce hypoglycemia. Markedly elevated glucose levels, however, warrant treatment.
3. Administer thiamine (100 mg) empirically to all cachectic, malnourished, or chronic alcoholic patients with suspected stroke.
4. Ensure adequate tissue oxygenation. Determine oxygen saturation for all patients with acute stroke and provide supplemental oxygen if desaturation is present. Routine use of supplemental oxygen conveys no benefit to patients with acute stroke who have normal oxygen saturation.
5. Fever can damage the ischemic brain. Use antipyretics early while the source of fever is being ascertained.
6. Record the volume of infused fluids and urinary output. Most stroke patients do not require an indwelling bladder catheter. Avoid placing one if possible. During the first few hours after a stroke, do not give the patient food or drink. Paralysis of bulbar muscles, decreased alertness, and vomiting can all increase the risk of aspiration or airway obstruction.

Management of Elevated Blood Pressure

Management of blood pressure after acute ischemic and hemorrhagic stroke is controversial. Current recommendations are based on the type of stroke (hemorrhagic or ischemic) and whether the patient is a candidate for fibrinolytic therapy.

Many patients develop hypertension after either ischemic or hemorrhagic stroke, but few require emergency treatment. Elevated blood pressure after stroke does not constitute a hypertensive emergency unless the patient has other medical indications, such as AMI or left ventricular failure. In most patients blood pressure will fall spontaneously as pain, agitation, vomiting, and increased ICP are controlled.

The following are AHA consensus recommendations for blood pressure management in acute ischemic stroke:

- Do not routinely treat elevated blood pressure in patients with acute ischemic stroke.
- Treat elevated blood pressure in patients who are candidates for fibrinolytic therapy (see sections below).
- Treat patients with specific medical indications. The major indications include
  - — AMI
  - — Aortic dissection
  - — True hypertensive encephalopathy
  - — Severe left ventricular failure
- Treat patients with severely elevated blood pressures at these levels:
  - — Systolic pressure greater than 180 to 185 mm Hg
  - — Diastolic pressure greater than 105 to 110 mm Hg
  - — Mean arterial pressure greater than 130 mm Hg
- Labetalol is the preferred antihypertensive agent because it is easy to titrate and has a limited effect on cerebral blood vessels.
- Do not use sublingual nifedipine; it can produce a precipitous drop in blood pressure that could extend an acute ischemic stroke.

Treatment of Elevated Blood Pressures if Fibrinolytic Therapy Is Planned

- Stringent control of blood pressure is necessary to decrease the chance of bleeding after administration of fibrinolytics.
- Fibrinolytic therapy is *contraindicated* for patients with a systolic blood pressure greater than 185 mm Hg or a diastolic pressure greater than 110 mm Hg at the time fibrinolytic therapy is started.
- Fibrinolytic therapy can be administered, however, if clinicians can bring acute blood pressure below 185 mm Hg systolic and 110 mm Hg diastolic in the ED with simple measures and medications.

Recommended Approach

- ***Nitroglycerin*** paste (because it can be titrated and easily removed).

or

- ***Labetalol*** 10 to 20 mg IV; may repeat 1 or 2 times.

or

- ***Enalapril*** 0.625 to 1.25 mg IV push.

- If nitroglycerin and labetalol are unsuccessful in reducing blood pressure below *185/110 mm Hg* within the *3-hour* time window for tPA, do not give fibrinolytics.
- If labetalol and nitroglycerin reduce blood pressure below 185/110 mm Hg, start fibrinolytics.
- Once tPA is started, monitor blood pressure closely. If blood pressure is unstable or hypertension develops, treat the problem aggressively.

7. *Drugs:* Fibrinolytic Therapy for Ischemic Stroke

The National Institute of Neurologic Disorders and Stroke (NINDS) Trial

In 1996 the US Food and Drug Administration (FDA) approved IV tPA for use in selected patients with ischemic stroke. The FDA based this approval on the positive results of the 2-part NINDS Trial, which was the only prospective, randomized controlled trial to show that the benefits of fibrinolytic therapy outweigh the risks. Many experts, including reviewers from the FDA, consider the positive results of the NINDS Trial more compelling than the negative results from several other trials. Their reasoning is that the NINDS trials "finally got it right" in terms of stronger study design and methods. In addition, the NINDS investigators used a safer dosing schedule and limited the trial to "early" stroke patients only, ie, those who could receive the fibrinolytic agent in less than 3 hours after stroke symptoms started.

Improved Outcomes

Patients enrolled in the NINDS 2-part studies who were treated with tPA within 3 hours of symptom onset were at least 30% more likely to have minimal or no disability at 3 months compared with those treated with placebo. However, there were 10-fold increases in the risk of fatal intracranial hemorrhage in the treated group (3% vs 0.3%) and a 10-fold increase in the frequency of all symptomatic hemorrhage (6.4% vs 0.6%).

Success and Disappointments

Clinical experience with fibrinolytics since 1996 has been good. Widespread predictions of excessive morbidity from intracranial bleeding have not proved accurate. Disappointments include the failure of some stroke patients and their families to seek immediate care when signs and symptoms of stroke appear. Some healthcare professionals have adopted a "wait and see" attitude toward fibrinolytic therapy for patients with acute stroke and have been reluctant to establish hospital- or community-based stroke teams. Clinical leaders and EMS system managers must attempt to bring local EMS systems into the planning and implementation of stroke care to reduce delay in treatment for stroke patients.

IV tPA represents the first FDA-approved therapy for acute ischemic stroke. *All patients presenting within 3 hours of the onset of signs and symptoms consistent with an acute ischemic stroke should be aggressively evaluated as candidates for IV fibrinolytic therapy.* The following section focuses on specific issues that all clinical caregivers, including ACLS providers, must consider when evaluating stroke patients for fibrinolytic therapy.

Advance Planning for Stroke Victims Is Required

All hospitals must develop and have in place policies and protocols for the identification and management of stroke patients. These policies and protocols must include specific strategies to achieve rapid diagnosis and therapy. Multidisciplinary input is required from emergency physicians, neurologists, neurosurgeons, internists, nurses, pharmacists, and prehospital personnel. As a minimum, care planning should address these issues:

- **Identification of patients** with possible acute stroke in the prehospital setting
- **Notification of hospitals** about patients with possible acute stroke before their arrival
- Designation of personnel to perform **rapid triage and medical evaluation** in the ED
- An agreed-upon plan for radiology to perform **noncontrast CTs of the head** quickly and effectively
- A plan for notification of a skilled physician to read the CT in a timely fashion (less than 20 minutes from completion of the CT)
- Designation of responsibility for determining **contraindications to fibrinolytic therapy**
- A plan for stocking, compounding, and administering fibrinolytic **agents**
- A plan for obtaining **urgent consultation** for atypical cases or hemorrhagic complications
- Agreement about which service will be the **admitting service**

Current AHA Recommendations: Use of Fibrinolytic Agents in Treatment of Acute Ischemic Stroke

Alteplase (tPA): Strict Adherence to Protocol

The fibrinolytic agent alteplase (tPA) should be administered to only carefully selected patients with strict adherence to treatment protocols. As noted above, fibrinolytic therapy can be provided when a physician experienced in diagnosing stroke is involved, when a physician trained to assess CT scans is part of the decision, and when they agree that the diagnosis of acute ischemic stroke is established and other contraindications to fibrinolytic therapy have been ruled out (see Table 7).

Resources must be available to handle potential bleeding complications in a timely fashion. These resources must be immediately available at either the treating hospital or another hospital accessible by ground or aeromedical transport.

Administration Guidelines

1. Dose

tPA is given IV (0.9 mg/kg, maximum 90 mg), with 10% of the dose given as a bolus followed by the remainder as an infusion lasting 60 minutes.

2. Timing

The 10% initial bolus of tPA must be administered within 3 hours of onset of ischemic symptoms. tPA *cannot* be recommended for a person who had onset of stroke symptoms more than 3 hours before therapy except in approved investigational settings. *Do not* give tPA when the start of stroke symptoms cannot be reliably ascertained. This includes strokes recognized on awakening but probably present before awakening. The time of onset should be when the patient was last seen normal.

3. Strict inclusion and exclusion criteria

These are listed in Table 7.

4. Informed consent

Always discuss the risks and potential benefits of tPA with the patient and family before treatment begins.

- Fibrinolytic agents may cause major bleeding.
- Use caution when treating severe stroke (NIHSS greater than 22).
- Use *extreme* caution when treating patients if their acute CT shows signs of a recent large cerebral infarction (eg, sulcal effacement, mass effect, or edema). These findings are associated with an increased risk of hemorrhage from administration of tPA.

5. Hospital admission

- Give fibrinolytic therapy only when emergency ancillary care and facilities for handling bleeding complications are available.
- Admit patients treated with tPA to a skilled care facility (intensive care or stroke unit) that can provide close observation, frequent neurologic assessments, and cardiovascular monitoring.

6. Management of hypertension

- Control blood pressure carefully.
- Elevated blood pressure predisposes fibrinolytic patients to bleed.
- Aggressive lowering of blood pressure worsens ischemic symptoms.

7. Central vein access; lumbar and arterial punctures

Avoid central IV lines, lumbar punctures, and arterial punctures before, during, and for 24 hours after fibrinolytic therapy.

8. Foley catheters; nasogastric tubes

- Avoid placement of an in-dwelling bladder catheter during drug infusion and for at least 30 minutes after the infusion ends.
- Avoid insertion of a nasogastric tube if possible during the first 24 hours after treatment.

9. Avoid these medications

- Patients receiving IV tPA should not receive ***aspirin, heparin, warfarin, ticlopidine,*** or other ***antithrombotic*** or ***anti–platelet-aggregating drugs*** during the first 24 hours of stroke treatment.
- People who have taken **aspirin** are eligible for treatment with tPA if they meet all other criteria. No data exist regarding **prior** use of ticlopidine or other antiplatelet agents.

10. Management of bleeding

If the patient deteriorates and bleeding is suspected as the cause, do the following:

- Stop the fibrinolytic agent.
- Order emergency CT of the brain to rule out intracranial hemorrhage.
- Draw blood; check the hematocrit, platelet count, PTT, PT, and fibrinogen.
- Watch for a picture similar to that of disseminated intravascular coagulation (DIC) (fibrinolytic therapy can produce such a reaction for several hours after infusion).
- Prepare for transfusion, cryoprecipitate, and platelets:
  - Type and crossmatch
  - Blood: 4 U packed cells
  - 4 to 6 U cryoprecipitate or fresh frozen plasma
  - 1 U single-donor platelets
- Request neurosurgical consultation.

Anticoagulant Therapy for Acute Ischemic Stroke

Heparin

Heparin has often been prescribed for patients with acute ischemic stroke, but as of 2000 its value is unproved.

- No data has established the efficacy of anticoagulants to reverse the deficits of an acute ischemic stroke.
- A theoretical reason to give heparin to a patient with acute ischemic stroke is to help prevent recurrent embolism or propagation of a thrombus. Heparin may, however, lead to bleeding complications, including brain hemorrhage.
  - Do not give heparin until a CT scan has ruled out intracranial bleeding.
  - If heparin is administered, there is no consensus about the desired level of anticoagulation, when it should be started, or whether a loading bolus should be given.
- In light of the uncertainty about the use of heparin after stroke, the most prudent course for an emergency physician is *not* to start heparin therapy unless the patient's neurologist or the responsible attending physician concurs with the decision.
- Heparin should not be given for the first 24 hours after fibrinolytic therapy.

Low-Molecular-Weight Anticoagulants, Antiplatelets, and Alternative Agents

Low-molecular-weight anticoagulants have more selective antithrombotic actions than heparin and may offer some advantages in stroke management. In one recent study, treatment with low-molecular-weight heparin administered within 48 hours of stroke onset was associated with improvement in survival rate and increased rates of independent function compared with placebo. Subsequent studies using low-molecular-weight heparins, however, have found no benefit.

Aspirin, warfarin, and ***ticlopidine*** have all been shown to reduce the risk of subsequent stroke in patients with TIA. These agents should be started within the first few days after TIA. Their usefulness in the treatment of acute stroke is unknown.

Other Treatments for Ischemic Stroke

Calcium channel blocking drugs, volume expansion, hemodilution, and low-molecular-weight dextran have not been shown to be beneficial in improving clinical outcome after ischemic stroke. A number of cytoprotective agents have been investigated for acute ischemic and hemorrhagic stroke after having shown benefit in animal models. To date, none has been proven effective in humans.

Streptokinase

Three large, randomized trials of streptokinase in stroke have recently been reported. All 3 studies were suspended because of increased hemorrhage and mortality in the group treated with streptokinase. *Streptokinase should not be used in stroke patients except in clinical studies approved by the Institutional Review Board.*

TABLE 7. Fibrinolytic Therapy Checklist for Ischemic Stroke

All boxes must be checked before tPA can be given.

***Inclusion Criteria** (all **Yes** boxes in this section must be checked):*

Yes

- ☐ Age 18 years or older?
- ☐ Clinical diagnosis of ischemic stroke with a measurable neurologic deficit?
- ☐ Time of symptom onset (when patient was last seen normal) well established as <180 minutes (3 hours) before treatment would begin?

***Exclusion Criteria** (all **No** boxes in "Absolute Contraindications" section must be checked):*

Absolute Contraindications:

No

- ☐ Evidence of intracranial hemorrhage on pretreatment noncontrast head CT?
- ☐ Clinical presentation suggestive of subarachnoid hemorrhage even with normal CT?
- ☐ Active internal bleeding
- ☐ Acute bleeding diathesis, including but not limited to
  - — Platelet count <100 000/mm^3?
  - — Heparin received within 48 hours, resulting in an activated partial thromboplastin time (aPTT) that is greater than upper limit of normal for laboratory?
  - — Current use of anticoagulant (eg, warfarin sodium) that has produced an elevated international normalized ratio (INR) of 1.7 or prothrombin time (PT) >15 seconds?*
- ☐ Within 3 months of intracranial or intraspinal surgery, serious head trauma, or previous stroke?
- ☐ Within 14 days of major surgery or serious trauma?

Relative Contraindications:

Recent experience suggests that under some circumstances—with careful consideration and weighing of risk to benefit ratio—patients may receive fibrinolytic therapy despite one or more relative contraindications. Consider the pros and cons of tPA administration carefully if any of these relative contraindications are present:

- ☐ Only minor or rapidly improving stroke symptoms
- ☐ At the time treatment should begin, systolic pressure remains >185 mm Hg or diastolic pressure remains >110 mm Hg despite repeated measurements; or patient has required aggressive treatment to reduce blood pressure to within these limits.
- ☐ Recent lumbar puncture (within previous 21 days)
- ☐ History of intracranial hemorrhage
- ☐ Known arteriovenous malformation, neoplasm, or aneurysm
- ☐ Witnessed seizure at stroke onset
- ☐ Recent gastrointestinal or urinary tract hemorrhage (within previous 21 days)
- ☐ Recent acute myocardial infarction (within previous 21 days)
- ☐ Postmyocardial infarction pericarditis
- ☐ Abnormal blood glucose level (<50 or >400 mg/dL [<2.8 or >22.2 mmol/L])

**In patients without recent use of oral anticoagulants or heparin, treatment with tPA can be initiated before availability of coagulation study results but should be discontinued if the INR is >1.5 or the partial thromboplastin time is elevated by local laboratory standards.*

Workbook Review

1. **You are walking through a shopping mall when you encounter a 65-year-old woman who stumbled and fell as she walked out of a store. She complains of a severe headache, has a facial droop, and slurs her words. She also complains of numbness in her right arm and leg. She has difficulty raising her right arm, although her left arm moves freely. When you ask if she takes medications, she says she has "high blood pressure." Which of the following actions would be most appropriate to take at this time?**

   a. phone 911 immediately and tell the dispatcher that you are with a conscious woman who may be demonstrating signs of a stroke

   b. suggest that the woman sit down for a few minutes and see if the symptoms disappear

   c. offer to drive the woman to the ED of the local hospital

   d. suggest that the woman contact her physician immediately

   Read more about it in the ECC Guidelines 2000, *page 204: "Early Recognition" and "Role of EMS in Stroke Care"*

2. **A 70-year-old woman presents to the ED with acute onset of garbled speech and weakness in her right arm and leg, which started 15 minutes ago. Which of the following neurologic evaluation sequences should be performed for this patient over the next 45 minutes?**

   a. obtain a patient history, perform a physical and neurologic examination, obtain a noncontrast CT scan, and ensure that it is read within 45 minutes of the patient's arrival in the ED

   b. obtain a noncontrast CT scan of the head, and if the scan is positive for a stroke, begin fibrinolytic treatment

   c. obtain a targeted history and perform a physical exam and immediate lumbar puncture to rule out meningitis; obtain a noncontrast CT scan of the head

   d. obtain a noncontrast CT scan of the head, wait until the neurologic symptoms start to improve, then begin fibrinolytic treatment

   Read more about it in the ECC Guidelines 2000, *page 206: "Brief Emergency Neurological Evaluation"; page 208: "Emergency Diagnostic Studies"; and page 209: Table 7: NINDS-Recommended Stroke Evaluation Targets for Potential Fibrinolytic Candidates*

3. **Which of the following conditions can mimic the signs and symptoms of an acute stroke?**

   a. hypoglycemia

   b. cardiac arrest

   c. pneumothorax

   d. Wolff-Parkinson-White syndrome

   Read more about it in the ECC Guidelines 2000, *page 206: "Stroke Screen or Scale"; and page 208: "Differential Diagnosis" and Table 6: Differential Diagnosis of Stroke*

4. **The following patients were given a diagnosis of an acute ischemic stroke. Which of the patients as described has no apparent contraindications to IV fibrinolytic therapy?**

   a. an 80-year-old man presenting within 2 hours of onset of symptoms

   b. a 65-year-old woman who lives alone and was found unresponsive by a relative

   c. a 54-year-old man presenting within 4 hours of onset of symptoms

   d. a 40-year-old woman diagnosed with bleeding ulcers 2 weeks before onset of stroke symptoms

   Read more about it in the ECC Guidelines 2000, *page 211: "Fibrinolytic Therapy" and Table 10: Contraindications to tPA Therapy for Acute Ischemic Stroke. Also see the* ECC Handbook: *"Fibrinolytic Therapy Checklist for Ischemic Stroke"*

5. **A 56-year-old woman arrives at the ED with new onset of facial droop when she smiles, arm drift when she holds both arms out, and inability to speak clearly. Before beginning fibrinolytic therapy, the *most* important question you need to answer is**

   a. have her vital signs remained stable?

   b. when exactly did the neurologic signs begin?

   c. does she have a history of heart attack?

   d. does she have any medication allergies?

   Read more about it in the ECC Guidelines 2000, *page 207: "Time of Onset of Symptoms"; and page 211: "Fibrinolytic Therapy"*

Read More About It

See the *ECC Guidelines 2000,* pages 204-216: "Acute Ischemic Stroke" or Chapter 18 of the *ACLS Reference Textbook.*

See the *Acute Ischemic Stroke* video (product code 70-2521) and the ACLS Provider Course slides.

Basic ACLS Skills: CPR and AED

Overview

This appendix covers 3 topics: basic adult CPR, operation and use of an automated external defibrillator (AED), and the combined use of CPR and an AED. This represents the "default ACLS scenario"—a single ACLS-trained rescuer responding alone, equipped only with access to an AED.

Learning and Skills Objectives

The major objective of this appendix is to prepare you for the *CPR-AED skills evaluation station* in the ACLS course. You will be expected to successfully meet the performance guidelines of the *CPR and AED Skills Checklist* at the end of this appendix. This appendix helps you learn the CPR and AED Skills Checklist by dividing the task into 3 parts: CPR only, AED only, and both. The learning and skills objectives of the 3 parts are listed at the beginning of each part.

Why Basic CPR in an ACLS Provider Course?

This appendix is modified for ACLS providers from the textbook *Heartsaver AED,* which was introduced in 1998 to teach lay rescuers how to use the AED.

It could be argued that ACLS providers should not be evaluated on the basic skills of CPR and use of an AED. Nothing could be further from the truth. Effective CPR must be performed before, during, and frequently after any ACLS intervention.

Educational studies have shown that many ACLS providers, when evaluated only on CPR skills, perform miserably. The first ACLS providers to arrive at a rescue attempt will often need to assume command of the scene, both in-hospital and out of hospital. If ACLS providers lack knowledge of effective CPR, they will be unable to identify and correct poor performance by others.

Why AEDs in an ACLS Provider Course?

The use of AEDs is not limited to BLS. Any ACLS provider who works outside a specialized unit such as an Emergency Department or a coronary care unit is much more likely to use an AED than a conventional defibrillator. This is especially true in the present era of widespread use of AEDs in programs of public access defibrillation and defibrillation at home. News reports of the use of AEDs during commercial air travel, at sporting events, and in private health and exercise clubs testify to the need for ACLS providers to know CPR and how to use an AED.

Part 1

CPR: The Second Link in the Chain of Survival

Learning and Skills Objectives for CPR

CPR skills combine *rescue breathing (blowing)* and *chest compressions (pumping).* You will also perform CPR between AED shocks (usually after every 3 shocks). At the end of the ACLS Provider Course you will be evaluated on your performance of 1-rescuer CPR skills using a manikin.

At the end of Part 1 you should be able to

1. Describe and demonstrate the steps of 1-rescuer CPR (at the end of this appendix)
2. Describe and demonstrate how to use a barrier device (face shield and pocket mask) and bag mask during CPR
3. Describe the major signs of choking from a foreign-body airway obstruction
4. Describe and demonstrate how to treat choking from foreign-body airway obstruction in these scenarios:
   - Conscious choking victim (see the end of this appendix)
   - The choking victim becomes unresponsive/unconscious (see the

end of this appendix). *Note: As a result of the ECC Guidelines 2000 these action steps have been eliminated from the training of lay responders.*

- You respond to a cry for help and find someone lying unresponsive on the floor of a hospital room *(unknown to you, a foreign body is totally blocking the trachea).* See the end of this appendix.

Responding to an Emergency: Detailed, Annotated Steps of Basic Adult CPR

The ABCs of CPR

When you encounter an emergency—in your professional role as a healthcare provider, at home, or in the community—move quickly yet calmly. If you are alone, follow the steps noted below. If you are with others who can help, *tell them what to do.*

First, check to see whether the victim is unresponsive by tapping or gently shaking the victim and shouting "Are you OK?"

- *If the victim does not respond, send someone to phone 911 and get the AED!* This activates the EMS system and ensures that professional help is on the way. In hospital settings the same principles apply except that the in-hospital response team rather than EMS professionals will respond in the hospital setting.
- If you are alone and find an unresponsive victim, you will have to leave the victim to phone 911 and get the AED. As standard practice the AED should be stored next to a telephone. You should be able to phone 911 while reaching for the AED in its carrying case.
- After sending someone to phone 911 and get the AED, kneel at the victim's *left* side near the head to start CPR (the left side is preferred when using an AED). The victim should be on his or her back. If not, carefully turn the victim onto his or her back.

A. **Airway: open the airway with the head tilt–chin lift maneuver.**

- ◆ Lift up with 2 fingers on the chin while pushing down on the forehead with the other hand.

B. **Breathing: head tilt–chin lift; look, listen, and feel; give 2 slow breaths.**

- ◆ To check for breathing, look, listen, and feel.
  - — Place your ear next to the victim's mouth and nose (Figure 1) and listen for breathing, turning your head to observe the chest.
  - — Look for the chest to rise. Listen and feel for air movement on your cheek.
- ◆ If the victim is not breathing or not breathing adequately, give 2 slow rescue breaths (Figure 2).
- ◆ *To perform rescue breathing:* Use a barrier device when performing rescue breathing in the workplace.

FIGURE 1. Check for breathing. If no trauma is suspected, open the airway with a head tilt–chin lift, place your face near the victim's nose and mouth, and look, listen, and feel for breathing.

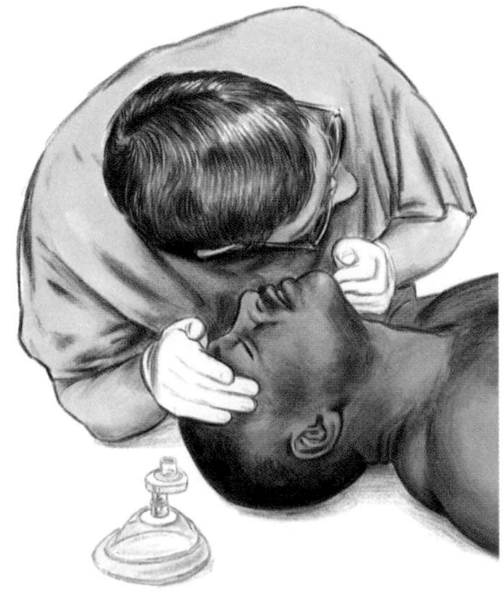

FIGURE 2. **A,** Mouth-to-mouth breathing. **B,** Mouth-to-mask technique.

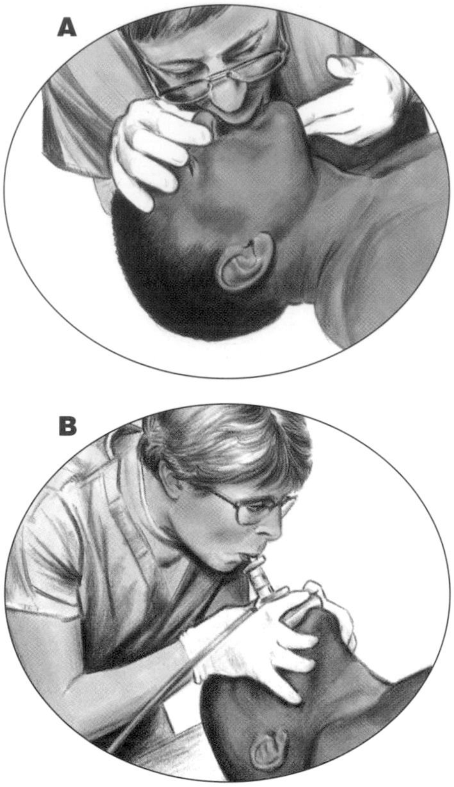

When performing CPR for an acquaintance or a loved one, rescuers may be less likely to use barrier devices because they probably know the victim's prearrest infectious status. Persons living with the victim may have already been exposed to any infectious organism. For anyone performing CPR the risk of acquiring an infectious disease is extremely small. In fact, there has never been a documented case of transmission of HIV, hepatitis, or tuberculosis during mouth-to-mouth or mouth-to-mask ventilation.

- — Place your mouth around the victim's mouth and pinch the nose closed or place the barrier device on the victim's face and place your mouth on the breathing piece or opening.
- — Continue to tilt the head and lift the chin.

— Give 2 slow breaths. Take 2 seconds to deliver each breath.

— Be sure the victim's chest clearly rises each time you give a rescue breath. If not, reopen the airway and try again.

- *To perform rescue breathing in the workplace or a public setting:*

— Quickly assemble the pocket face mask (kept in the AED case); if one is not available, perform rescue breathing with a barrier device as above.

— Place the mask over the victim's nose and mouth.

— Continue to tilt the head and lift the chin.

— Provide 2 slow breaths into the opening of the pocket face mask. Take 2 seconds to deliver each breath.

— Adjust the mask as needed to ensure a tight seal. Be sure the victim's chest clearly rises each time you blow into the mask.

C. Circulation: Check for a pulse or other signs of circulation (see details below).

- Since 2000, lay rescuers have not been taught to check for a pulse as an indicator for starting chest compressions. *(See the* ECC Guidelines 2000, *pages 39-40, for the scientific rationale behind this new recommendation.)* Instead lay responders are taught to "look for signs of circulation," which most commonly will be normal (adequate) breathing, coughing, or movement.

- Healthcare providers, however, should check for a pulse and other signs of circulation (normal breathing, coughing, or movement in response to the 2 rescue breaths). If no signs of circulation and no pulse are detected, start chest compressions (see details below). If the victim has a pulse but is not breathing, provide rescue breathing. Give 1 breath every 5 seconds (approximately 12 breaths per minute).

- If the victim has a pulse and is breathing adequately and has no signs of head or neck trauma, place the victim in the recovery position. See Figure 3 and sidebar.

Barrier Devices and Masks

When you perform CPR, you have almost no chance of becoming infected with a disease such as AIDS or hepatitis. Nevertheless many rescuers prefer to avoid direct mouth-to-mouth contact with another person, especially a stranger. ACLS providers should practice delivery of rescue breaths with a barrier device so that they will be able to use the device in an emergency.

Barrier devices should be available in all healthcare settings and should be available to any rescuer who is expected to perform CPR in the workplace. If a barrier device is not available, rescuers can make either of 2 decisions. First, the rescuer can deliver mouth-to-mouth ventilations without a barrier device. Barrier devices are not required to deliver the rescue breaths. Second, the rescuer can perform chest compressions only, without mouth-to-mouth ventilations. Laboratory studies and 1 clinical trial suggest that rescue breaths may not be required during the first minutes of a sudden, witnessed VF arrest in adults. Rescuers, particularly lay rescuers, are under no moral, ethical, or legal obligation to perform mouth-to-mouth ventilations if they feel uncomfortable. The best way to avoid feeling uncomfortable, however, is to ensure that barrier devices are always available. Healthcare providers should also be equipped to provide bag-mask ventilation.

There are 2 types of barrier devices: face shields and face masks.

Face Shields

Face shields are clear plastic or silicon sheets placed over the victim's face to keep the rescuer's mouth from directly touching the victim. All face shields have an opening or tube in the center of the plastic sheet. This allows your rescue breaths to enter the victim's airway. Face shields are small, flexible, and portable. A shield will fit easily on a key ring, where it is much more likely to be available when you need it.

Face Masks

Face masks are hard plastic devices that fit over the victim's mouth and nose. Much more effective than face shields, face masks are bulkier and cost more. A drawback is that face masks are less likely to be available.

Bag-Mask Ventilation

Bag-mask ventilation is a critical skill for all healthcare providers. It is a complex technique that requires considerable skill and practice. Such skill is difficult to maintain when used infrequently. However, recent studies suggest that prehospital

FIGURE 3. Recovery position. This stable, modified lateral position maintains alignment of the back and spine while allowing the rescuer to observe and maintain access to the victim.

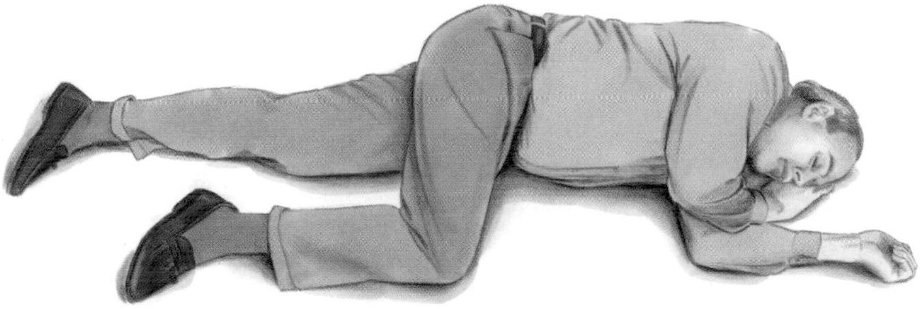

The Recovery Position

How to Place a Person in the Recovery Position if Unconscious but Breathing

If there is no evidence of trauma, place the victim on his or her side in the recovery position. The recovery position keeps the airway open.*

The following steps are recommended:

1. Kneel beside the victim; straighten the victim's legs.
2. Place the victim's arm nearer you in a "waving good-bye" position, that is, at right angles to the victim's body, elbow bent, palm up.
3. Place the victim's other arm across the chest (see Figure 3). If the victim is small, bring this arm farther across the victim's chest so that the back of the hand can be held against the victim's nearer cheek.
4. Grasp the victim's far-side thigh above the knee; pull the thigh up toward the victim's body.
5. Place your other hand on the victim's far-side shoulder and roll the victim toward you onto his or her side. Begin moving the victim's uppermost hand toward the victim's nearer cheek (the hand must not get trapped under the body).
6. Adjust the upper leg of the knee you are holding until both the hip and knee are bent at right angles.
7. Tilt the victim's head back to keep the airway open. Bring the back of the uppermost hand under the victim's cheek. Use this hand to maintain head tilt. Use chin lift if necessary.

- Continue to check the victim.
- Check breathing regularly ("look, listen, and feel").
- If the victim stops breathing, turn the victim onto his or her back, be sure that 911 has been called and that the AED is nearby, and begin the ABCs of CPR.
- *Memory aid:* Victim is waving good-bye with an arm that has a sore shoulder. He or she decreases the discomfort by holding the shoulder with the other hand.

*During transport of a comatose patient on a gurney, a left- or right-sided decubitus position is the safest position to reduce the risk of aspiration if vomiting occurs. The Trendelenburg position is preferred to the patient's lying flat. If the patient is obtunded and vomits while in a lateral decubitus or the Trendelenburg position, the risk of aspiration is lower than if the patient is lying flat.

intubation may be associated with an unacceptably high rate of undetected tube misplacement and displacement, with fatal results. As a result, bag-mask ventilation may be the preferred technique of ventilatory support in the prehospital setting, particularly when transport time is short. Bag-mask ventilation is also a fundamental method of respiratory support for patients with respiratory arrest and insufficiency. For all of these reasons, it is essential that all healthcare providers be able to demonstrate effective bag-mask ventilation as part of their BLS skills.

How to Perform the Pulse Check

Remember, the pulse check is not taught to lay rescuers (laypeople learning CPR). Citizens should instead "look for signs of circulation."

1. Maintain head tilt.
2. Place 2 or 3 fingers on the Adam's apple.
3. Slide your fingers into the groove between the Adam's apple and the muscle (sternocleidomastoid). Pull your fingers toward you. (See Figure 4A and 4B.)
4. When your fingers are in the correct position, determine if a pulse is present by feeling for it. This should take no more than 10 seconds.
5. If there is no pulse, start chest compressions.

How to Perform Chest Compressions

1. Find a position on the lower half of the sternum right between the nipples.
2. Place the heel of one hand on this location.
3. Place the heel of the second hand on top of the first hand.
4. Position your body directly over your hands. Your shoulders should be above your hands, and you should look down on your hands (Figure 5).
5. Provide 15 compressions at a rate of 100 compressions per minute. This rate is fast. It is much faster than 60 times per minute ("one-one-thousand, two-one-thousand") or 80 times per minute ("one-and-two-and-three-and-four-and . . ."). We strongly suggest using a much faster, sharper, 1-syllable mnemonic such as the first 15 letters of the alphabet: *"a, b, c, d, e, f, g, h, i, j, k, l, m, n, off."*
6. Compressions and ventilations: Provide cycles of 15 chest compressions, then 2 rescue breaths, but the rescue breaths must be "long and slow." Each breath should take about 2 seconds and should make the chest rise clearly. Note that if rescue breaths are delivered with supplemental oxygen through a pocket mask or bag mask, smaller tidal volumes can be delivered over 1 to 2 seconds (instead of somewhat larger breaths delivered over 2 seconds).
7. Continue 1-rescuer CPR with 15 chest compressions and 2 slow breaths.

FIGURE 4. Checking the carotid pulse. **A,** Locate the trachea. **B,** Gently feel for the carotid pulse.

A

B

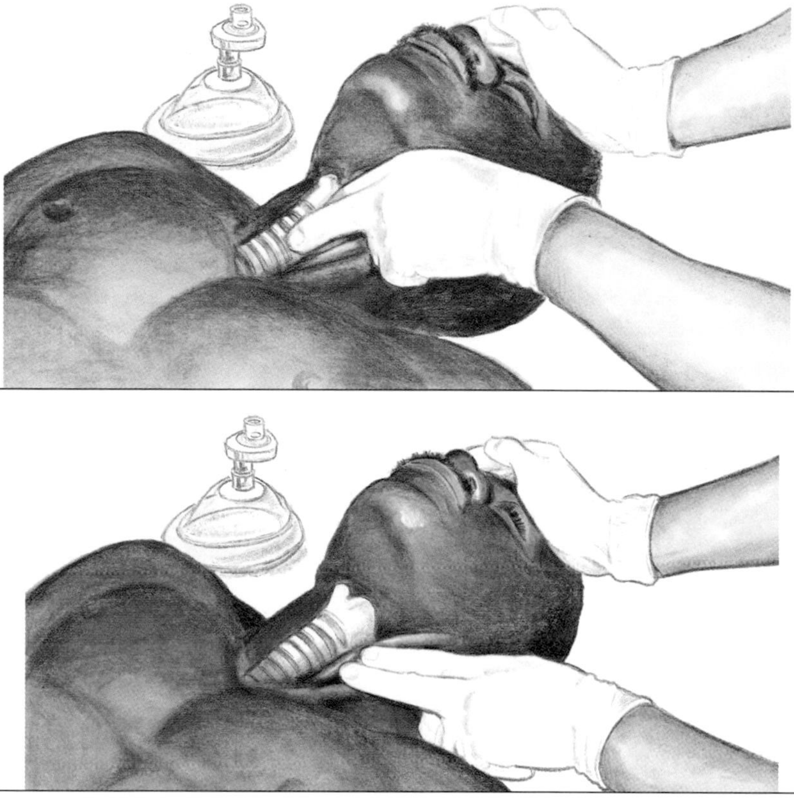

FIGURE 5. Position of the rescuer during chest compressions.

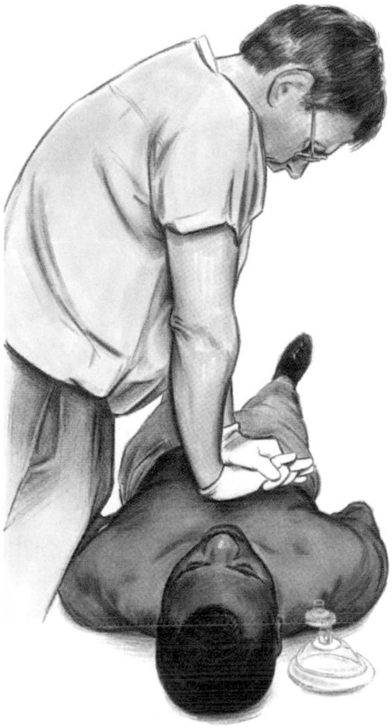

After about 1 minute of CPR (4 cycles of 15 compressions and 2 breaths), check the pulse to see whether circulation has been restored. Check the pulse every few minutes. If a pulse returns, stop chest compressions and continue providing rescue breaths if needed (1 breath every 5 seconds).

Choking: Airway Obstruction by a Foreign Body

Sudden choking alarms everyone. The desperate efforts of the choking person to clear the airway heightens the drama and increases the pressure on the rescuer to take immediate and correct actions. Foreign bodies may partially block the airway but still allow good air movement. In such cases choking victims remain conscious, can cough forcefully, and usually can speak. Breath sounds may be noisy. These victims require no immediate actions from you, but you should prepare to act if the airway obstruction worsens.

Victims with severe airway obstruction remain conscious at first but will be unable to move enough air to cough forcefully. You must be prepared to help relieve the obstruction with abdominal thrusts.

- To determine whether a conscious victim has an obstructed airway, ask "Are you choking?" If the victim nods, ask "Can you speak?" If the airway obstruction is complete or severe, the choking victim will not be able to speak.
- In a conscious, choking person the following are red flags or major warning signs of severe airway obstruction that require you to act:
  - The universal choking sign: the victim clutches his or her neck with the thumb and index finger. Note the following:
    1. You do not need to act if the victim can cough forcefully and speak. A strong cough is the most effective way to remove a foreign body.
    2. Stay with the victim; monitor the victim's condition.
    3. If the partial obstruction persists, activate the EMS system.
  - Inability to speak (ask "Can you speak?")
  - Poor, ineffective coughs
  - High-pitched sounds while inhaling (stridor)
  - Increasing difficulty breathing
  - Bluish skin color (cyanosis)
  - Loss of consciousness if not treated immediately

First Aid for Airway Obstruction by a Foreign Body

Use the Heimlich maneuver (abdominal thrusts) to relieve severe or complete airway obstruction caused by a foreign body. The Heimlich maneuver quickly and vigorously forces air from the victim's lungs. This expels the blocking object like a cork from a bottle. Protocols distinguish between the conscious and the unconscious choking victim:

1. If the victim is conscious (but not speaking) and standing, use the Heimlich maneuver.
2. If the victim is unconscious, use CPR skills A (open the airway) and B (give rescue breaths) plus abdominal or chest thrusts (straddle the victim), tongue-jaw lift, and finger sweeps.

If the Choking Victim Is Conscious and Standing

Perform the Heimlich maneuver:

1. Make a fist with one hand.
2. Place the thumb side of the fist on the victim's abdomen, slightly above the navel and well below the breastbone.
3. Grasp the fist with the other hand and provide quick upward thrusts into the victim's abdomen.
4. Repeat the thrusts and continue until the object is expelled or the victim becomes unconscious.
5. If the foreign-body airway obstruction is not relieved, the victim will stop breathing. Then the brain and heart will lack oxygen-rich blood. The victim will lose consciousness and become unresponsive. When the victim loses consciousness, activate the EMS system—phone 911 and get the AED. Then perform the unconscious-choking maneuver described below.

If the Choking Victim Becomes Unconscious

The *ECC Guidelines 2000* provide different recommendations for the lay rescuer than for the healthcare provider. The following sequence of actions is far too complicated for lay responders to learn or remember after an initial basic CPR course. Few healthcare providers can perform this entire sequence from memory. Therefore, this complex sequence of actions, which remains a requirement for healthcare providers, is not expected of or taught to the layperson. (Furthermore, recently published studies suggest that routine chest compressions performed by rescuers from the side may be superior to the Heimlich maneuver for removing a foreign body from obstructing the airway of an unconscious victim.)

Perform a finger sweep, straddle the victim, and use the Heimlich maneuver (healthcare providers only):

1. Place the victim on his or her back.
2. Grasp the jaw and lift the jaw and tongue with one hand (tongue-jaw lift).
3. Perform a finger sweep with the index finger of the other hand.
4. Attempt slow rescue breathing.
5. If the chest does not rise, reposition the victim's head and reattempt rescue breath(s)

If the victim's chest still does not rise with your breaths, perform the Heimlich maneuver for an unconscious victim:

1. Straddle the victim.
2. Place the heel of one hand on the abdomen just above the navel and well below the breastbone. Place the heel of the other hand on top of the first. Give up to 5 quick abdominal thrusts.
3. Repeat finger sweeps, rescue breaths, and abdominal thrusts until the obstruction is cleared.

If the Choking Victim Is Pregnant or Obese, Conscious or Unconscious

When choking victims are in the later stages of pregnancy or are very obese, you must position your hands *on the chest* rather than *on the abdomen* to deliver thrusts.

Obese or Pregnant Choking Victim—Conscious

1. Stand behind the victim and put your arms around the victim's chest.
2. Place your fist on the middle of the victim's breastbone between the nipples (take care to avoid the lower tip of the breastbone).
3. Grab your fist with your other hand and perform firm backward thrusts.
4. Repeat thrusts until the object is removed or the victim becomes unconscious.

Obese or Pregnant Choking Victim—Unconscious

1. Place the victim on his or her back.
2. Grasp the victim's tongue and jaw with one hand. Perform a finger sweep with the index finger of the other hand.
3. Try to give slow rescue breaths.
4. If the victim's chest does not rise, reposition the victim's head and try again.
5. If the victim's chest still does not rise with your breaths, perform chest thrusts:
   - Do not straddle the pregnant victim. Work from the side.
   - Place the heel of one hand on top of the other. Then place the heel of the lower hand on the center of the breastbone at the nipple line (like the chest compressions in CPR).
   - Position your body directly over your hands (as for the chest compressions of CPR).
   - Give up to 5 firm chest thrusts.
6. Repeat tongue-jaw lift, finger sweeps, breathing attempts, and chest thrusts until the obstruction is cleared.

Summary

The ABCs of CPR are an important first aid skill that everyone should know. In your professional career you will probably encounter emergencies in which your ability to perform the ABCs will help save someone's life or prevent an urgent problem from becoming a life-threatening emergency. Problems with the airway are common.

Know the steps to take for

1. Opening the airway of an unconscious victim
2. Rescuing a choking victim who is distressed but still conscious
3. Rescuing a choking victim who becomes unconscious
4. Rescuing pregnant or obese choking victims, both conscious and unconscious

Problems with breathing occur in many emergencies. To *manage* these breathing problems you must know how to open the airway and give rescue breaths in the following emergencies:

1. Respiratory and cardiac arrest
2. Stroke and seizure
3. Head trauma
4. Drowning and near-drowning
5. Medication overdoses and drug intoxication

Part 2

Automated External Defibrillators (AEDs)

Learning and Skills Objectives

At the end of Part 2: AEDs you should be able to

1. Describe what an AED does
2. List the 4 universal steps of operating an AED
3. Describe in detail the 4 universal steps
4. Describe how to attach AED electrode pads in the correct position on the victim's chest
5. Explain why no one should touch the victim while the AED is analyzing, charging, or shocking the victim
6. List at least 3 special conditions that when present will modify your approach to using an AED
7. List the proper actions to take when the AED prompts *"no shock indicated"* (or *"no shock advised"*)
8. List 3 maintenance actions that depend on the operator rather than the manufacturer

How AEDs Operate

Description and Indications

An AED is a computerized defibrillator that can

- Analyze the heart rhythm of a person in cardiac arrest
- Recognize a shockable rhythm
- Advise the operator (through voice prompts and lighted indicators) whether the rhythm should be shocked

AEDs should be used if a victim has signs of cardiac arrest:

- Unresponsive
- Not breathing
- No pulse or other signs of circulation

AED adhesive electrode pads are placed on the victim's bare chest and connected to the AED. AED electrode pads have 2 functions:

- To sense the cardiac electric signal and send it to the computer
- To deliver a shock through the electrodes if a shock is indicated

AEDs have been tested and are very accurate for use with adults. AEDs contain computer chips that analyze the rate, size, and wave shape of the human cardiac rhythm, among other criteria. The AED examines the ECG signal for "matches" with the preprogrammed criteria of a shockable rhythm.

AEDs are relatively inexpensive and need little maintenance. They can be operated easily with very little training. Because of their effectiveness and ease of use and care, they are now being placed on airplanes and in public buildings, homes, and worksites.

Major Automated Functions

Analyze

AEDs analyze the victim's heart to see whether its rhythm can be shocked. If the AED detects a shockable rhythm, the AED will tell you through synthesized voice components and flashing indicator lights that a *shock is advised.*

Charge and Shock

All AEDs must charge before they can deliver a shock. Some AEDs charge automatically upon recognition of VF. The operator presses the SHOCK button only when prompted to do so by the AED. Some AEDs will detect VF but then require you to press a CHARGE button before they will charge. Then you push another button to deliver the shock.

How to Operate an AED

4 Universal Steps

Like automobiles, AEDs are available in different models. There are small differences from model to model, but again like cars all AEDs operate basically the same way. Do not be distracted by minor differences. Focus instead on the 4 universal steps you must perform with all AEDs. They are listed below.

4 Universal Steps of AED Operation

1. POWER ON the AED first!
2. ATTACH the AED to the victim's chest with electrode pads.
3. ANALYZE the rhythm.
4. SHOCK (if a shock is indicated).

Special Conditions That May Require Additional Actions

When you arrive with an AED at the scene of a possible cardiac arrest or if you are doing CPR and someone else arrives with an AED, quickly look for "special conditions" that may change how you use the AED. These are presented in more detail in the sidebar.

1. Children less than 8 years of age: AEDs may be used in children 1 to 8 years of age. Use child pads when available.
2. Victim immersed in water or with water covering the chest: Remove the victim from water and dry the chest.
3. Implantable defibrillator: Do not place an AED electrode directly over the implantable defibrillator.
4. Transdermal medications: If the victim has a medication patch positioned where you would normally place an AED electrode, remove the patch, wipe the skin dry, and place the electrode in the proper location.

General Rules for Use of an AED During Attempted Resuscitation

- Make sure you have enough room to perform CPR and operate the AED.
- Do not attempt CPR in a soft bed, for example, or with the victim slumped over in a car or a chair.
- Place the victim on a firm surface, such as the floor.
- If possible, place the AED next to the victim's left ear. This position allows you to reach the AED controls easily, place the adhesive electrode pads in the proper location without long reaches, and to direct CPR.

Details of the Universal Steps of AED Operation

This section covers specific details you should know about using an AED in a

Special Situations in AED Use

1. **Children:** The AHA now recommends the use of AEDs for children 1 to 8 years of age (approximately 9 to 25 kg) with prehospital cardiac arrest. Ideally the AED has *child* pads and delivers a *child* dose. The AHA does not recommend for or against the use of AEDs in infants <1 year of age.

   Actions:

   - Use *child* pads when available for children 1 to 8 years of age.
   - Use *adult* pads for adults or for children >8 years of age. *Do not use child pads* for this age.

2. **Water:** *Is the victim immersed in water, or is water covering the victim's chest? Do not deliver a shock while the victim's chest is covered with water.* Water on the victim's chest may cause the current to arc between the electrodes and bypass the heart, preventing defibrillation or reducing its effectiveness. But if the victim is lying on water that is not near the electrodes (eg, victim lying supine on wet pavement) or water is not on the chest (eg, victim lying supine in the snow), the water poses little danger to the victim or rescuers.

   Actions:

   - Remove the victim from water. Drag the victim gently by the arms or legs or use a blanket drag.
   - Quickly dry the victim's chest before attaching the AED pads.

3. **Implanted pacemakers or defibrillators:** *Does the victim have a pacemaker or implanted cardioverter-defibrillator?* These devices create a hard lump beneath the skin of the upper chest or abdomen (usually on the victim's left side). The lump is about half the size of a deck of cards and usually has a small overlying scar. Placing an AED electrode pad directly over an implanted medical device may reduce the effectiveness of defibrillation.

   Actions:

   - Do not place an AED electrode pad directly over an implanted device.
   - Place an AED electrode pad at least 1 inch to the side of any implanted device.

4. **Transdermal medications:** *Do patch medications interfere with placement of electrode pads on the victim's chest?* Placing an AED electrode pad on top of a medication patch may block delivery of shocks or cause small burns to the skin.

   Action:

   - Remove the patch and wipe the area clean before attaching the AED.

real situation. Remember, these steps start only *after* you have verified that the victim is unresponsive, is not breathing, and has no pulse and you have placed the AED near the victim's left ear.

Step 1. POWER ON the AED first!

a. ***Open the AED.*** This automatically turns the power on in some devices.

b. ***Press the POWER ON button first.***

This is critical because sound alerts, lights, and voice prompts will tell you that the power is on and will direct you through the steps of using the AED. Always turn the AED on as the first step. Do not wait until you have opened the package of adhesive electrode pads or attached the electrode pads to the victim's chest.

Step 2. ATTACH adhesive electrode pads to the victim's chest (stop CPR chest compressions).

a. ***Remove clothing from the victim's chest.*** Place 2 adhesive electrode pads directly on the skin of the victim's chest. The chest should be bare to the skin. Remove clothing and undergarments as needed, even for women. Do not hesitate—remember that you are trying to save the victim's life. Bandage scissors can be stored in the AED carrying case to cut clothing that is hard to remove.

b. ***Dry the victim's chest if necessary.*** Be sure the victim's chest is bare and wiped dry. This will help the AED electrode pads stick firmly so that they will not shift or fall off during defibrillation. Keep a cloth or gauze in the AED carrying case for drying.

c. ***Open the package of adhesive electrode pads in the AED carrying case.*** Some defibrillation electrode pads are preconnected to the cables. For others, attach one end of the cable to the AED. Then attach the other end of the cable to the electrode pads.

d. ***Join ("snap") the connecting cables to the electrode pads (in some AEDs the cables are preconnected to the electrode pads).*** First put the electrode pads on the floor or the ground. Then snap the cables down on the pad connecting posts *before* you place the pads on the victim's chest.

e. ***Attach the adhesive electrode pads to the victim's chest (stop CPR chest compressions during this step to ensure proper pad placement).***

Critical Sequence

- Peel away the protective plastic backing from the electrode pads to expose the adhesive surface.
- Attach the AED electrode pads, adhesive side down, directly to the skin of the victim's chest.
- Place the pads just as pictured on the nonsticky side of the pads.

Follow the example pictured on the pad packaging. It is not essential to match position and cable alignment exactly, but try to place the pads no more than 1 or 2 inches from what is shown in the illustrations. The first pad goes on the *upper right side* of the victim's chest, to the right of the breastbone, between the nipple and collarbone. The second pad goes to the outside of the left nipple, with the top margin of the pad several inches below the left armpit.

Step 3. ANALYZE the victim's rhythm.

a. ***Stop CPR. Do not touch the victim.*** When you are ready to analyze the victim's rhythm, stop CPR completely. *Do not touch the victim or have any physical contact with the victim.* Such contact could interfere with AED analysis. Some AEDs start to analyze the rhythm as soon as the electrode pads are attached. Others require you to push an ANALYZE button to start rhythm analysis. From this point forward—whenever the machine is analyzing, preparing to shock, or actually delivering the shock to the victim—it is critical that you, the team members, and all bystanders avoid *all* contact with the victim.

Electrode Pad Placement

- Practice opening the electrode pad package and attaching the cables while your partner performs CPR, including rescue breathing and chest compressions. When you are ready to attach the electrode pads, remove the adhesive backing of the first pad. Then stop CPR chest compressions. Quickly attach the pads and allow the AED to analyze the rhythm.
- With some AEDs you may have to press the ANALYZE button. Other AEDs will automatically analyze as soon as the electrode pads are properly attached.
- You may receive a voice prompt or alarm if the electrode pads are not securely attached to the chest or if the cables are not fastened properly. The voice warning will state *"check pads"* or *"check electrodes,"* or words to that effect.
- Troubleshoot by checking the following:
  1. If the victim has a hairy chest, try removing and reattaching the pads or shaving the chest (see "The Hairy Chest Problem").
  2. Are the electrode pads stuck firmly and evenly to the skin of the chest?
  3. Are the cables correctly connected to the adhesive electrode pads?
  4. Are the cables correctly connected to the AED?
  5. When you correct the problem, most AEDs will automatically go into the analyze mode.

The Hairy Chest Problem

If the victim has a hairy chest, the adhesive electrode pads may stick to the hair of the chest, preventing contact with the skin on the chest. This will lead to a *check electrodes* or *check electrode pads* message on the AED.

Try the following:

- Press down firmly on each pad. That may solve the problem.
- Quickly pull off the electrode pads. This will remove much of the chest hair. Dry the chest and attach a second set of electrode pads. See if the AED will now analyze.
- If you still cannot get a good connection, pull off the second set of electrode pads. Shave the area for pad placement with a few strokes of the prep razor in the AED carrying case. Then open and attach a new (third) set of electrode pads.

Professional responders are given plastic disposable razors to quickly shave a suitable area of chest hair so that the electrode pads stick directly to the skin. After practicing the Heartsaver AED scenarios, consider whether you are comfortable with the idea of shaving someone's chest. Two of these razors should be packed in the AED storage case with 2 extra sets of electrode pads.

b. ***Announce "Stand clear of the victim!"*** The rescuer operating the AED should state clearly *"Stand clear of the victim! Analyzing rhythm! Stand clear!"* You do not need to use these exact words, but make sure the message gets across. *No one should touch the victim during analysis or shock.* If anyone is touching the victim, refuse to push the ANALYZE or SHOCK buttons until contact with the victim stops.

Step 4. Charge the AED and deliver the SHOCK (if indicated).

a. ***Stay clear while charging.*** When the AED recognizes a shockable rhythm, voice messages will prompt you to "stay clear." Most AED models begin charging automatically. You must make sure that no one is touching the victim.

b. To prepare for shock delivery, announce and verify (with a visual check) ***"I'm clear, you're clear, we're all clear."***

c. ***Push to shock.*** When charging is complete, the machine will advise you to *"push to shock"* or *"press the SHOCK button."* Just before you press the SHOCK button, *"clear" the victim* (make one last check to confirm that no one is touching the victim). Then press the SHOCK button to deliver the shock to the victim.

d. ***Follow the shock sequence:***

- ***Analyze, shock***
- ***Analyze, shock***
- ***Analyze, shock***

The number of shocks an AED delivers and the energy level for each shock are preset by the manufacturer. Let the AED follow the shock sequence it has been programmed to deliver. Follow the AED voice and visual prompts. Continue to follow the sequence of actions outlined in this appendix until the code team or EMS personnel arrive. Transfer the care of the victim to other in-hospital or out-of-hospital personnel after the AED has completed the shock cycles.

Subsequent Analysis and Actions

Leave AED electrode pads attached. Check ABCs. If the victim's heart is no longer in ventricular fibrillation/ventricular tachycardia, the AED will signal *"no shock indicated"* (or *"no shock advised"*) or *"check breathing and pulse."* Leave the AED electrodes attached to the victim's chest. Check for a pulse. Then follow the ABCs of CPR.

If the victim is breathing adequately and has a pulse, place the victim in the *recovery position* and monitor breathing until EMS personnel arrive.

If the victim is not breathing but has a pulse, give rescue breaths (1 breath every 5 seconds). Check the pulse frequently.

If the victim is not breathing and has no pulse, resume CPR.

Care after shock. Leave the AED electrode pads in place and the AED turned ON. *Do **NOT** remove the electrode pads or turn the AED off until instructed to do so by EMS personnel.* The victim may "rearrest" and lose spontaneous respirations and pulse. If the AED is always ready for use, you and your rescue team can resume the *AED action sequence* as soon as it is needed.

Making the Connections

AEDs require that 4 objects be connected in a line: from the AED, to the connecting cable, to the AED electrode pads, to the victim's chest. Remember

→ The AED is joined to the

→ Connecting cables, which are joined to the

→ AED electrode pads, which are attached to the

→ Victim's chest

AED manufacturers have not yet standardized these connections. Learn the details about your particular AED. In newer AED models the electrode pads are preattached to the connecting cables and the connecting cables are preattached to the AED. All the operator has to do is open the electrode pad package and attach the pads to the victim's chest. Learn exactly how much of the AED "circuit" you must put together for your AED before you need it in an emergency. Remember that you can figure out the connections by recalling the 4 elements that must be joined: **AED → cables → electrode pads → victim.**

AED Maintenance and Troubleshooting

Newer AED models require almost no maintenance. AEDs are programmed to run "self-tests" or "readiness-for-use" tests to see whether they are working and ready for use. All operators, however, must still check daily to make sure the AED is ready for use at a moment's notice. AED manufacturers provide specific recommendations about checking maintenance and readiness. See the handout *Manufacturer's Instructions and Guide to Maintenance* for more details.

Summary

- POWER ON the AED first. Listen to the voice and visual prompts.
- ATTACH the electrode pads (paying attention to the figures for pad location and stopping chest compressions).
- ANALYZE the rhythm (this may occur automatically).
- Press the SHOCK button if a shock is indicated (clear the victim first).

These are the only defibrillation steps most rescuers, lay or professional, will ever need to know. Performing these same steps during an actual VF arrest will get the job done.

Other responders, however, will appreciate the details about defibrillation presented in this appendix. If you are curious about the rich variety of "what if?" situations that can arise during defibrillation, this appendix will help answer your questions. It will also enrich your understanding of defibrillation.

Part 3

ABCD: Putting CPR and AED Together

Learning and Skills Objectives

At the end of this section you should be able to

1. List the 3 criteria for when to start chest compressions and when to use the AED
2. Describe the 3 factors that you must assess and support as needed when you find a collapsed person
3. Describe the steps of the Heartsaver AED protocol:
   - What you do at the first assessment of ***"Unresponsive"***
   - What you do at the ***start of the ABCDs***
   - What you do during the ***5-step AED treatment protocol***
4. Describe what your next actions would be if you were offering your help to a collapsed fellow passenger on a commercial airliner flying at 30,000 feet. The flight attendant has asked you to take charge, stating *"We have an AED and a doctors-only advanced medical kit kit on board."*

The Heartsaver AED Rescuer Treatment Algorithm

This algorithm (Figure 6) guides you whether you respond to a cardiac arrest alone as a lone rescuer or with others who can help. For the ACLS rescuer the major learning task is to become familiar with the steps you will perform during the "pump and blow" of CPR and how to open, attach, and use the AED.

When Should I Start Chest Compressions? When Should I Use the AED?

There are 3 major cues for starting chest compressions and using the AED. All 3 conditions must be present:

a. ***Unresponsive:*** This prompts you to take 2 actions: phone 911 and get the AED.

b. ***Not breathing:*** This prompts you to give rescue breathing.

c. ***No pulse:*** This prompts you to take 2 actions: get the AED and start chest compressions.

At this point just recognize the 3 conditions: ***unresponsive, not breathing, no pulse.*** Know what actions you must take in response.

When the AED is turned on, attached to the victim, and set in analyze mode, it

AED Maintenance

- Become familiar with your AED and how it operates.
- Check the AED for any visible problems, such as an open case or signs of damage.
- Check the "ready-for-use" indicator on your AED (if so equipped) daily.
- Perform any other user-based maintenance according to the manufacturer's recommendations.
- Check to see that the AED carrying case contains the following minimum accessories:
  - — 2 sets of spare defibrillator electrode pads (3 total)
  - — 2 pocket face masks
  - — 1 extra battery (if appropriate; some AEDs have batteries that last for years)
  - — 2 prep razors (supplied by manufacturers)
  - — 5 to 10 alcohol wipes
  - — 5 sterile gauze pads (4 × 4 inches), individually wrapped
  - — 1 absorbent cloth towel

Remember: AED malfunctions are extremely rare. Most reported problems have been caused by failure to perform user-based maintenance of the AED.

FIGURE 6. AED algorithm for out-of-hospital use of AEDs until EMS personnel arrive.

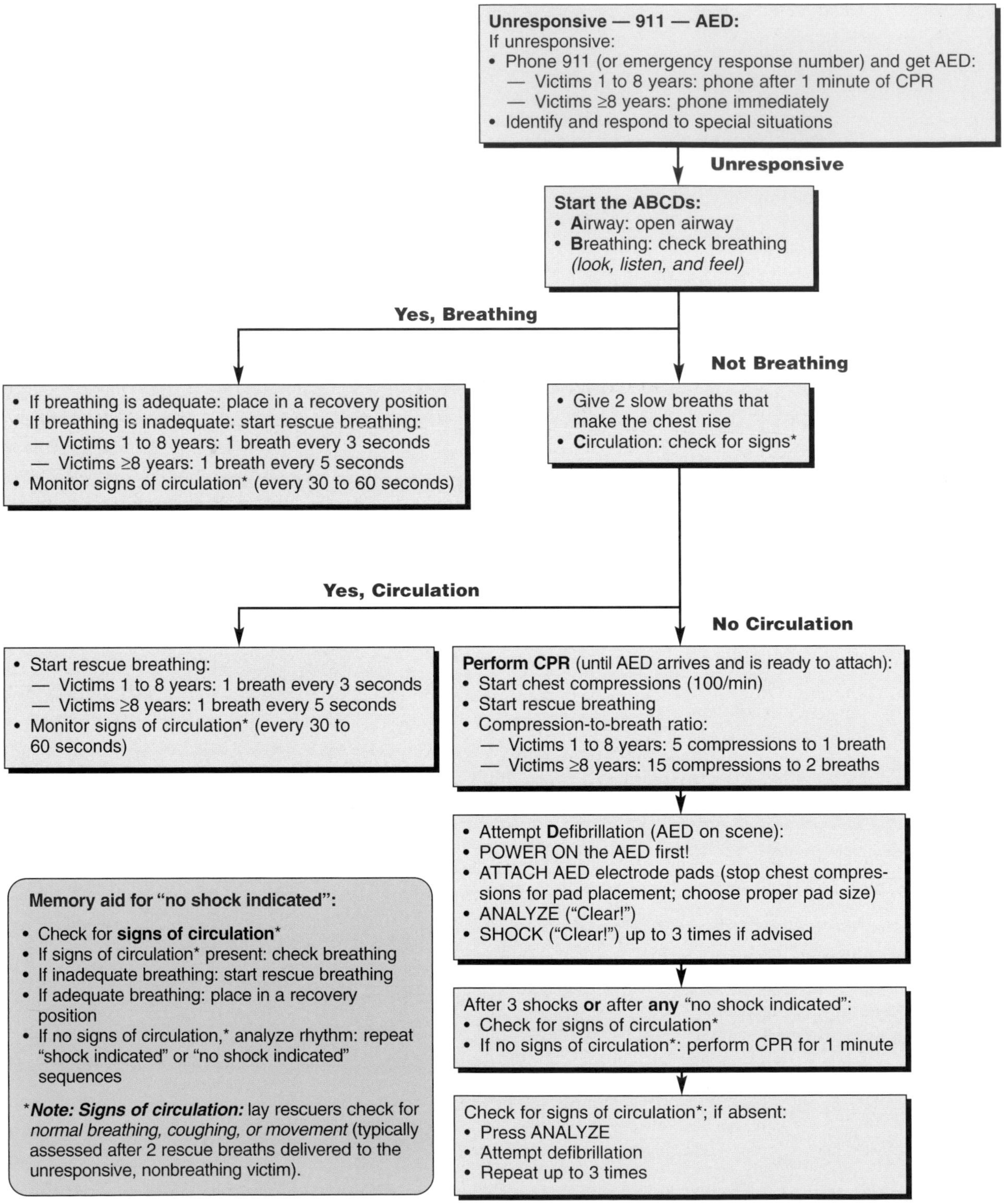

will identify 1 of 2 conditions: *shockable rhythm present* or *shockable rhythm absent.* You respond to the AED prompts by "clearing" the victim, pressing the ANALYZE button (this is done automatically in some models), and pressing the SHOCK button when indicated. That's all there is to the use of the AED.

The Heartsaver AED Protocol: Combining CPR With Using an AED

When you see a person who may be in cardiac arrest, act quickly but calmly. Follow the sequences you learned for CPR and AED operation.

CPR and AED With 2 or More Rescuers

The Heartsaver Rescuer With an AED

Consider yourself the *rescue director.* You have the skills to do CPR and operate an AED. In many rescue situations you may be the only witness who has either of these abilities. The tasks are simple—tell other witnesses to *"phone 911—get the AED located by the telephone"*; tell other rescuers to *"help with CPR."* You will ensure that actions are taken in the proper sequence as quickly as possible and that they are well coordinated.

Witnessed Arrest With 2 People Responding

In the 1-rescuer scenario *a single person witnesses a collapse and performs the entire Heartsaver AED action sequence.* Another common scenario is the 2-rescuer scenario: a witnessed arrest in a public place, such as a worksite, with several bystanders. To avoid conflicts and confusion, the AHA recommends the following roles for each rescuer:

2-Rescuer Heartsaver AED Action Sequence

- ***Check unresponsiveness:*** Shout "Are you OK?"

If unresponsive:

- **Phone 911!** Point to another witness: "You! Go phone 911!"
- **AED:** Get the AED located next to the telephone: ". . . and get the AED next to the phone!"
- The person who phones 911 gets the AED.
- The person who will use the AED stays with the victim.

(These roles may be reversed in many circumstances.)

- The Heartsaver AED rescuer starts CPR during the phone call to 911.

The Heartsaver AED Rescuer With 2 or More People to Help

What happens when a cardiac arrest is witnessed by several people? They all want to help but may be unsure of what to do. In some worksites all employees will be trained as Heartsaver AED rescuers. Almost everyone will be knowledgeable and have a sense of what to do.

The answer—*you direct them.* The Heartsaver AED rescuer will perform *both* the initial assessment and CPR and will *operate* the AED when it arrives. The AED rescuer should not leave the victim's side. If other witnesses are present, particularly other CPR-AED trained rescuers, *use them.* Direct them to perform one of these tasks:

- ***Phone 911.***
- ***Get the AED.***
- ***Do CPR: Do rescue breathing. Do chest compressions.***

Instructors may teach these roles another way: *whoever calls 911 and gets the AED will operate the AED.* This means that the second rescuer must be able to perform the initial ABCs and CPR. Either approach is acceptable. The preferred approach is for the AED rescuer to always remain with the victim.

AED Prompts and Messages

The AED is a remarkable electric device. One of its most useful features is the audio voice prompts that provide feedback to the Heartsaver AED rescuer. All AED models provide at least 4 types of voice messages:

- *Analysis indicator:* when the AED is analyzing the rhythm *("analyzing: do not touch the victim")*
- *Shockable rhythm indicator:* whether or not the AED identifies a shockable rhythm during analysis *("shock indicated"* or *"no shock indicated")*
- *Loose electrode indicator: "check electrodes"* sounds when there is any break in the connections between the victim's skin and the AED. Most often this break occurs where the electrode pad is attached to the skin, but the break can also occur at the cable-to-pad connections or the cable-to-AED connections.
- *Sequencing information:* AEDs provide sequencing steps *("connect electrodes"* or *"check airway, check breathing, check pulse"* or *"perform CPR if no pulse").*

Summary

All ACLS providers must know how to perform CPR, how to use an AED, and how to do the two together. Most expert observers predict that AEDs are well on the way to becoming standard-of-care equipment in US hospitals. Ease of use and training will result in designation of the trained healthcare provider closest to the patient as the person to perform defibrillation.

The AHA added AED training to the ACLS Provider Course to help prepare healthcare professionals for this future. Most in-hospital ACLS providers will respond with others to a witnessed cardiac arrest. In the near future, however, they will often find that the patient has

FIGURE 7. The first rescuer begins CPR. The second rescuer gets the AED and places it beside victim's left ear.

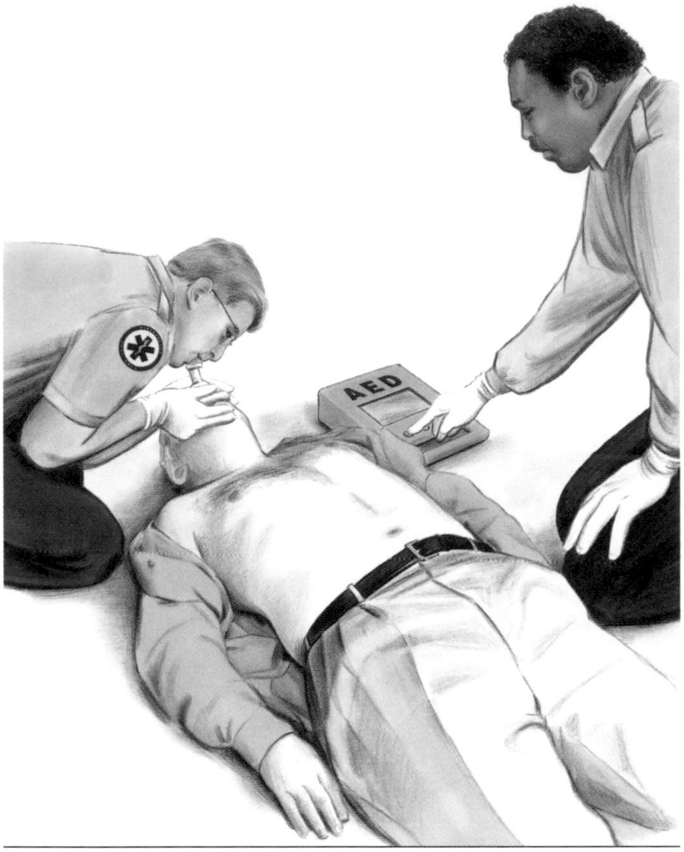

FIGURE 8. Operator turns AED on.

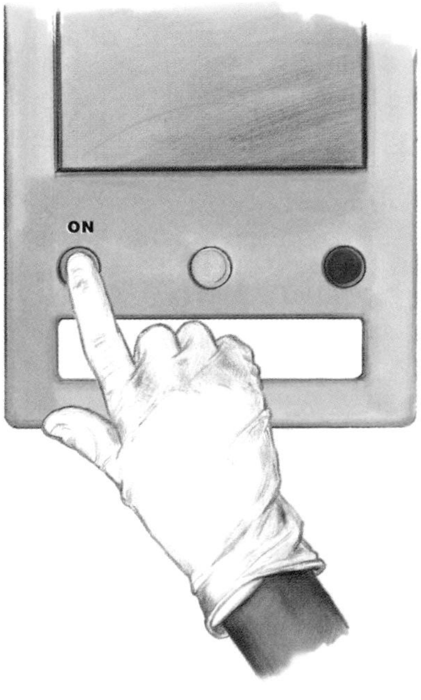

already received defibrillation from a floor nurse using an AED. Many, many arrests, however, occur at home or in a public setting outside the hospital. You may not have other trained rescuers to help you. You may be in situations where the only available defibrillator is the AED the flight attendant brings you at 30,000 feet.

The AHA approach in this appendix teaches ACLS providers to respond in the worst-case scenario: you are alone, no one hears your call for help, and you have only an AED. If you can manage this situation, you can manage any situation requiring CPR and AED.

Two-Rescuer AED Sequence of Action

1. **Verify unresponsiveness:** if victim is unresponsive:
   - Call 911 (or other emergency access number).
   - Get the AED located next to the telephone:
     - — The person who calls 911 gets the AED.
     - — The person who will use the AED stays with the victim and performs CPR until the AED arrives. (In many circumstances these roles may be reversed.)
2. **Open airway:** head tilt–chin lift (or jaw thrust if trauma is suspected)
3. **Check for effective breathing:** provide breathing if needed:
   - Check for breathing *(look, listen, and feel).*
   - If not breathing, give 2 slow breaths:
     - — A face shield is more likely to be available to the first rescuer outside the hospital.
     - — A mouth-to-mask device should be available in the AED carrying case.
     - — A bag-mask device is often available in the healthcare setting.
4. **Check for signs of circulation:** if no signs of circulation are present:
   - Perform chest compressions and prepare to attach the AED:
     - — If there is any doubt that the signs of circulation are present, the first rescuer initiates chest compressions while the second rescuer prepares to use the AED.
     - — Remove clothing covering the victim's chest to provide chest compressions and apply the AED electrode pads.
5. **Attempt defibrillation with the AED:** if no signs of circulation are present:
   - The caller delivers the AED to the person performing CPR. The preferred placement of the AED is beside the victim's left ear (Figure7), but this may not be possible in all cases.
   - The caller begins performing CPR while the rescuer who was performing CPR prepares to operate the AED. (It is acceptable to reverse these roles.)

The AED operator takes the following actions:

- **POWER ON** the AED first (some devices will turn on automatically when the AED lid or carrying case is opened) (Figure 8).

FIGURE 9. Electrodes are attached to victim and then to AED.

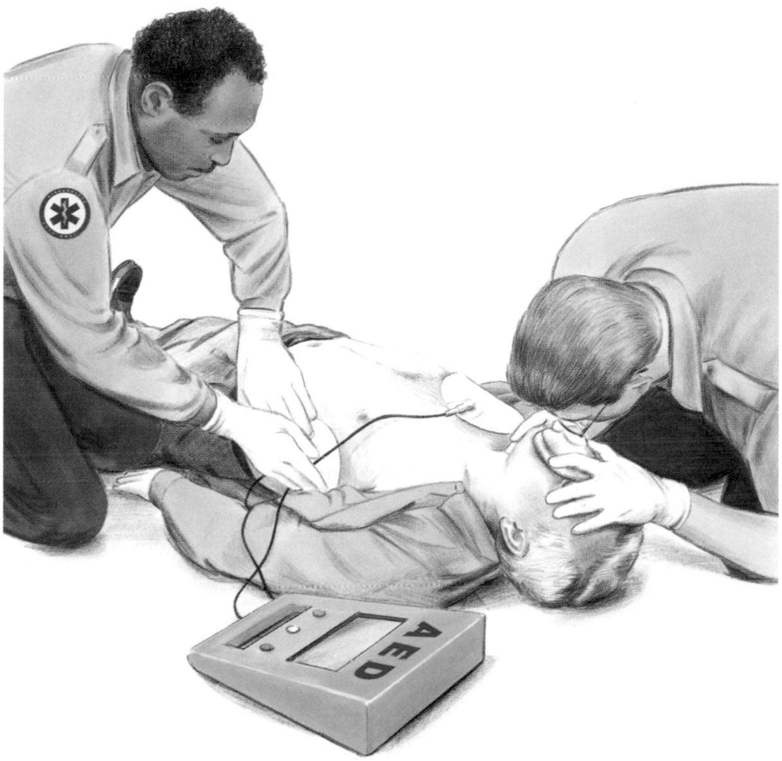

- **ATTACH** the AED to the victim (Figure 9):
  - — Attach the AED to the AED connecting *cables* (cables may be preconnected).
  - — Attach the AED connecting *cables* to the adhesive *electrode pads* (pads may be preconnected).
  - — Attach the adhesive *electrode pads* to the victim's bare chest.
  - — Ask the rescuer performing CPR to interrupt chest compressions just before attaching pads.
- **ANALYZE** rhythm:
  - — Clear the victim before and during analysis (Figure 10A).
  - — Check that no one is touching the victim.
  - — Press the ANALYZE button (Figure 10B) to start rhythm analysis (some brands of AEDs do not require this step).

FIGURE 10. **A,** The operator "clears" the victim before rhythm analysis. **B,** If needed, the operator then activates the ANALYZE feature of the AED.

A

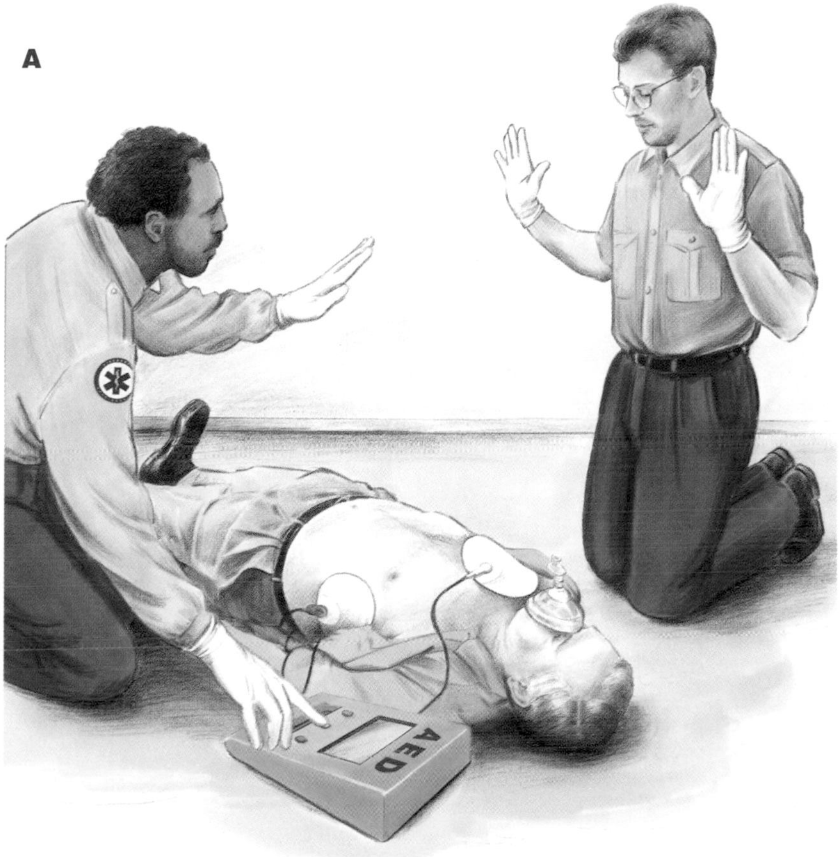

B

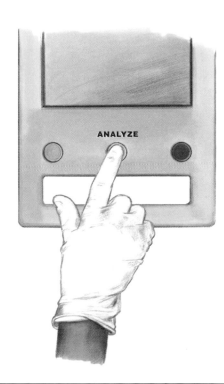

FIGURE 11. **A,** The operator "clears" the victim before delivering a shock. **B,** When everyone is "clear" of the victim, the operator presses the SHOCK button.

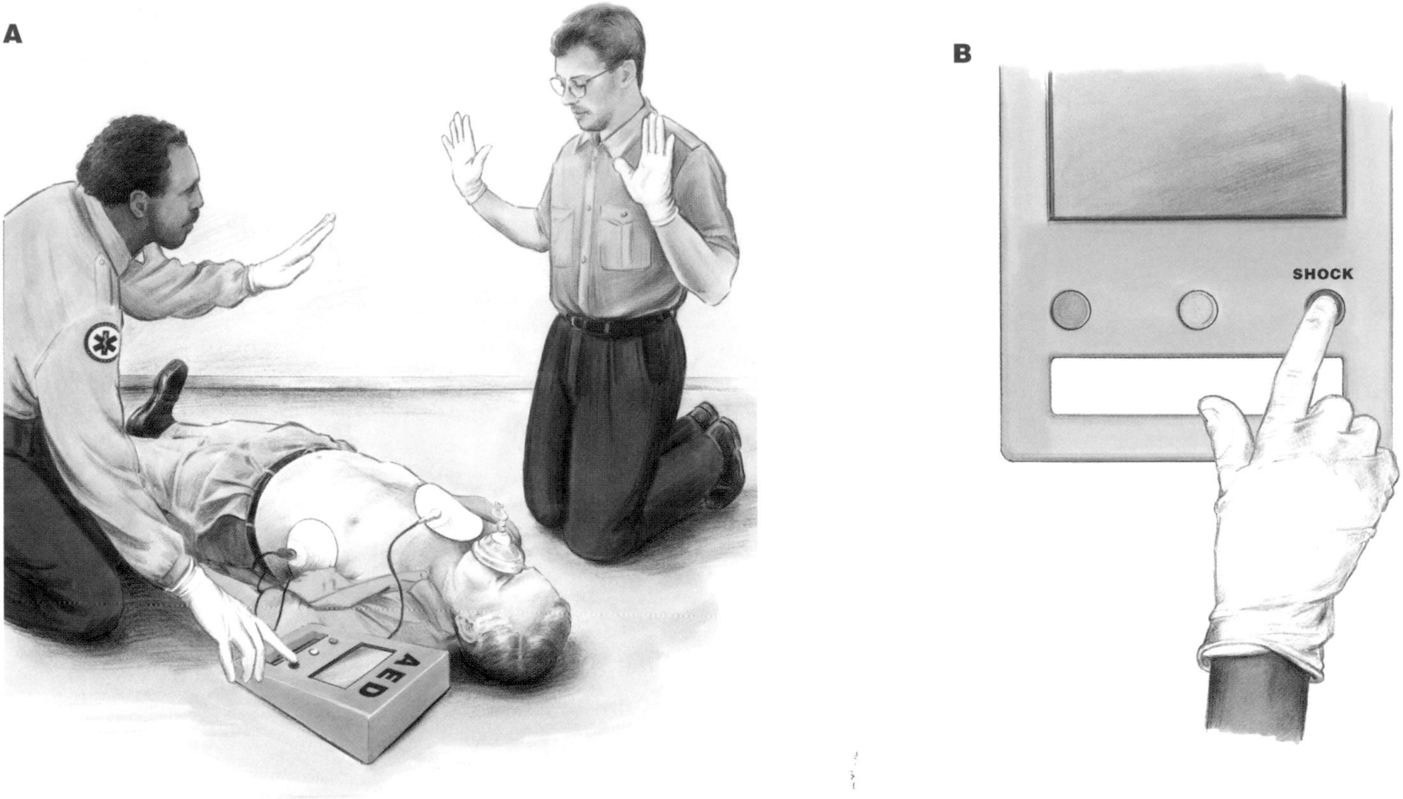

FIGURE 12. If no shock is indicated, the rescuer checks for signs of circulation, including a pulse.

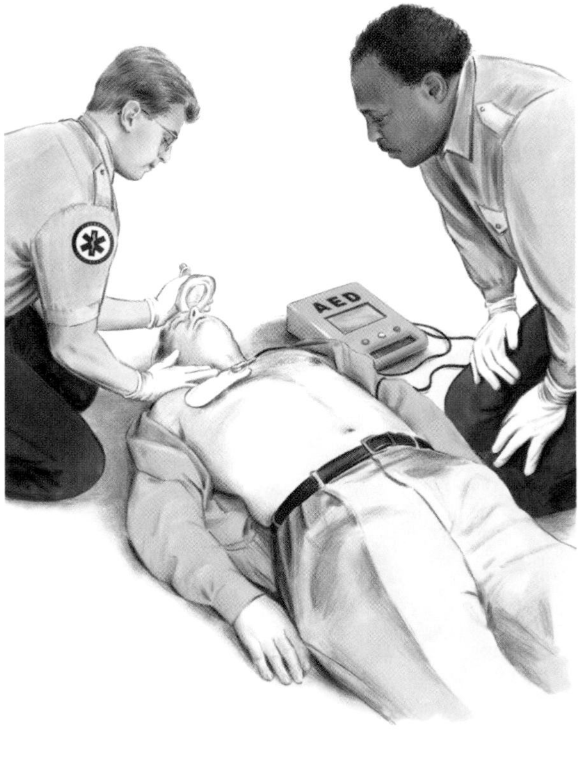

- *"Shock Indicated"* **message:**
  - — Clear the victim once more before pushing the SHOCK button (*"I'm clear, you're clear, everybody's clear"*) (Figure 11A).
  - — Check that no one is touching the victim.
  - — Press the SHOCK button (victim may display muscle contractions) (Figure 11B).
  - — Press the ANALYZE and SHOCK buttons up to 2 more times if the AED signals *"shock advised"* or *"shock indicated."* (Clear the victim before each analysis and shock.)
- *"No Shock Indicated"* **message:**
  - — Check for signs of circulation (including a pulse) (Figure 12). If signs of circulation are present, check breathing:
    - If breathing is inadequate, assist breathing.
    - If breathing is adequate, place the victim in the recovery position, with the AED attached.
  - — If no signs of circulation are present, resume CPR for 1 minute, then recheck for signs of circulation.
    - If there are still no signs of circulation, analyze rhythm, then follow the *"shock indicated"* or *"no shock indicated"* steps as appropriate.

Final Evaluation Skills Sheet for Adult Victims (CPR-AED)

American Heart Association®
Fighting Heart Disease and Stroke

Participant Name Date

Case Scenario: You are called to a clinic office and find a 52-year-old man who has collapsed to the floor. Another healthcare provider is in the room with you. The nearest AED is down the hall. Please proceed to help this victim.

Performance Guidelines	Performance	
	Satisfactory	Remediate
1. Establish unresponsiveness—direct colleague to activate the emergency response system and get the AED.		
2. Open the airway (head tilt–chin lift or, if trauma is suspected, jaw thrust)—check breathing (look, listen, and feel).		
3. If breathing is absent or inadequate, give 2 slow breaths (2 seconds per breath) that cause the chest to rise.		
4. Check carotid pulse and other signs of circulation ***(no signs of circulation).*** Start chest compressions (ratio of 15 to 2 breaths at 100 compressions per minute).		
AED Skills (AED arrives after 2 cycles of CPR)		
5. Place the AED next to the victim; POWER ON the AED and begin timing for collapse-to-shock interval.		
6. Attach electrode pads in the proper position (as pictured on each of the AED electrodes, sternum and apex, with proper contact and no overlap of pads).		
7. Clear the victim and press the ANALYZE button (if present). ***(AED advises shock and charges electrodes.)***		
8. Clear the victim and press the SHOCK button, if not automated. Stop timing for collapse-to-shock interval. (May repeat 1 to 2 more analyze-shock cycles. End when AED gives *"no shock indicated"* message.)		
9. Check carotid pulse and other signs of circulation ***(no signs of circulation present).*** Check breathing (no breathing present).		
10. Continue CPR until advanced life support personnel arrive.		

Critical Actions	Performance Satisfactory	Remediate
• Assess responsiveness.		
• Activate the emergency response system (or send second rescuer); get the AED.		
• Open the airway, check breathing.		
• If breathing is absent or inadequate, provide 2 breaths (must cause chest to rise).		
• Check pulse and other signs of circulation.		
• Begin chest compressions (must have proper hand placement).		
• When AED arrives: POWER ON the AED.		
• Attach electrode pads to patient's bare chest in proper location with adequate skin contact and no overlap of pads.		
• "Clear" victim before ANALYZE and SHOCK.		
• Push SHOCK button (if not automated) to attempt defibrillation.		
• Check breathing and signs of circulation after *"no shock indicated"* message.		
• Interval from collapse to first shock is less than 3 minutes; interval from AED arrival to first shock is less than 90 seconds.		
• Rescuer should be prepared to continue CPR if nonshockable rhythm is present.		

Comments ______________________________

Instructor ______________________________

Circle one: Complete Needs more practice

Appendix 2

Workbook Review Questions and Annotated Answers

Case 1: Respiratory Compromise: From Shortness of Breath to Respiratory Arrest (With a Pulse)

1. If there is continued doubt about correct placement of a tube after tracheal intubation and 5-point auscultation of breath sounds, the rescuer should visually check to see that the tube passes through the _______ ______.

The correct answer is vocal cords.

The *ECC Guidelines 2000* indicate the need for primary and secondary confirmation of tracheal tube placement. The *ECC Guidelines 2000* suggest 5-point auscultation during hand ventilation, and if there is doubt about proper tube placement, remove and replace the tube. According to the *ECC Guidelines 2000,* "If there is continued doubt about correct tube placement, use the laryngoscope and look directly to see whether the tube is passing through the vocal cords." The *ECC Guidelines 2000* also provide important information about secondary confirmation in the section immediately following the quoted passages.

Read more about it in the ECC Guidelines 2000, *pages 101-102: "How to Confirm Accurate Placement of Tracheal Tube: Primary Confirmation" and "How to Confirm Accurate Placement of Tracheal Tube: Secondary Confirmation"*

2. To confirm proper placement of tracheal tube or advanced airway device through 5-point auscultation, which of the following observations are appropriate? (Check all that apply.)

___ check breath sounds in the left and right lateral chest and lung bases

___ auscultate breath sounds in the left and right anterior sides of the chest

___ listen for gastric bubbling noises from the epigastrium

___ ensure equal and adequate chest expansion bilaterally

The correct answer is all 4 choices.

The *ECC Guidelines 2000* suggest that the rescuer perform 5-point auscultation during hand ventilation as follows: "As the bag is squeezed, listen over the epigastrium and observe the chest wall for movement. If you hear stomach gurgling and see no chest wall expansion, you have intubated the esophagus. Deliver no further ventilations. Remove the tracheal tube at once. Reattempt intubation. If the chest wall rises appropriately and stomach gurgling is not heard, listen to the lung fields: left and right anterior, left and right midaxillary, and once again over the stomach."

Read more about it in the ECC Guidelines 2000, *page 101: "How to Confirm Accurate Placement of Tracheal Tube: Primary Confirmation"*

3. Which of the following is true about an oropharyngeal airway?

a. it eliminates the need to position the head of the unconscious patient

b. it eliminates the possibility of an upper airway obstruction

c. it is of no value once a tracheal tube is inserted

d. it may stimulate vomiting or laryngospasm if inserted in the semiconscious patient

The correct answer is d.

An oropharyngeal airway may stimulate vomiting or laryngospasm in the semiconscious patient. A semiconscious patient may maintain an intact gag reflex, so insertion of the airway can cause vomiting or laryngospasm. Use of an oropharyngeal airway is recommended to help hold the tongue from the back of the pharynx in an unconscious victim. Answer **a** is incorrect because you must still maintain proper head positioning in an unconscious patient even when an oropharyngeal airway is in place. Answer **b** is incorrect because incomplete upper airway obstruction can occur despite an oropharyngeal airway.

Monitor the victim closely. Answer **c** is incorrect because oropharyngeal airways help prevent intubated patients from biting down on the tracheal tube.

Read more about it in the ECC Guidelines 2000, *page 98: "Airway Adjuncts"*

4. You have just attempted tracheal intubation. You hear stomach gurgling over the epigastrium, you see no chest expansion, and you are unable to hear breath sounds on either side of the chest during hand ventilation with a bag. Pulse oximetry indicates that the hemoglobin saturation has failed to rise. Which of the following is the most likely explanation of this finding?

a. intubation of the esophagus

b. intubation of the left main bronchus

c. intubation of the right main bronchus

d. unilateral tension pneumothorax

The correct answer is a.

Intubation of the esophagus is the most likely explanation because you *do* hear gurgling over the epigastrium, but you don't hear breath sounds during hand ventilation. In addition, the hemoglobin saturation has failed to rise. The guidelines suggest that the rescuer perform 5-point auscultation during hand ventilation as follows: "As the bag is squeezed, listen over the epigastrium and observe the chest wall for movement. If you hear stomach gurgling and see no chest wall expansion, you have intubated the esophagus." Answer **b** is incorrect because if you intubated the left main bronchus you are likely to hear breath sounds and see chest expansion over the left side but not the right side of the chest. Answer **c** is incorrect because intubation of the right main bronchus should produce breath sounds and chest expansion in the right side of the chest but not the left side. Answer **d** is not the most likely explanation because a unilateral tension pneumothorax typically results in the presence of breath sounds and chest expansion on the side opposite the side of the pneumothorax. In the scenario above no breath sounds are heard on either side of the chest.

Read more about it in the ECC Guidelines 2000, *pages 101-102: "How to Confirm Accurate Placement of Tracheal Tube: Primary Confirmation" and "How to Confirm Accurate Placement of Tracheal Tube: Secondary Confirmation"*

5. Which of the following is an indication for tracheal intubation?

a. difficulty encountered by qualified rescuers in ventilating an apneic patient with a bag-mask device

b. a respiratory rate of less than 20 breaths per minute in a patient with severe chest pain

c. presence of premature ventricular contractions

d. to provide airway protection in a responsive patient with an adequate gag reflex

The correct answer is a.

If adequate chest expansion and breath sounds cannot be achieved, tracheal intubation should be performed to ensure adequate ventilation. This answer closely matches specific statements in the guidelines, page 100: "Indications for tracheal intubation include: (1) inability of the rescuer to ventilate the unconscious patient with less invasive methods and (2) absence of protective reflexes (coma or cardiac arrest)." Answer **b** is incorrect because a respiratory rate of less than 20 in a patient with severe chest pain is not in itself an indication of the need for intubation. Tracheal intubation secures an unprotected airway and facilitates adequate ventilation. There is no indication that this patient with chest pain has an unprotected airway or inadequate ventilation. Answer **c** is incorrect because the presence of premature ventricular contractions does not indicate the need for control of the airway. In comparison, the treatment algorithms for both asystole and pulseless electrical activity call for immediate intubation because of the gravity of the patient's condition and inadequate ventilation. Answer **d** is incorrect because it describes a conscious patient with an adequate airway.

Read more about it in the ECC Guidelines 2000, *page 100: "Tracheal Intubation," right column*

6. You are treating a victim of trauma who is in shock and a deep coma. Which of the following is the airway of choice for this patient?

a. a tracheal tube

b. the patient's own airway

c. a nasopharyngeal airway

d. an oropharyngeal airway

The correct answer is a.

This patient would fall within those indications for tracheal intubation specifically listed in the guidelines, page 100: "Indications for tracheal intubation include: (1) inability of the rescuer to ventilate the unconscious patient with less invasive methods and (2) absence of protective reflexes (coma or cardiac arrest)." This trauma patient is deeply comatose and is at risk for compromise of oxygen delivery because of potential blood loss, potential hypoventilation, and possible cardiothoracic injury. The guidelines cite indications for intubation of the trauma patient (page 245), 2 of which would describe this patient: severe head injury or inability to protect the upper airway (eg, loss of gag reflex, depressed level of consciousness, coma). Answer **b** is incorrect because a deeply comatose patient who is at risk for other injuries requires establishment and protection of a patent airway and support of oxygenation and ventilation. Answers **c** and **d** are incorrect because although they will assist in supporting a patent airway, they cannot be used to support oxygenation and ventilation that may be required by the injured and deeply comatose patient.

Read more about it in the ECC Guidelines 2000, *pages 100-101: "Tracheal Intubation"; and page 245: "ACLS for Cardiac Arrest Associated with Trauma: Airway"*

7. Once a tracheal tube is inserted and the position verified (with both primary and secondary confirmation) during CPR, which of the following best describes the ventilations that should be provided?

a. an average of 12 to 15 ventilations per minute without pauses for chest compressions

b. ventilations should provide prompt hyperventilation to correct acidosis, with a pause after every fifth compression

c. ventilations should be delivered with an estimated tidal volume of 3 to 5 mL/kg

d. ventilations should be delivered with room air to avoid hyperoxygenation

The correct answer is a.

The number of ventilations should average 12 to 15 per minute without pauses for chest compressions. This is the correct (physiologic) number of ventilations to provide for the typical adult patient. In fact, this respiratory rate is specifically proposed in the guidelines, page 102: "The respiratory rate during cardiac or respiratory arrest when the patient has been intubated should be 12 to 15 breaths per minute (1 breath every 4 to 5 seconds). Once the tracheal tube is in place, ventilation need not be synchronized with chest compressions." Answer **b** is incorrect. Although in the past there was a perception that hyperventilation was required to correct metabolic acidosis during attempted resuscitation, it is now clear that hyperventilation may actually worsen cerebral ischemia (the *ECC Guidelines 2000,* page 168: Respiratory System). Answer **c** is incorrect because a tidal volume of 6 to 7 mL/kg is recommended when oxygen is administered; 10 mL/kg is recommended when oxygen is not administered. Answer **d** is incorrect because 100% oxgyen should be administered during attempted resuscitation.

Read more about it in the ECC Guidelines 2000, *page 102: top left column*

8. You are providing hand ventilations with a bag mask for a patient with no spontaneous ventilation. You are explaining the use of bag-mask ventilation to a group of new nurses and residents who are observing your technique. Which of the following statements would most accurately describe the use of bag-mask ventilation during resuscitation?

a. bag-mask ventilation can be performed effectively with minimal training and little practice

b. bag-mask ventilation will deliver nearly 100% oxygen if a reservoir with a high oxygen flow rate is used

c. bag-mask ventilation cannot be performed effectively by one person during resuscitation

d. bag-mask ventilation should not be used if the patient makes any spontaneous respiratory effort

The correct answer is b.

Bag-mask ventilation will deliver nearly 100% oxygen if a reservoir with a high oxygen flow rate is used. One of the qualities of a "satisfactory bag-mask unit" stated in the guidelines (page 95: Bag-Valve Devices) includes "a system for delivering high concentrations of oxygen through an ancillary oxygen reservoir." Answer **a** is incorrect because in fact the guidelines (page 38) state, "Bag-mask ventilation technique requires instruction and practice. The rescuer should be able to use the equipment effectively in a variety of situations." Answer **c** is incorrect because bag-mask ventilation can be performed effectively by one person during resuscitation. The guidelines (page 38) do acknowledge that bag-mask ventilation is a complex technique, and "Effective ventilation is more likely to be provided when 2 rescuers use the bag-mask system." Answer **d** is incorrect because bag-mask ventilation should be provided even if spontaneous respiratory effort is present but ventilations are inadequate.

Read more about it in the ECC Guidelines 2000, *page 95: "Bag Valve Devices"; and page 97: Figure 2 (legend). Bag-mask ventilation is also presented on page 38*

9. Which of the following is the *most important* step to restore oxygenation and ventilation for the unresponsive, breathless submersion (near-drowning) victim?

a. attempt to drain water from breathing passages by performing the Heimlich maneuver

b. begin chest compressions

c. provide cervical spine stabilization because a diving accident may have occurred

d. open the airway and begin rescue breathing as soon as possible, even in the water

The correct answer is d.

Open the airway and begin rescue breathing as soon as possible, even in the water. This information is almost verbatim from the guidelines, page 234: Rescue Breathing: "The first and most important treatment of the near-drowning victim is provision of immediate mouth-to-mouth ventilation. Prompt initiation of rescue breathing has a positive association with survival." Answer **a** is incorrect because the drainage of water is unnecessary and will delay provision of rescue breathing. The guidelines state "There is no need to clear the airway of aspirated water. Some victims aspirate nothing .... At most only a modest amount of water is aspirated by the majority of drowning victims, and it is rapidly absorbed." In addition the abdominal thrusts can cause injuries. Answer **b** is incorrect because chest compressions should be performed only if there are no signs of circulation after delivery of 2 breaths if the victim is unresponsive and not breathing. Answer **c** is incorrect because providing cervical spine stabilization will not restore oxygenation and ventilation.

Read more about it in the ECC Guidelines 2000, *pages 234-235: "Modifications to Guidelines for BLS for Resuscitation From Submersion"*

10. You have completed a tracheal intubation attempt for a patient in cardiac arrest. The tracheal tube appears to be in place after primary confirmation: you hear no stomach gurgling over the epigastrium, and breath sounds and chest expansion are equal and adequate bilaterally over the chest. You check the end-tidal carbon dioxide and do not detect exhaled carbon dioxide. Which of the following actions would be appropriate at this time?

- **a.** immediately remove the tracheal tube because the absence of exhaled carbon dioxide always indicates esophageal placement of the tube
- **b.** use an esophageal detector device, because low pulmonary blood flow during cardiac arrest can result in low exhaled carbon dioxide despite correct tracheal placement of the tube
- **c.** check pulse oximetry and remove the tube unless the hemoglobin saturation rises above 95%
- **d.** leave the tube in place and do not attempt further verification of tube placement because no confirmatory device is accurate for the patient in cardiac arrest

The correct answer is b.

Use an esophageal detector device, because low pulmonary blood flow during cardiac arrest can result in a low exhaled carbon dioxide despite correct tracheal placement of the tube. Answer **a** is incorrect for the same reason that answer **b** is correct: absence of exhaled carbon dioxide may be caused by the cardiac arrest and low pulmonary blood flow and may not necessarily indicate esophageal placement of the tracheal tube. Answer **c** is incorrect because in the absence of a pulsatile circulation the pulse oximeter may fail to function properly. The hemoglobin saturation may be low in the presence of cardiac arrest. Answer **d** is incorrect because the rescuer must be able to verify that the tube is in place. The esophageal detector device is often reliable in the presence of cardiac arrest.

Read more about it in the ECC Guidelines 2000, *pages 101-102: "How to Confirm Accurate Placement of Tracheal Tube: Primary Confirmation" and "How to Confirm Accurate Placement of Tracheal Tube: Secondary Confirmation"*

Case 2: Witnessed VF Arrest: Treatment by a Lone Rescuer With CPR and an AED

1. Which of the following choices lists *in correct order* the major steps of CPR and AED operation for an unresponsive victim

- **a.** send someone to phone 911, check for a pulse, attach the AED electrode pads, open the airway, provide 2 breaths if needed, then turn on the AED
- **b.** wait for the AED and barrier device to arrive, then open the airway, provide 2 breaths if needed, check for a pulse, and if no pulse is present, attach the AED and follow the sequence of AED prompts
- **c.** send someone to phone 911 and get the AED, open the airway, provide 2 breaths if needed, check for a pulse, and if no pulse is present attach the AED and follow the sequence of AED prompts
- **d.** provide 2 breaths, check for a pulse, call for the AED, provide chest compressions until the AED arrives, attach the AED

The correct answer is c.

Send someone to phone 911 and get the AED, open the airway, provide 2 breaths if needed, check for a pulse, and if no pulse is present, attach the AED and follow the sequence of AED prompts. These steps are listed in the guidelines, page 67: Figure 4, the AED treatment algorithm. Answer **a** is incorrect because in this answer the rescuer checks for a pulse before opening the airway and providing 2 breaths. The AED should be used only if the victim is unresponsive, is not breathing, and has no signs of circulation. Answer **b** is incorrect because the rescuer should **not** wait for the AED to arrive before acting. CPR should be provided while another rescuer phones 911 and gets the AED. CPR improves the victim's chance of survival at any interval to defibrillation. Answer **d** is incorrect because the rescuer should send another rescuer to phone 911 and get the AED as soon as the victim is found to be unresponsive. The lone rescuer should leave the victim to phone 911 and get the AED as soon as the victim is found to be unresponsive.

Read more about it in the ECC Guidelines 2000, *page 67: Figure 4: The AED Treatment Algorithm*

2. In correct order, what are the 4 "universal steps" required to operate an AED?

a. POWER ON the AED, attach the AED to the victim, analyze the rhythm, deliver a shock if indicated

b. attach the AED to the victim, POWER ON the AED, analyze the rhythm, deliver a shock if indicated

c. attach the electrode pads to the victim, attach the electronic cables to the AED, POWER ON the AED, analyze the rhythm, deliver a shock if indicated

d. POWER ON the AED, attach the AED to the victim, deliver the first shock, analyze the rhythm

The correct answer is a.

POWER ON the AED, attach the AED to the victim, analyze the rhythm, deliver a shock if indicated. This is the order of steps as listed in the guidelines, page 65. The first step in AED use is to turn the AED on so that the AED can provide voice prompts to assist the rescuer. Answers **b** and **c** are incorrect because the first rescuer action should be to turn on the AED. The AED should always be turned on first before it is attached to the victim or before the electrode cables are attached to the AED. Answer **d** is incorrect because the AED will not allow you to deliver a shock before the victim's rhythm is analyzed.

Read more about it in the ECC Guidelines 2000, *page 65: "The 'Universal AED': Common Steps to Operate All AEDs"*

3. A 12-year-old child collapses in a crowded museum. A museum employee is first on the scene and has an AED. She finds the victim unresponsive, so she immediately tells a bystander to activate EMS. The victim is not breathing, so the employee delivers 2 rescue breaths, checks for signs of circulation, and finds none. Next she POWERS ON the AED and attaches it correctly to the victim. She "clears" the victim and the AED analyzes the rhythm. The AED advises a shock, and the employee clears the victim and delivers a shock. What should the employee do next?

a. immediately give 2 rescue breaths to provide oxygen to the circulation

b. allow the AED to analyze the rhythm and deliver a shock up to 2 more times

c. provide chest compressions for approximately 1 minute

d. check for signs of circulation; if signs of circulation are present, begin rescue breathing

The correct answer is b.

Allow the AED to analyze the rhythm and deliver a shock up to 2 more times. The rescuer should do nothing that will interrupt the ability of the AED to analyze the rhythm immediately after the first and second shock and to charge to deliver a second and third shock if needed. This will allow delivery of up to 3 "stacked shocks" if VF continues. After analysis of the rhythm if the AED does not recommend a shock, the rescuer should check signs of circulation and provide chest compressions and ventilations if signs of circulation are absent.

Answer **a** is incorrect because defibrillation is the more important treatment to offer if VF continues. Answer **c** is incorrect because chest compressions should be provided only if VF continues after the delivery of a total of 3 shocks in succession. Answer **d** is incorrect because nothing should be done to interrupt the rapid delivery of a total of 3 shocks in succession if VF continues.

Read more about it in the ECC Guidelines 2000, *page 66: top left paragraph*

4. You respond with 2 other rescuers to a 50-year-old man who is unresponsive, pulseless, and not breathing. What tasks would you assign the other rescuers while you set up the AED?

a. one rescuer should phone 911 and the other rescuer should begin CPR

b. both rescuers should help set up the AED and provide CPR

c. one rescuer should open the airway and begin rescue breathing, and the second rescuer should begin chest compressions

d. recruit additional first responders to help

The correct answer is a.

One rescuer should phone 911 and the other rescuer should begin CPR. The rescuers should act simultaneously to ensure rapid EMS activation and immediate initiation of CPR. These simultaneous actions are listed in the *ECC Guidelines 2000,* page 66: "Integration of CPR and AED Use." Answers **b** and **c** are incorrect because if both rescuers assist with setting up the AED or performing CPR, no one is activating the EMS system. Answer **d** is incorrect because 2 rescuers are already available to help.

Read more about it in the ECC Guidelines 2000, *page 66: "Integration of CPR and AED Use"; and page 67: Figure 4: The AED Treatment Algorithm*

5. You are participating in the attempted resuscitation of a man who collapsed in the airport. You are operating the AED. After 3 successive shocks the victim is still pulseless. What should you do next?

   a. resume delivering shocks immediately

   b. do not attempt to shock again until EMS personnel arrive

   c. perform CPR for 1 minute and reanalyze the victim's rhythm

   d. remove the AED and transport the victim to the ED

   The correct answer is c.

   Perform CPR for 1 minute and reanalyze the victim's rhythm. AEDs are programmed to pause after each group of 3 shocks to allow 1 minute of CPR. The purpose of this pause is to enable circulation of some oxygenated blood to increase the likelihood of defibrillation success. When ACLS providers arrive, they will use this interval after 3 shocks to administer epinephrine or vasopressin and perform CPR to increase coronary artery perfusion and perfusion pressure to increase the likelihood of defibrillation success. Answer **a** is incorrect because the AED is programmed to pause for 1 minute. Answer **b** is incorrect because analysis should be performed and up to 3 shocks delivered if indicated after 1 minute of CPR. This cycle should be repeated (analysis and up to 3 shocks, 1 minute of CPR) until no shock is advised (other than after the third shock) or EMS personnel arrive. Answer **d** is incorrect because the AED should remain attached to the patient and "on" throughout transport. If the victim refibrillates during transport, the AED will typically prompt the rescuer to check the patient.

   Read more about it in the ECC Guidelines 2000, *pages 65-66: "Step 4: Clear the victim and press the SHOCK button"*

6. You attach an AED to a 43-year-old victim who is pulseless and not breathing, and the AED advises *"no shock indicated."* What should you do?

   a. reanalyze immediately

   b. perform CPR for 1 minute and reanalyze

   c. perform CPR until EMS personnel arrive

   d. remove the AED

   The correct answer is b.

   Perform CPR for 1 minute and reanalyze. Answer **a** is incorrect because AEDs are very accurate. The rescuer should perform CPR and reanalyze the rhythm every minute or so. Answer **c** is incorrect because the rhythm should be analyzed every minute or so in case VF returns. Answer **d** is incorrect because the patient may develop a shockable rhythm, and if you remove the AED you will not detect it.

   Read more about it in the ECC Guidelines 2000, *page 66: "'No Shock Indicated' Message"*

7. An AED hangs on the wall in the radiology suite where you work. Suddenly a code is called. You grab the AED and run to the room where the resuscitation attempt is ongoing. A colleague has begun CPR and confirms that the patient is in pulseless arrest. As you begin to attach the AED to the victim, you see a transdermal medication patch on the victim's upper right chest, precisely where you were going to place an AED electrode pad. What is your most appropriate *next* action?

   a. ignore the medication patch and place the electrode pad in the usual position

   b. avoid the medication patch and place the second electrode pad on the victim's back

   c. remove the medication patch, wipe the area dry, and place the electrode pad in the correct position

   d. place the electrode pad on the victim's right abdomen

   The correct answer is c.

   Remove the medication patch, wipe the area dry, and place the electrode pad in the correct position. This answer is taken almost verbatim from the *ECC Guidelines 2000,* page 65. Answer **a** is incorrect because if you place the electrode pad over the medication patch, it may result in reduced current delivery to the heart and reduced effectiveness of the shock. Answers **b** and **d** are incorrect because the guidelines do not suggest alternative sites for placement of AED pads to avoid a medication patch. Instead, the guidelines recommend that the medication patch be removed, the area wiped dry, and the electrode pad placed in the correct location.

   Read more about it in the ECC Guidelines 2000, *pages 64-65: "Transdermal Medications"*

Case 3: VF/Pulseless VT: Persistent/ Refractory/Recurrent/ Shock Resistant

1. A patient develops sudden VF arrest during evaluation for chest pain in an outpatient clinic. The patient has just received the first shock from the clinic AED. The monitor screen on the AED displays VF. What is the next action rescuers should take?

   a. resume CPR for approximately 1 minute; then reanalyze the rhythm

   b. establish IV access for medication administration

   c. press the ANALYZE control on the AED to reanalyze the rhythm

   d. administer epinephrine 1 mg IV as soon as the IV is established

The correct answer is c.

Press the ANALYZE control on the AED to reanalyze the rhythm. The VF/pulseless VT algorithm calls for up to 3 shocks to be delivered as "stacked shocks." This means that if VF/VT persists after the first shock, a second shock should be delivered without delay. If VF/VT persists after the second shock a third shock should be delivered without delay. Answer **a** is incorrect because if a defibrillator is available you should withhold CPR until the AED has delivered up to 3 shocks as close together as possible. There is no period of CPR prescribed between the first and second and the second and third shocks. Of course CPR must be performed continuously and at all times other than analysis and delivery of shocks by the AED. Provision of CPR should not interrupt the rapid delivery of shocks. Answer **b** is incorrect because rapid defibrillation attempts take precedence over establishment of IV access. If IV access can be established without delaying defibrillation, it should be accomplished. Answer **d** is incorrect because if a defibrillator is available, epinephrine should be delivered if the patient remains in cardiac arrest despite 3 shocks or if the patient converts to asystole.

Read more about it in the ECC Guidelines 2000, *page 129: "Epinephrine"; page 146: "Newly Recommended Agent: Vasopressin for VF/VT"; and pages 147-150: Figure 3: VF/Pulseless VT Algorithm and text*

2. The patient in question 1 has failed to respond to 3 shocks (VF persists). Paramedics arrive, start an IV, and insert a tracheal tube, confirming proper placement. Which of the following drugs should this patient receive *first?*

a. amiodarone 300 mg IV push

b. lidocaine 1 to 1.5 mg/kg IV push

c. procainamide 30 mg/min up to a total dose of 17 mg/kg

d. epinephrine 1 mg IV push or vasopressin 40 U single dose

The correct answer is d.

Epinephrine 1 mg IV push ***or*** vasopressin 40 U single dose. If VF/pulseless VT persists after 3 shocks, either epinephrine or vasopressin should be administered. These drugs produce vasoconstriction, elevating aortic end-diastolic pressure, and may improve coronary artery perfusion pressure. A shock should be delivered within 30 to 60 seconds after either drug is administered. Answers **a** and **b** are incorrect because antiarrhythmics should be considered only after administration of 1 mg epinephrine IV ***or*** 40 U vasopressin plus a fourth shock. Answer **c** is incorrect because antiarrhythmics should be considered only after administration of epinephrine or vasopressin plus a fourth shock. The antiarrhythmics to be considered should not include procainamide because procainamide is not indicated for refractory VF.

Read more about it in the ECC Guidelines 2000, *page 129: "Epinephrine"; page 146: "Newly Recommended Agent: Vasopressin for VF/VT"; and pages 147-150: Figure 3: VF/Pulseless VT Algorithm and text*

3. The patient in questions 1 and 2 remains in VF after epinephrine 1 mg IV and a fourth shock. You want to continue to administer epinephrine at appropriate doses and intervals if the patient remains in VF. Which epinephrine dose is *recommended* under these conditions?

a. give the following epinephrine dose sequence, each 3 minutes apart: 1 mg, 3 mg, and 5 mg

b. give a single "high dose" of epinephrine: 0.1 to 0.2 mg/kg

c. give epinephrine 1 mg IV, then in 5 minutes start vasopressin 40 U IV every 3 to 5 minutes

d. give epinephrine 1 mg IV; repeat 1 mg every 3 to 5 minutes

The correct answer is d.

If epinephrine 1 mg IV fails, higher doses are acceptable but not recommended. Large clinical trials have failed to show benefit for higher doses of epinephrine. In fact, high cumulative doses may be associated with worse neurologic outcome and postresuscitation hyperadrenergic states. Epinephrine should be administered every 3 to 5 minutes during cardiac arrest. If the initial standard dose fails, administration of a single higher dose, eg, 5 mg or 0.1 mg/kg, is left to the discretion of the clinician. Answers **a** and **b** are incorrect because the ACLS Subcommittee does not recommend high-dose or escalating-dose epinephrine because of lack of demonstrated benefit and because of potential for harm. As noted above, administration of a single higher dose is at the discretion of the clinician. Answer **c** is incorrect because vasopressin is administered in a single dose. Epinephrine should be administered every 3 to 5 minutes during cardiac arrest.

Read more about it in the ECC Guidelines 2000, *pages 129-130: "Epinephrine"; page 149: "New Class of Recommendation for Epinephrine and Lidocaine: Indeterminate"; and page 147: Figure 3: VF/Pulseless VT Algorithm*

4. Which of the following therapies is the *most important intervention* for VF/pulseless VT, with the greatest effect on survival to hospital discharge?

a. epinephrine

b. defibrillation

c. oxygen

d. amiodarone

The correct answer is b.

Treatment of VF/pulseless VT requires defibrillation. CPR prolongs the duration of VF and therefore the time the heart will be responsive to a shock.

CPR also increases the probability that the postshock rhythm will be a perfusing rhythm and not asystole or persistent VF. By these mechanisms bystander CPR is associated with twice as high a survival rate from VF as that for the no-bystander CPR groups. Answers **a** and **d** are incorrect because their effects on survival are minor compared with defibrillation. Vasopressors (epinephrine) and antiarrhythmics (amiodarone) come into play only when a patient with VF fails to respond to 3 "stacked" shocks. The vast majority of VF patients who are successfully resuscitated respond with the first 3 shocks. Answer **c** is incorrect because, although oxygen is important, patients can be successfully ventilated with room air. The key to successful resuscitation is time from collapse to defibrillation.

Read more about it in the ECC Guidelines 2000, *page 116: "VF/Pulseless VT"; and pages 147-150: Figure 3: VF/Pulseless VT Algorithm and text*

5. The *ECC Guidelines 2000* recommend vasopressin as a new adrenergic-like agent for treatment of cardiac arrest. Which algorithms recommend vasopressin?

- **a.** VF/pulseless VT
- **b.** asystole
- **c.** PEA
- **d.** bradycardia

The correct answer is a.

The VF/pulseless VT algorithm recommends vasopressin. In doses many times higher than the natural antidiuretic hormone, it produces the vasoconstrictive effects of epinephrine but without the cardiac toxicity. Reported (human) clinical trials have examined the value of vasopressin only for VF/pulseless VT. It is an alternative therapy to epinephrine in the VF/pulseless VT algorithm. Answers **b** and **c** are incorrect because vasopressin has not been studied in the treatment of asystole or PEA, and no published data is available to support its use in the treatment of asystole or PEA. Answer **d** is incorrect because there is no indication or rationale for using vasopressin, a peripheral vasoconstrictor, in the treatment of bradycardia.

Read more about it in the ECC Guidelines 2000, *page 130: "Vasopressin"; and page 146: "Newly Recommended Agent: Vasopressin for VF/VT"*

6. A 53-year-old man has suffered sudden VF arrest in the ED. He remains in VF after 3 "stacked" shocks, epinephrine, and a fourth shock. The team leader asks for amiodarone 300 mg IV. Which of the following statements is true about amiodarone for refractory VF?

- **a.** amiodarone is a Class IIb–recommended therapy for treatment of patients who have not responded to 3 stacked shocks, IV epinephrine, and a fourth shock
- **b.** amiodarone is associated with better 1-year survival than that for any other therapy for people who remain in VF after 3 shocks, 1 mg epinephrine, and a fourth shock
- **c.** amiodarone is not recommended for refractory VF
- **d.** amiodarone should be administered as soon as an IV is available and at least 1 shock has failed to achieve defibrillation

The correct answer is a.

The mainstay of treatment for VF is electrical therapy, not chemical therapy. But if patients fail to respond to 3 shocks, epinephrine 1 mg, and a fourth shock, consider antiarrhythmics. Amiodarone received a Class IIb recommendation in the *ECC Guidelines 2000* with only fair evidence to support its use. Although in one prospective, randomized controlled clinical trial the drug improved survival to hospital admission, it did not improve survival to hospital discharge. Success with a short-term outcome but no benefit for an intermediate or long-term outcome was a reason for the IIb (rather than, eg, IIa) recommendation.

Answer **b** is incorrect because amiodarone was associated with improved survival only to hospital admission. The ARREST trial found no improvement in hospital discharge rates or 1-year survival. This limitation was responsible for the Class IIb recommendation despite a good short-term outcome demonstrated with a prospective, randomized placebo-controlled clinical trial. Answer **c** is incorrect because a vasoconstrictor is recommended before use of antiarrhythmic drugs. Increased aortic diastolic pressure increases coronary artery perfusion pressure and drug delivery to the myocardium as well as the likelihood of defibrillation—the next fourth shock. Answer **d** is incorrect because vasoconstrictors should be administered before antiarrhythmics. Antiarrhythmics are considered after the patient fails to respond to 3 shocks, epinephrine or vasopressin, and a fourth shock.

Read more about it in the ECC Guidelines 2000, *page 116: "VF/Pulseless VT"; page 120: "Amiodarone (IV)"; and page 148: Figure 3: VF/Pulseless VT*

7. A 60-year-old man persists in VF arrest despite 3 stacked shocks at appropriate energy levels. Your code team, however, has been unable to start an IV or insert a tracheal tube. Therefore administration of IV or tracheal medications will be delayed. What is the most appropriate immediate next step?

- **a.** deliver additional shocks in an attempt to defibrillate
- **b.** deliver a precordial thump
- **c.** perform a venous cut-down to gain IV access
- **d.** administer intramuscular epinephrine 2 mg

The correct answer is a.

Deliver additional shocks in an attempt to defibrillate. Repeated shocks for VF/VT should continue regardless of inability to deliver epinephrine, antiarrhythmics, or other medications. The most important treatment for VF is always prompt defibrillation. In fact, definitive evidence is lacking that medications, either vasoconstrictors or antiarrhythmics, make a significant difference in VF resuscitation independent of more shocks. That is why lidocaine and epinephrine are Class Indeterminate and no antiarrhythmic has a higher recommendation than Class IIb based on the evidence. Answer **b** is incorrect because a precordial thump would be very unlikely to achieve defibrillation in a patient who continues in VF after 3 shocks. Answer **c** is incorrect because it would be inappropriate to delay additional shocks to perform a surgical procedure (or, for that matter, any other nonessential function).

Answer **d** is incorrect because there is no human evidence regarding the use of intramuscular epinephrine in cardiac arrest. Animal evidence suggests that intramuscular agents would not be adequately absorbed by that route during cardiac arrest.

Read more about it in the ECC Guidelines 2000, *page 90: "Defibrillation"; and page 91: the paragraph beginning "The most important determinant of survival in adult VF is rapid defibrillation"*

8. A 75-year-old homeless man is in cardiac arrest with pulseless VT at a rate of 220 bpm. After CPR, 3 shocks in rapid succession, 1 mg IV epinephrine, plus 3 more shocks, the man continues to be in polymorphic pulseless VT. He appears wasted and malnourished. The paramedics recognize him as a chronic alcoholic known in the neighborhood. Because he remains in VT after 6 shocks, you are considering an antiarrhythmic. Which of the following agents would be *most appropriate* for *this* patient at *this* time?

a. amiodarone

b. procainamide

c. magnesium

d. diltiazem

The correct answer is c.

Low levels of magnesium sulfate are very common in chronic malnourished people and alcoholics, and this man combines both risk factors. At certain levels of low magnesium, patients with refractory VF/pulseless VT will simply not convert without emergency replacement of magnesium. No other antiarrhythmic will be effective, and magnesium alone may be sufficient to render the fibrillating myocardium responsive to the next shock. In addition, magnesium is the agent of choice for treating torsades de pointes even when the torsades is not associated with hypomagnesemia. This man's VT, described as polymorphic VT, may well be torsades.

Answer **a** is not incorrect, but it is not the *most appropriate* choice for a patient who is very likely to have hypomagnesemia. Answer **b** is incorrect because procainamide is not recommended for the treatment of cardiac arrest (the patient does not have a perfusing rhythm). Procainamide is among the recommended antiarrhythmics to consider if the patient displays *recurrent* VF/VT. Recurrent VF/VT is present when defibrillatory shocks succeed in converting VF/VT to a perfusing rhythm, but then VF/VT recurs. The periods of intermittent non-VF/VT provide the only time when procainamide can be administered in 100-mg boluses every 5 minutes due to the hypotensive effects. Answer **d** is incorrect because calcium channel blockers can cause further cardiovascular collapse in patients with VT. In addition, calcium channel blockers affect only reentry tachycardias, not the automatic focus tachycardias, the problem for this patient.

Read more about it in the ECC Guidelines 2000, *page 116: "VF/Pulseless VT"; page 120: "Amiodarone (IV)"; page 123: "Magnesium"; and page 148: Figure 3: VF/Pulseless VT*

9. Which statement is true about the use of antiarrhythmics for patients with shock-refractory VF/pulseless VT?

a. antiarrhythmic agents are indicated because of the well-documented long-term benefits of increasing 1-year survival for VF/VT victims

b. antiarrhythmic agents can replace the need for continued shocks if infused fast and early

c. antiarrhythmic agents reduce the myocardial damage from continued shocks

d. in prospective, randomized trials, antiarrhythmic agents have not yet been found to improve survival to hospital discharge of patients with VF/pulseless VT

The correct answer is d.

In prospective, randomized trials antiarrhythmic agents have not yet been found to improve survival to hospital discharge in patients with VF/pulseless VT. In the ARREST trial amiodarone compared with placebo improved survival to hospital admission but not survival to hospital discharge. Answer **a** is incorrect because some antiarrhythmics have increased return of spontaneous circulation and survival to hospital admission, and none has prospectively been shown to improve 1-year survival. Answer **b** is incorrect because although antiarrhythmics should be considered early rather than late in the course of recurrent VF/pulseless VT, defibrillation is what restores a perfusing rhythm. The effect of antiarrhythmic therapy in theory is to prevent refibrillation but only *after* defibrillation. Answer **c** is incorrect because there is no evidence that significant myocardial damage occurs from defibrillation attempts until the shocks reach double-digit range. There is no evidence that antiarrhythmics prevent such damage.

Read more about it in the ECC Guidelines 2000, *page 116: "VF/Pulseless VT"; and page 148: Figure 3: VF/Pulseless VT*

10. A 55-year-old man running in his first marathon collapses after 15 miles. Paramedics on the scene attempt defibrillation with an AED and report a pattern of "in-and-out" VF in which a perfusing rhythm resumes after 1 or more shocks but then VF recurs. Upon arrival in the ED the man continues to go into VF, respond briefly to a shock, then return to VF. Currently he has hypotensive tachycardia (BP = 80/50; HR = 120 to 140 bpm). What would be the most appropriate action to take to prevent VF from recurring?

a. institute transvenous pacing

b. search for and treat conditions that can be risk factors for recurrent VF, such as unstable angina, hypoxia, hypovolemia, hypoglycemia, and electrolyte disorders

c. administer epinephrine 1 mg IV every 3 to 5 minutes for at least 3 doses

d. begin a slow, prophylactic infusion of amiodarone 360 mg IV over 6 hours (1 mg/min) or procainamide 250 mg IV push every 3 minutes

The correct answer is b.

Patients who repeatedly return to VF after successful defibrillation usually do so for a reason. If that reason can be identified and corrected, the prognosis is much better. The blood pressure and heart rate between VF recurrences can supply a clue. The low blood pressure and rapid heart rate in this man fit with significant hypovolemia produced by the long period of running and perhaps associated electrolyte imbalances. Repeated assessments of the patient are critical. Volume infusions and correction of electrolytes could completely eliminate recurring VF.

Answer **a** is incorrect because the patient has an adequate heart rate. Answer **c** is incorrect because the epinephrine dose indicated is a resuscitation dose and much too high for this patient, who is already tachycardic. Answer **d** is incorrect, although the use of prophylactic antiarrhythmics during periods of perfusion is a good idea. The amiodarone dose is too low to have any effect during the critical acute period. The procainamide dose is too high and would produce unacceptable side effects.

Read more about it in the ECC Guidelines 2000, *pages 116-117: "VF/Pulseless VT"; page 120: "Antiarrhythmic Drugs and the Arrhythmias They Treat"; and pages 147-150: Figure 3: VF/Pulseless VT Algorithm and text*

Case 4: Pulseless Electrical Activity

1. You are called to assist in the attempted resuscitation of a patient who is demonstrating PEA. As you hurry to the patient's room, you review the information you learned in the ACLS course about management of PEA. Which one of the following statements about PEA is *true?*

a. chest compressions should be administered only if the patient with PEA develops a ventricular rate of less than 50 bpm

b. successful treatment of PEA requires identification and treatment of reversible causes, such as the 5 H's and 5 T's

c. atropine is the drug of choice for treatment of PEA, whether the ventricular rate is slow or fast

d. PEA is rarely caused by hypovolemia, so fluid administration is contraindicated and should not be attempted

The correct answer is b.

Successful treatment of PEA requires identification and treatment of reversible causes, such as the 5 H's and 5 T's. PEA is the absence of a pulse in the presence of organized cardiac electrical activity other than VT or VF. PEA, which can cause cardiac arrest, is often caused by reversible conditions that begin with either an "H" (hypovolemia, hypoxia, hydrogen ion or acidosis, hyperkalemia/hypokalemia, or hypothermia) or a "T" (tablets causing intentional or unintentional overdose, tamponade, tension pneumothorax, thrombosis of a coronary artery, or thrombosis in the pulmonary artery). If the rescuer can identify and treat the reversible cause of PEA, the patient may regain a perfusing cardiac rhythm (on producing pulses).

Answer **a** is incorrect because chest compressions should be provided to the patient in PEA regardless of the rate of the ventricular complexes: the patient is in pulseless cardiac arrest, and chest compressions should be administered until the patient regains a perfusing (with pulses) cardiac rhythm. Answer **c** is incorrect because atropine is recommended if the PEA rate is *slow* or *relatively slow.* Administration of atropine is not recommended for PEA with a rapid ventricular rate. PEA with a rapid rate is often caused by a heart responding appropriately to hypovolemia, infection, pulmonary emboli, or cardiac tamponade, so efforts should be made to rule out or treat these conditions. Answer **d** is incorrect because hypovolemia is one of the *most common* causes (not an uncommon cause) of electrical activity without a pulse, so empiric fluid administration should be considered and may be helpful.

Read more about it in the ECC Guidelines 2000, *pages 150-152: Figure 4: Pulseless Electrical Activity and PEA Algorithm*

2. You are called to the ED to assist in the attempted resuscitation of a patient in pulseless cardiac arrest from unknown causes. When the patient arrives in the ED, chest compressions are being performed, and the patient is receiving ventilations through a tracheal tube placed by EMS personnel in the field. The patient is transferred to a gurney; you confirm that chest compressions are producing palpable femoral pulses, but no pulses are palpable between administered compressions. The patient is attached to a cardiac monitor that confirms the presence of organized QRS complexes. What is the *first* thing you should assess in an attempt to identify a reversible cause of cardiac arrest in this patient?

a. check tracheal tube placement with primary and secondary techniques and evaluate breath sounds to rule out tension pneumothorax

b. check arterial blood gases

c. check serum electrolytes to rule out imbalances

d. obtain a serum sample to identify drug overdose

The correct answer is a.

Treatment of cardiac arrest begins with good basic life support: establishment of airway, breathing, and circulation. The rescuer should always evaluate the airway in place and verify that effective ventilations are provided. This evaluation is particularly important when the patient initially arrives in the ED after placement of a tracheal tube in the field. The position of the tube should also be verified if the patient is moved (eg, from the ED to the unit). The Primary and Secondary ABCD Surveys in ACLS require establishment and verification of placement of an advanced airway. Finally, 2 potentially reversible causes of PEA listed in the "5 H's and 5 T's" are hypoxia and tension pneumothorax. The rescuer can rule these out by verifying that the tracheal tube is in the trachea and producing bilateral chest expansion and adequate bilateral breath sounds.

Answer **b** is incorrect because there is no point in evaluating arterial blood gases if the tracheal tube is misplaced or a tension pneumothorax is present. The results of the arterial blood gas analysis will not be available for several minutes, and identification of a misplaced tube or a tension pneumothorax should be accomplished without delay. Answers **c** and **d** are incorrect because they are part of the Secondary ABCD Survey, "differential diagnosis." The rescuer should search for the cause of the arrest, but the Primary ABCD Survey and the ABCs of the Secondary Survey should be accomplished first.

Read more about it in the ECC Guidelines 2000, *page 151: PEA Algorithm, Secondary ABCD Survey*

3. You are participating in the attempted resuscitation of a 62-year-old woman who collapsed suddenly at her home 3 weeks after cardiovascular surgery for aortic and mitral valve replacement. She recently began taking anticoagulants. Chest compressions are being performed, a tracheal tube is in place (proper placement was confirmed using primary and secondary confirmation techniques), and the patient is receiving 100% oxygen. Ventilation is producing bilateral chest expansion and adequate breath sounds. The ECG reveals narrow QRS complexes with a rate of 80 bpm, but no pulses are present. Ultrasound reveals no cardiac tamponade. Which of the following sequences of therapy is most appropriate for this patient?

a. atropine 1 mg IV every 3 to 5 minutes to a total dose of 0.04 mg/kg, followed by vasopressin 40 U IV single dose

b. sodium bicarbonate 1 mEq/kg every 3 to 5 minutes for empiric treatment of hyperkalemia

c. epinephrine 1 mg, followed by a fluid bolus and search for reversible causes

d. send blood for coagulation screening profile, and send patient for immediate CT scan to rule out intracranial hemorrhage

The correct answer is c.

Give epinephrine 1 mg, followed by a fluid bolus. Epinephrine is a nonspecific intervention for pulseless cardiac arrest that will improve coronary artery perfusion pressure. The narrow-complex PEA at a rate of 80 bpm is consistent with hypovolemia, so an empiric fluid bolus would be appropriate. This is the only answer option that includes the phrase "search for reversible causes" that is essential for the treatment of PEA. A reasonable theory of the cause of the PEA is gastrointestinal or other occult bleeding after initiation of anticoagulation. However, all other potential causes (the 5 H's and 5 T's) should be considered and ruled out.

Answer **a** is incorrect for 2 reasons. First, atropine is recommended only if the PEA is associated with a slow complex rate (the complex rate in this patient is 80 bpm, which is too fast for atropine administration). Second, there is no evidence to justify the use of vasopressin for PEA. Although this drug is an alternative to epinephrine in the pulseless VT/VF algorithm, it does not appear in the PEA algorithm. The best treatment for PEA is treatment of reversible causes while providing good BLS and epinephrine every 3 to 5 minutes. Answer **b** is incorrect because no evidence is offered to support the diagnosis of hyperkalemia. If this were a patient with known renal failure or other likely cause of hyperkalemia, administration of calcium chloride, then sodium bicarbonate, then glucose plus insulin would be indicated. Answer **d** is incorrect because although you should check the patient's coagulation panel, you cannot send the patient for the CT scan until she has a perfusing cardiac rhythm.

Read more about it in the ECC Guidelines 2000, *pages 150-152: Figure 4: Pulseless Electrical Activity and PEA Algorithm, particularly page 152: top paragraph, right column.*

4. You are participating in the attempted resuscitation of a patient with PEA. The patient has been intubated (with tube position confirmed) and is receiving 100% oxygen and effective ventilation with bilateral breath sounds and good chest expansion. Epinephrine 1 mg was administered 2 minutes ago. PEA continues, with a ventricular rate of 45 bpm. While you search for reversible causes of the PEA, which of the following therapies would now be appropriate?

a. monophasic defibrillation up to 3 times at 200 J, 200 to 300 J, and 360 J, or biphasic defibrillation at approximately 150 J

b. synchronized cardioversion

c. epinephrine 10 mL of 1:10 000 solution IV bolus

d. atropine 1 mg IV

The correct answer is d.

Atropine 1 mg IV should be administered for the patient with PEA if the rate is slow. This is the most appropriate of the therapies listed to be administered while you search for reversible causes. Answer **a** is incorrect because defibrillation is *not* indicated or recommended for PEA and should not be performed unless pulseless VT or VF develop. Answer **b** is incorrect because the patient does not have a tachycardia that would respond to synchronized cardioversion, and there is no evidence that cardioversion would improve the mechanical action of the heart. Answer **c** is incorrect because epinephrine was administered only 2 minutes ago. It is appropriate to administer epinephrine every 3 to 5 minutes for treatment of pulseless cardiac arrest.

Read more about it in the ECC Guidelines 2000, *pages 150-152: Figure 4: Pulseless Electrical Activity and PEA Algorithm*

5. For which of the following patients with PEA is sodium bicarbonate therapy (1 mEq/kg) most likely to be *most* effective?

a. the patient with hypercarbic acidosis and tension pneumothorax treated with decompression

b. the patient with a brief arrest interval

c. the patient with documented severe hyperkalemia

d. the patient with documented severe hypokalemia

The correct answer is c.

The patient with documented severe hyperkalemia should be treated with the hyperkalemia sequence that begins with administration of calcium chloride and includes sodium bicarbonate and glucose plus insulin. Answer **a** is incorrect because sodium bicarbonate is contraindicated for the patient with hypercarbic acidosis and inadequate ventilation. The metabolism of the sodium bicarbonate results in formation of carbon dioxide, so ventilation must be adequate if bicarbonate is administered. Tension pneumothorax should be treated immediately. Administration of sodium bicarbonate to the patient with inadequate ventilation or ventilation compromised by a tension pneumothorax will result in greater hypercarbia and worsening of the respiratory acidosis. Answer **b** is incorrect because most patients with a brief arrest interval will not require sodium bicarbonate because the best way to correct any mild acidosis from a brief arrest interval is to restore a perfusing rhythm with effective ventilation. Answer **d** is incorrect because hypokalemia will be worsened by administration of sodium bicarbonate. Sodium bicarbonate alkalinizes the serum, which produces an intracellular shift of potassium so that serum potassium falls.

Read more about it in the ECC Guidelines 2000, *pages 150-152: Figure 4: Pulseless Electrical Activity and PEA Algorithm, particularly page 152: top left column, sodium bicarbonate. Information about treatment of hyperkalemia is presented on page 217: "Life-Threatening Electrolyte Abnormalities; Hyperkalemia."*

Case 5: Asystole

1. Which of the following potential causes of prehospital asystole is most likely to respond to immediate treatment?

a. prolonged cardiac arrest

b. prolonged submersion in warm water

c. drug overdose

d. blunt multisystem trauma

The correct answer is c.

Drug overdose is one of the atypical clinical features listed in the final box of the asystole algorithm as a feature that should be considered before ceasing resuscitative efforts. Specific references to the need to consider poisoning or drug overdose and the fact that poisoning or drug overdose can justify prolonged resuscitative efforts are made in the algorithm review in Part 6: Advanced Cardiovascular Life Support, in Part

2: Ethical Aspects of CPR and ECC, and in the Toxicology section of Part 8: Advanced Challenges in Resuscitation.

Answer **a** is incorrect because the 3 references cited note that in the absence of mitigating factors (such as drug overdose or prearrest hypothermia), patients are unlikely to survive after a long arrest interval. Answer **b** is incorrect because only submersion in *icy* water has been associated with improved survival after submersion. Warm water would not exert any protective effect when hypoxia develops after submersion. Answer **d** is incorrect because survival from out-of-hospital cardiac arrest associated with blunt trauma is uniformly low in children and adults.

Read more about it in the ECC Guidelines 2000, *page 154: Notes for Figure 5: Asystole Algorithm; and page 227: "Prolonged CPR and Resuscitation." Issues to be considered before termination of resuscitative efforts are also presented on page [illegible]: "Criteria for Terminating Resuscitative Efforts." Prognostic factors associated with poor outcome following submersion are presented on page 233: "Definitions, Classifications, and Prognostic Indicators." The outcome of cardiac arrest associated with trauma is presented on page 244: "Cardiac Arrest Associated With Trauma"*

2. Which of the following is the correct *initial* drug and dose for treatment of asystole?

a. epinephrine 2 mg IV

b. atropine 0.5 mg IV

c. lidocaine 1 mg/kg IV

d. epinephrine 1 mg IV

The correct answer is d.

Epinephrine 1 mg IV is traditionally recommended for the treatment of asystole and is listed in the asystole algorithm. Answer **a** is incorrect because this dose of epinephrine is noted as "may be used but is not recommended" and should be considered only if the patient fails to respond to the conventional dose. It should not be administered as the initial dose of epinephrine. Answer **b** is incorrect because atropine 1 mg IV should be administered *after* a dose of epinephrine. Answer **c** is incorrect because lidocaine is not included in the asystole algorithm.

Read more about it in the ECC Guidelines 2000, *pages 152-154: Figure 5: Asystole: The Silent Heart Algorithm and notes*

3. Paramedics have arrived with an asystolic 42-year-old man who was found unconscious, breathless, and pulseless in the hallway of his apartment. CPR is ongoing. The patient is intubated. He has bilateral breath sounds and equal and adequate chest expansion. IV access has been successfully established, with fluid infusion at a "keep open" rate. The patient's vital signs are as follows: PaO_2 = 85 mm Hg; $PaCO_2$ = 32 mm Hg; pH = 7.3; serum potassium = 4.5 mEq/L; core body temperature = 37°C. In this scenario, which is the most likely reversible cause to consider before stopping the resuscitation attempt?

a. tracheal tube in the esophagus

b. drug overdose

c. tension pneumothorax

d. hypothermia

The correct answer is b.

It is noted several times in the guidelines that the prognosis for asystole caused by drug overdose or poisoning can justify more prolonged resuscitative efforts (Part 6: Advanced Cardiovascular Life Support; Part 2: Ethical Aspects of CPR and ECC; and Part 8: Advanced Challenges in Resuscitation, Toxicology in ECC). Answer **a** is incorrect because a tracheal tube in the esophagus is unlikely to be associated with equal and adequate bilateral breath sounds and effective oxygenation and ventilation (as indicated by the arterial oxygen tension of 85 mm Hg and normocarbia). Answer **c** is incorrect because a tension pneumothorax is unlikely to be associated with equal and adequate bilateral breath sounds and effective oxygenation. Answer **d** is incorrect because hypothermia is an unlikely diagnosis in a patient found inside an apartment building with a core body temperature of 37°C.

Read more about it in the ECC Guidelines 2000, *pages 153-154: Figure 5: Asystole Algorithm and notes; and page 227: "Prolonged CPR and Resuscitation"*

4. You are considering transcutaneus pacing for a patient in asystole. Which of the following candidates would be most likely to respond to such a pacing attempt?

a. the patient in asystole who has failed to respond to 20 minutes of BLS and ACLS therapy

b. the patient in asystole following blunt trauma

c. the patient in asystole following a defibrillatory shock

d. the patient who has just arrived in the ED following transport and CPR in the field for persistent asystole after submersion

The correct answer is c.

Transcutaneous pacing is most likely to be effective in the patient in asystole following a defibrillatory shock if performed immediately. If the patient developed asystole immediately after defibrillation, that asystole would be short-lived. Answers **a** and **d** are incorrect because both characterize patients who have been in cardiac arrest for a prolonged time. Answer **b** is incorrect because reversible causes of cardiac arrest associated with blunt trauma include conditions such as hypovolemia, neurologic injury, tension pneumothorax, or major organ damage. It is unlikely that any of these causes would respond to transcutaneous pacing.

Read more about it in the ECC Guidelines 2000, *pages 153-154: Figure 5: Asystole Algorithm and notes; and page 244: "Cardiac Arrest Associated With Trauma." Also see the* ECC Handbook.

5. Which of the following should be checked as part of the flat line protocol to confirm the presence of asystole and rule out operator or monitoring error as the reason for the isoelectric ECG?

a. check power switch, all connections between the monitor and patient, monitor/defibrillator battery, sensitivity or gain and lead choice

b. obtain a 12-lead ECG

c. push the SYNCHRONIZE button on the cardioverter/defibrillator

d. administer a trial defibrillatory shock to rule out occult VF

The correct answer is a.

Check the power switch, all connections between the monitor and patient, monitor/defibrillator battery, sensitivity or gain, and lead choice. Items to be checked to confirm true asystole are listed in the discussion of the asystole algorithm. The rescuer must rule out the possibility that the isoelectric ECG is the result of a faulty monitor or connection between the patient and the monitor. Answer **b** is incorrect because you should not halt chest compressions and resuscitative efforts to obtain a 12-lead ECG. Answer **c** is incorrect because there is no need to push the SYNCHRONIZE button on the cardioverter/defibrillator unless you are preparing for synchronized cardioversion. Such therapy is not warranted for asystole. Answer **d** is incorrect because there is no evidence that attempting to "defibrillate" asystole is beneficial. Although in rare patients occult VF may be present in some leads in patients with an apparent isoelectric ECG, examination of the ECG in 2 leads will be sufficient to determine if VF is present.

Read more about it in the ECC Guidelines 2000, *page 154: "Confirm True Asystole"; and page 93: "'Occult' Versus 'False' Asystole." This information is also presented in the box: "The Flat Line Protocol" in Case 5.*

6. You are in the ED assisting in a resuscitation attempt for a normothermic patient who was transported in asystolic cardiac arrest. You are providing a trial of BLS and ACLS. The patient has been successfully intubated, and you have confirmed proper tube placement. IV access has been obtained. Which of the following interventions would be most likely to have the greatest therapeutic effect at this time?

a. ask the family if they would like to be present during the resuscitation attempt

b. administer escalating doses of epinephrine

c. administer fibrinolytics to treat a possible myocardial infarction

d. administer an empiric defibrillatory shock of 200 J

The correct answer is a.

This scenario documents what is likely to be an unsuccessful resuscitative effort—the patient has failed to respond to a course of BLS and ACLS and has no hypothermia. Unless additional mitigating factors are identified and reversed, this patient is unlikely to survive. Whenever possible, family members should be offered the option of being present during resuscitation. This is particularly important when your resuscitative efforts are unlikely to be effective; under these conditions the needs of family members should be strongly considered. Although family presence can be potentially beneficial in many resuscitative situations, the strongest evidence of benefit has been documented in studies of family members following the death of a loved one. Family members who were given the option of being present during the resuscitation attempt showed less anxiety and depression and more constructive grief behavior than family members who were not given the option.

Answer **b** is incorrect because there is no evidence that escalating doses of epinephrine are effective in the treatment of asystole that persists in a normothermic patient. Answer **c** is incorrect because this patient has none of the indications for fibrinolytic therapy, and fibrinolytic therapy is not provided during cardiac arrest. Answer **d** is incorrect because there is no evidence that attempting to "defibrillate" asystole is beneficial. Although in rare patients occult VF may be present in some leads in patients with an apparent isoelectric ECG, examination of the ECG in 2 leads will be sufficient to determine if VF is present.

Read more about it in the ECC Guidelines 2000, *pages 153-155: Figure 5: Asystole Algorithm and notes; pages 14-15: "Criteria for Terminating Resuscitative Efforts"; page 19: "Family Presence During Resuscitation Attempts"; and page 93: "'Occult' Versus 'False' Asystole"*

Case 6: Acute Coronary Syndromes

1. You are an EMS paramedic evaluating a 50-year-old man at his home. He complains of crushing substernal chest pain, profuse sweating, and shortness of breath. His vital signs are as follows: temperature = 37°C; HR = 100 bpm; BP = 170/110 mm Hg; resp = 32; oxygen saturation = 90%. Which of the following includes the best immediate treatment for this patient?

a. oxygen, morphine, aspirin, followed by sublingual nitroglycerin if morphine fails to relieve pain

b. oxygen, sublingual nitroglycerin, morphine, but withhold aspirin unless the ST segment is elevated more than 3 mm

c. oxygen, sublingual nitroglycerin, followed by morphine if nitroglycerin fails to relieve pain, aspirin

d. oxygen, sublingual nitroglycerin, no morphine because of the high blood pressure, no aspirin until admitted to the hospital

The correct answer is c.

Oxygen, sublingual nitroglycerin, followed by morphine if nitroglycerin fails to relieve the pain, and aspirin is the correct sequence. The acute coronary syndrome cases teach the use of the memory aid *"MONA greets all patients"* to help the rescuer remember the immediate general treatment with *morphine, oxygen, nitroglycerin,* and *aspirin.* This is not, however, the *sequence* in which these agents are usually given. *Oxygen* is a critical therapy for all chest pain patients: it should always be given as the first agent. Sublingual *nitroglycerin* should be given next; it is quick, easy to administer, and frequently effective. *Morphine* is held in reserve until the response to nitroglycerin is determined. If nitroglycerin does not provide complete pain relief, morphine should be used. *Aspirin* can be given at any time because the sequence is inconsequential if given in the first 15 to 30 minutes.

Answer **a** is incorrect because nitroglycerin should be given *before* morphine, a point specifically stated in the acute coronary syndromes algorithm. Answer **b** is incorrect because the aspirin instructions are incorrect—aspirin is not limited to only patients with ST-segment elevation. Answer **d** is incorrect because morphine is not withheld from patients with high blood pressure. In fact, morphine helps lower blood pressure. Aspirin is also not withheld until admission to the hospital.

Read more about it in the ECC Guidelines 2000, *page 25: "Out-of-Hospital Care for ACS" and the algorithm on page 26; and pages 176-180: "Initial General Measures"*

2. You are an ED physician evaluating the recently arrived 50-year-old man in question 1. The 12-lead ECG shows 3-mm ST-segment elevation in leads V_2 through V_4. Despite prehospital administration of oxygen, aspirin, nitroglycerin, and morphine, the man continues to have severe chest pain, which is now of more than 20 minutes' duration. His blood pressure is 170/110 mm Hg; his heart rate is 120 bpm. Which of the following treatments would be most appropriate for this patient at this time?

a. calcium channel blocker PO plus bolus of heparin

b. ACE inhibitor IV plus lidocaine infusion

c. magnesium sulfate plus aspirin

d. IV β-blocker, tPA, heparin

The correct answer is d.

IV β-blocker, tPA, and heparin are appropriate treatments for this patient at this time. This case describes classic indications for using β-blockers and fibrinolytic therapy in a patient with an AMI. Use of β-adrenergic blockers is recommended for all patients with ST-elevation infarction and continuing or recurrent ischemic pain (and all patients with non–ST-elevation MI and patients with tachyarrhythmias). The β-adrenoreceptor blocking agents will decrease myocardial oxygen consumption, reduce mortality and nonfatal reinfarction, and decrease the primary incidence of VF. Indications for fibrinolytic therapy include chest pain suggesting MI, ST-segment elevation greater than 1 mm in 2 or more contiguous leads, time to therapy less than 12 hours, and age less than 75 years (age more than 75 years is a Class IIa recommendation). The need for an urgent reperfusion strategy is obvious. Potential contraindications to fibrinolytic therapy should be ruled out.

Answer **a** is incorrect because calcium channel blockers have not been shown to reduce mortality after AMI and in some patients may be harmful. They should be considered an alternative or additional therapy if β-blockers are contraindicated or the maximum dose has been achieved. Heparin is indicated as an adjunct to fibrin-specific lytics. The dose, however, has been reduced to decrease the incidence of intracerebral hemorrhage, particularly in the elderly. The current ACC/AHA–recommended dose of heparin includes a bolus of 60 U/kg (maximum bolus of 4000 U), followed by infusion at a rate of 12 U/kg per hour (maximum infusion of 1000 U/h) for patients weighing more than 70 kg.

Answer **b** is incorrect. ACE inhibitors are valuable in limiting infarct expansion, improving the structural remodeling of the ventricle, reducing the neurohormonal impact on the heart, and increasing collateral flow to the peri-infarct ischemic area. They should be given on the first day of MI but should not be given within the first 6 hours. They should be given when the patient is stable after reperfusion, initial measures, and other therapies have been provided. Lidocaine is not recommended for primary VF prophylaxis or treatment of asymptomatic "warning" arrhythmias in patients with AMI. The use of lidocaine is limited to the treatment of hemodynamically stable VT and prevention of *recurrent* VF (secondary prophylaxis).

Answer **c** is incorrect because magnesium is not indicated for routine use in management of an AMI unless the patient had documented low magnesium. Studies are now looking at its use in specific subgroups such as elderly patients ineligible for fibrinolytics.

Read more about it in the ECC Guidelines 2000, *pages 182-184: "ST-Segment Elevation MI"; and pages 191-194: "Adjunctive Therapy for ACS"*

3. You are a healthcare provider working in a community medical clinic. A 65-year-old man begins to experience "heavy chest pressure" and shortness of breath, and perspiration is trickling down his face. When you tell him you are calling 911 for care and transport to the ED, he protests, *"No lights and sirens! My wife will drive me to the hospital."* Which of the following would be the *best* reasons to give for transporting this patient to the hospital in an ACLS mobile unit?

- **a.** EMS personnel can radio ahead to the ED, activate the acute chest pain protocol, and make the ED aware of an incoming patient with a possible acute coronary syndrome
- **b.** EMS personnel can provide immediate assessment, including use of a 12-lead ECG if available and immediate treatment with prearrival notification of the receiving hospital
- **c.** EMS personnel can obtain a blood sample for evaluation of cardiac markers to diagnose the cause of the chest pain
- **d.** EMS personnel can admit the patient directly to the coronary care unit and not waste time in the ED

The correct answer is b.

The best reasons to transport this patient in an ACLS mobile unit are that EMS personnel can provide immediate assessment, including 12-lead ECG if available, and immediate treatment with prearrival notification of the receiving hospital. More than half of patients who have an AMI fail to contact the EMS system for care and evaluation; and more than half wait more than 3 hours before presenting for care. Many patients ignore their symptoms, rationalize them, or simply deny the possibility of an AMI. Mobile advanced care provided by EMS professionals offers many positive benefits. Patients can receive oxygen; pain control; hemodynamic benefits from morphine, nitroglycerin, and β-blockers, and prevention of arrhythmias. EMS professionals will monitor the patient closely for rhythm abnormalities and are prepared to treat VF and pulseless VT. Most deaths from AMI occur in the first hour, usually from VF. Finally, paramedics can obtain a 12-lead ECG and send the results ahead to the receiving hospital so that the patient can be classified for therapy before arrival. This reduces delays to definitive therapy and improves outcome. During this time paramedics can explain the need for transportation with monitor and defibrillator availability. The patient's wife can be brought into the discussion to encourage and reassure him. Lights and sirens are not mandatory and may adversely affect this patent.

Answer **a** is not the best answer because it does not cite the major benefit from ACLS transport. The information is true and often helpful but not the best answer. Answer **c** is incorrect because there is no benefit in obtaining a blood sample for cardiac markers in the field. This will only delay transport, and the sample will not be tested until the patient arrives at the hospital, where other tests will be run. In addition, cardiac markers (troponin, CK-MB mass) are not positive until 6 hours after the onset of symptoms in most patients. Answer **d** is incorrect because ability to ensure direct admission to the CCU is not the major benefit of ACLS transport to the hospital. In addition, stopping in the ED is not "a waste of time." Triage is most effective, and the entire range of therapeutic options is available in most EDs. In fact, admission to the CCU has been shown to delay administration of fibrinolytics by at least 1 hour.

Read more about it in the ECC Guidelines 2000, *pages 24-26: "Recognition and Actions for Acute Coronary Syndromes," including the algorithm on page 26; and pages 173-176: "Out-of-Hospital Management"*

4. A patient presents to the ED complaining of severe, crushing, midsternal chest pain of 30 minutes' duration. He has a history of smoking and diet-controlled diabetes. His blood pressure is 110/70 mm Hg; his heart rate is 90 bpm. The 12-lead ECG shows a regular sinus rhythm of 90 bpm. Aspirin is administered, and oxygen 2 L/min is provided through a nasal cannula. Nitroglycerin provides no relief for the chest pain. Which of the following drugs should be administered next?

- **a.** atropine 0.5 mg IV
- **b.** lidocaine 1 to 1.5 mg/kg
- **c.** furosemide 20 to 40 mg IV
- **d.** morphine sulfate 2 to 4 mg IV

The correct answer is d.

Morphine sulfate 2 to 4 mg IV is indicated for pain relief in patients who do not get complete relief from nitroglycerin. The patient's blood pressure is adequate (110/70 mm Hg), so there are no apparent contraindications to administration of morphine. Answer **a** is incorrect because atropine 0.5 mg is used in the treatment of bradycardia, not chest pain. Bradycardia is not a problem with this patient because the heart rate is 90 bpm. Atropine may produce an increase in heart rate and an increase in myocardial oxygen demand, which may worsen chest pain. Answer **b** is incorrect because lidocaine is an antiarrhythmic drug that is not appropriate for a patient in sinus rhythm with no history of VF/pulseless VT. Routine use of lidocaine is no longer recommended for primary VF prophylaxis in AMI. Answer **c** is incorrect because furosemide is used in the treatment of pulmonary edema, not chest pain.

Read more about it in the ECC Guidelines 2000, *pages 24-26: "Recognition and Actions for Acute Coronary Syndromes," including the algorithm on page 26; and pages 173-176: "Out-of-Hospital Management"*

5. Which of the following adjunctive therapies is a component of management of an uncomplicated ST-segment elevation AMI?

a. amiodarone

b. aspirin

c. epinephrine

d. heparin

The correct answer is b.

Aspirin is now recognized as an important component of the immediate general therapy for all patients with acute ischemic chest pain. Aspirin blocks the formation of thromboxane A_2, which causes platelets to aggregate. In the acute coronary syndromes platelet aggregation starts the cascade of acute clot formation in the coronary arteries. Aspirin and agents like it interfere with that process and reduce AMI mortality, reinfarction, and nonfatal stroke. Answer **a** is incorrect because amiodarone is an antiarrhythmic indicated for recurrent VT, refractory VF, and pulseless VT. Amiodarone is not routinely administered for treatment of uncomplicated AMI. Answer **c** is incorrect because there is no indication for epinephrine in uncomplicated AMI. Epinephrine would increase myocardial oxygen consumption at a time when myocardial oxygen delivery may be compromised. Epinephrine may also contribute to development of ventricular arrhythmias. Answer **d** is incorrect because routine heparin administration is not part of the management of uncomplicated MI unless the patient is going to undergo direct or adjunctive percutaneous coronary intervention (PCI) or will receive a fibrin-specific lytic (eg, alteplase, reteplase, or tenecteplase).

Read more about it in the ECC Guidelines 2000, *pages 24-26: "Recognition and Actions for Acute Coronary Syndromes," including the algorithm on page 26; and pages 173-176: "Out-of-Hospital Management"*

6. Which of the following answers includes the major components of therapy for the 60-year-old patient presenting with ST-segment elevation MI within 30 minutes of the onset of symptoms of acute ischemic chest pain?

a. reperfusion therapy (fibrinolytics or PCI), aspirin, heparin, IV β-blockers

b. antithrombin therapy with heparin, antiplatelet therapy with aspirin, glycoprotein IIb/IIIa inhibitors, IV β-blockers, and nitrates, monitoring for "high-risk" status

c. serial ECGs with ST-segment monitoring, serum cardiac markers, further risk assessment with perfusion radionuclide imaging and stress echocardiography, aspirin

d. administer prophylactic lidocaine, fluid bolus, and vasopressor infusion

The correct answer is a.

The reperfusion therapy selected will be determined by local resources, presence or absence of contraindications to fibrinolytic therapy, and presence or absence of signs of cardiogenic shock. Maximum myocardial salvage occurs if eligible patients receive fibrinolytics within a few hours after onset of symptoms. Answer **b** is incorrect because these therapies represent the approach to management of the patient with ST-segment depression or dynamic T-wave inversion strongly suspicious for ischemia. Answer **c** is incorrect because these therapies represent the approach to management of the patient with acute ischemic chest pain and a nondiagnostic or normal ECG. Answer **d** is incorrect for several reasons. Routine lidocaine administration for patients with AMI is no longer recommended for primary prophylaxis of VF. Fluid bolus and vasopressor therapy may be indicated for patients with shock and hypotension but are not part of the routine management of ST-segment elevation MI. Vasopressor infusion will increase aortic diastolic pressure, left ventricular afterload, and myocardial oxygen consumption and should not be used unless a specific indication exists (eg, hypotension).

Read more about it in the ECC Guidelines 2000, *pages 178-179: Figure 3: Acute Ischemic Chest Pain Protocol and Figure 4: Acute Coronary Syndromes Algorithm; and pages 180-193: "Risk Stratification, Initial Therapy, and Evaluation for Reperfusion in the ED," "ST-Segment Elevation MI," "ST-Segment Depression: Non–Q-Wave MI/High-Risk Unstable Angina," and "Nondiagnostic ECG"*

7. Which of the following includes the major components of *initial* therapy for the patient with acute ischemic chest pain and a nondiagnostic ECG?

a. reperfusion therapy, aspirin, heparin, β-blockers, and nitrates

b. antithrombin therapy with heparin, antiplatelet therapy with aspirin, glycoprotein IIb/IIIa inhibitors, β-blockers, and nitrates, monitoring for "high-risk" status

c. serial ECGs with ST-segment monitoring, serum cardiac markers, and further risk assessment with perfusion radionuclide imaging and stress echocardiography, aspirin

d. prophylactic lidocaine, fluid bolus, and vasopressor infusion

The correct answer is c.

If cardiac markers, radionuclide imaging, or stress echochardiography indicates that the patient has "high-risk criteria," then treatment with aspirin, glycoprotein IIb/IIIa inhibitors, unfractionated heparin, and IV β-blockers is indicated. This therapy is similar to that for patients who are at high risk on initial evaluation. But these therapies would not be indicated unless or *until* the patient becomes "high risk" with development of ST-segment depression, persistent symptoms or recurrent ischemia, diffuse or widespread ECG abnormalities, depressed left ventricular function, congestive heart failure, or serum marker release. Answer **a** is incorrect because these therapies represent the approach to management of the patient with ST-segment elevation MI. Answer **b** is incorrect because these therapies represent the approach to management of the patient with ST-segment depression, non–Q-wave MI. Answer **d** is incorrect for several reasons. Routine lidocaine administration for patients with AMI is no longer recommended for primary prophylaxis of VF. Fluid bolus and vasopressor therapy may be indicated for patients with shock and hypotension but are not part of the routine management of ST-segment elevation MI. Vasopressor infusion will increase aortic diastolic pressure, left ventricular afterload, and myocardial oxygen consumption and should not be used unless a specific indication exists (eg, hypotension).

Read more about it in the ECC Guidelines 2000, *pages 178-179: algorithms; and pages 180-193: "Risk Stratification, Initial Therapy, and Evaluation for Reperfusion in the ED," "ST-Segment Elevation MI," "ST-Segment Depression: Non–Q-Wave MI/High-Risk Unstable Angina," and "Nondiagnostic ECG"*

8. Which of the following patients with acute continuing ischemic chest pain is *most likely* to benefit from β-adrenoreceptor blocking agent therapy?

a. the patient with second- or third-degree heart block

b. the patient with severe left ventricular failure

c. the patient with a systolic arterial blood pressure of 90/60 mm Hg and sinus rhythm of 55 bpm

d. the patient with ST-segment elevation MI and blood pressure of 180/104 mm Hg

The correct answer is d.

All patients with ST-segment elevation MI should receive β-adrenoreceptor blocking agents unless contraindications exist. In this patient a β-blocker would also be an ideal agent for treatment of hypertension occurring with MI. Answers **a, b,** and **c** are incorrect because all are contraindications to β-adrenoreceptor blocking agents. These contraindications include heart rate less than 60 bpm, systolic arterial pressure less than 100 mm Hg, severe left ventricular failure, signs of hypoperfusion, and advanced second- or third-degree AV block. Patients with mild or moderate left ventricular failure benefit the most from β-blockade but should be monitored closely and serially. They may require therapy with diuretic agents as well.

Read more about it in the ECC Guidelines 2000, *pages 178-179: algorithms; and pages 180-193: "Risk Stratification, Initial Therapy, and Evaluation for Reperfusion in the ED," "ST-Segment Elevation MI," "ST-Segment Depression: Non–Q-Wave MI/High-Risk Unstable Angina," and "Nondiagnostic ECG"*

9. For which of the following patients would PCI, including angioplasty/stent, be a Class I recommendation and a better option than a conservative strategy with initial medical therapy?

a. a patient with non–ST-segment elevation MI but no "high-risk" characteristics

b. a patient less than 75 years of age with acute coronary syndromes and signs of severe left ventricular dysfunction and cardiogenic shock presenting within 16 hours of symptom onset

c. a patient with ST-segment elevation inferior MI, no signs of shock or left ventricular dysfunction, and no contraindications to fibrinolytic therapy, presenting within 2 hours of onset of symptoms

d. a patient with ST-segment depression who responds to initial treatment

The correct answer is b.

A patient less than 75 years of age with acute coronary syndromes and signs of severe left ventricular dysfunction and cardiogenic shock presenting within 16 hours of symptom onset would be most likely to benefit from prompt catheterization and revascularization. This patient is not presenting within the optimum 12-hour window for fibrinolytics. In addition, the presence of cardiogenic shock indicates the need for urgent restoration of perfusion to the myocardium. Answer **a** is incorrect because the care of the patient with non–ST-segment elevation MI and no "high-risk" factors is initially managed with antithrombin and antiplatelet therapy. Cardiac catheterization (invasive strategy) may be selected but is not emergent. Answer **c** is incorrect because this patient appears to be a good candidate for fibrinolytic therapy as well. Although a PCI can be performed for this patient, there are other options. PCI and fibrinolytic therapy are equivalent treatments in this patient. If signs of right ventricular infarction or hypotension develop, the recommendation would change. Answer **d** is incorrect because if the patient with ST-segment depression can be stabilized, urgent PCI is not needed.

Read more about it in the ECC Guidelines 2000, *pages 178-179: algorithms; and pages 180-193: "Risk Stratification, Initial Therapy, and Evaluation for Reperfusion in the ED," "ST-Segment Elevation MI," "ST-Segment Depression: Non–Q-Wave MI/High-Risk Unstable Angina," and "Nondiagnostic ECG"*

10. Which of the following patients presenting with AMI would be most likely to present with atypical, unusual, or vague signs and symptoms?

a. a 65-year-old woman with a past medical history of typical angina and moderate coronary artery disease according to prior angiogram

b. a 56-year-old man with no prior history of heart disease

c. a 45-year-old woman diagnosed with type I diabetes 22 years ago

d. a 48-year-old man in the intensive care unit after coronary artery bypass surgery

The correct answer is c.

The elderly, persons with diabetes, and women are more likely to present with atypical or vague symptoms of an ACS. An acute coronary syndrome should be suspected in a 45-year-old woman with long-standing diabetes who has vague complaints such as diffuse chest "discomfort" or "pressure" rather than "pain," pain between the shoulder blades, or other vague symptoms. Too often such a patient is thought to be too young to have an MI, yet her long-standing diabetes places her at risk for early development of coronary artery disease. Answer **a** is incorrect because a 65-year-old woman with a history of coronary artery disease and angina is more likely to present with typical signs and symptoms. Answer **b** is incorrect because a 56-year-old man is more likely to present with typical signs and symptoms. Answer **d** is incorrect because even after coronary artery bypass surgery, a man is more likely to demonstrate typical signs and symptoms.

Read more about it in the ECC Guidelines 2000, *page 24: "Recognition and Actions for Acute Coronary Syndromes"; and page 174: "Patient Education and Delays in Therapy"*

Advanced Question: Management of ACS for Experienced Providers

11. Which of the following includes the major components of therapy for the patient with ST-segment depression MI, good left ventricular function, and no prior MI?

a. reperfusion therapy, aspirin, heparin, β-blockers

b. antithrombin therapy with heparin, antiplatelet therapy with aspirin, glycoprotein IIb/IIIa inhibitors, β-blockers, and nitrates, and monitoring for "high-risk" status

c. serial ECGs with ST-segment monitoring, serum cardiac markers, further risk assessment with perfusion radionuclide imaging and stress echocardiography, aspirin

d. prophylactic lidocaine, fluid bolus, and vasopressor infusion

The correct answer is b.

Antithrombin therapy with IV heparin, antiplatelet therapy with aspirin, glycoprotein IIb/IIIa inhibitors, β-blockers, nitrates, and monitoring for "high risk" status are appropriate for initial management and therapy of this patient. If the patient meets "high-risk" criteria, treatment with aspirin, glycoprotein IIb/IIIa inhibitors, and unfractionated heparin is indicated. Low-molecular-weight heparin instead of IV heparin and glycoprotein IIb/IIIa inhibitors can be used in patients at intermediate risk. All patients without contraindications should receive β-blockers. Aspirin should be given to all patients.

Answer **a** is incorrect because these therapies represent the approach to management of the patient with ST-segment elevation MI. Patients with ST-segment depression will not benefit from fibrinolytic therapy. However, *high-risk* patients with recurrent ischemia, depressed left ventricular function, widespread ECG changes (ST depression), or prior MI should be considered for coronary angiography and possible revascularization. These characteristics do not apply to this patient. Answer **c** is incorrect because these therapies represent the approach to management of the patient with acute ischemic or atypical chest pain and a nondiagnostic or normal ECG. Answer **d** is incorrect for several reasons. Routine lidocaine administration for patients with AMI is not recommended for primary prophylaxis of VF. Fluid bolus and vasopressor therapy may be indicated for patients with shock and hypotension but are not part of the routine management of ST-segment elevation MI. Vasopressor infusion will increase aortic diastolic pressure, left ventricular afterload, and myocardial oxygen consumption and should not be used unless a specific indication exists (eg, hypotension).

Read more about it in the ECC Guidelines 2000, *pages 178-179: algorithms; and pages 180-193: "Risk Stratification, Initial Therapy, and Evaluation for Reperfusion in the ED," "ST-Segment Elevation MI," "ST-Segment Depression: Non–Q-Wave MI/High-Risk Unstable Angina," and "Nondiagnostic ECG"*

Case 7: Bradycardia

1. Which of the following bradycardias is most likely to be associated with clinical symptoms?

a. a heart rate of 53 bpm in an athlete

b. a heart rate of 53 bpm in a patient with cardiovascular disease, presenting with shortness of breath and decreased level of consciousness

c. a heart rate of 53 bpm in a patient who has just vomited after insertion of a nasogastric tube

d. a heart rate of 53 bpm in a patient with first-degree heart block receiving digoxin

The correct answer is b.

The patient with cardiovascular disease is likely to be dependent on an adequate heart rate to maintain an adequate cardiac output even in the face of a reduced ejection fraction or other compromise in cardiac function. The patient's presentation with shortness of breath and decreased level of consciousness are likely to indicate signs of symptomatic bradycardia (symptoms likely to be caused by the bradycardia). These 2 clinical signs are specifically mentioned in the *ECC Guidelines 2000,* page 155: Notes to Figure 6: Bradycardia.

Answer **a** is incorrect because a heart rate of 53 bpm is often normal in a well-conditioned athlete. Conditioned athletes have very high stroke volumes, so they can maintain adequate cardiac output with a lower heart rate. Answer **c** is incorrect because the patient who has had a nasogastric tube inserted and vomited may experience a brief drop in heart rate due to vagal effects. The healthcare provider should ensure that the heart rate returns to normal within a few minutes. Answer **d** is incorrect because a slight slowing of the heart rate and prolongation of the P-R interval is expected after administration of digitalis.

Read more about it in the ECC Guidelines 2000, *pages 155-157: Figure 6: Bradycardia Algorithm and notes*

2. Which of the following would be an appropriate indication for transcutaneous pacing?

a. asymptomatic sinus bradycardia

b. normal sinus rhythm with hypotension and shock

c. complete heart block with pulmonary edema

d. prolonged asystole

The correct answer is c.

Complete heart block with pulmonary edema is likely to cause bradycardia, and the development of pulmonary edema suggests that the bradycardia is *symptomatic*. Pulmonary congestion is specifically listed as one of the potential signs of symptomatic bradycardia in the *ECC Guidelines 2000:* page 155: Notes to Figure 6: Bradycardia. Answer **a** is incorrect because transcutaneous pacing is recommended for *symptomatic* bradycardia, not for *asymptomatic* bradycardia. Answer **b** is incorrect because transcutaneous pacing would not be recommended for the patient with normal sinus rhythm with hypotension and shock, because bradycardia is not present. This patient is likely to respond to therapy that improves cardiac function and ejection fraction rather than therapy that increases heart rate. Answer **d** is incorrect because transcutaneous pacing should be attempted early if it is attempted at all. It is unlikely to be effective if it is initiated after a period of prolonged asystole.

Read more about it in the ECC Guidelines 2000, *page 155: paragraph beginning "Transcutaneous pacing ...."*

3. You are evaluating a patient with a heart rate of 45 bpm; a complaint of dizziness; cool, clammy extremities; and prolonged capillary refill. What is the *first* drug of choice you would administer to this patient?

a. atropine 0.5 to 1 mg

b. epinephrine 1 mg IV push

c. isoproterenol infusion 1 to 10 μg/kg per minute

d. adenosine 6 mg rapid IV push

The correct answer is a.

Atropine 0.5 to 1 mg is the first drug recommended in the bradycardia algorithm for treatment of *symptomatic* bradycardia. This patient is bradycardic with a heart rate of 45 bpm and demonstrates symptoms of inadequate cardiac output, including dizziness; cool, clammy extremities; and prolonged capillary refill. It is likely that these symptoms are related to and caused by the slow heart rate. Answer **b** is incorrect because the bradycardia algorithm recommends an infusion of epinephrine rather than a bolus dose for symptomatic bradycardia. Answer **c** is incorrect because isoproterenol is no longer included in the bradycardia algorithm. This drug increases myocardial oxygen consumption and may increase ventricular ectopy. Answer **d** is incorrect because adenosine is not recommended for bradycardia; adenosine is the drug of choice for treatment of supraventricular tachycardia.

Read more about it in the ECC Guidelines 2000, *pages 155-156: Figure 6: Bradycardia Algorithm and notes*

4. Which of the following signs and symptoms are most likely to result from symptomatic bradycardia?

a. headache, pain or pressure in the center of the chest, palpitations

b. nausea, diaphoresis, pain radiating to the back and between the shoulder blades

c. chest pain, shortness of breath, hypotension, dizziness or altered level of consciousness, congestive heart failure, premature ventricular contractions

d. difficulty with speech, unilateral limb weakness, severe headache, facial droop

The correct answer is c.

Chest pain, shortness of breath, hypotension, dizziness or altered level of consciousness, congestive heart failure, and premature ventricular contractions are listed almost verbatim in the *ECC Guidelines 2000* discussion of the clinical manifestations of symptomatic bradycardia (page 155). Answer **a** is incorrect because headache is a nonspecific sign and could be caused by other problems, including stroke. Chest pain or pressure can be caused by acute coronary syndromes or inadequate cardiac output. Palpitations are more often associated with tachyarrhythmias rather than bradyarrhythmias, so this constellation of symptoms would not be the most common one associated with symptomatic bradycardia. Answer **b** is incorrect because nausea and pain radiating to the back and shoulder blades is more consistent with angina or signs of a heart attack listed in the *ECC Guidelines 2000*, page 25. Answer **d** is incorrect because these signs are the warning signs of stroke as listed in the *ECC Guidelines 2000*, pages 26 to 27.

Read more about it in the ECC Guidelines 2000, *pages 155-156: Figure 6: Bradycardia Algorithm and notes; and Part 3: "Adult Basic Life Support"*

5. You are treating a patient with a slow heartbeat. For which of the following patients would *atropine* be effective?

a. a 55-year-old man with severe, crushing chest pain and sinus bradycardia at 35 bpm

b. a 55-year-old man with weakness and fatigue on walking short distances and a third-degree AV block at 35 bpm

c. a 55-year-old man with weakness and fatigue on walking short distances and with a history of a heart transplant 6 months ago.

d. a 55-year-old man with weakness and fatigue following acute symptoms of nausea and vomiting and with a slow sinus rhythm at 35 bpm.

The correct answer is d.

Atropine is most effective in the treatment of patients with symptomatic bradycardia due to vagal nerve suppression of the SA node. If the patient has severe symptoms from the bradycardia (eg, severe hypotension with signs and symptoms of the shock syndrome), the rescuer should use an immediate infusion of epinephrine or dopamine, instead of atropine. The patient described in answer **d** is an ideal candidate for atropine. The weakness and fatigue is due to the slow heartbeat rather than to vomiting-induced hypovolemia. Gastrointestinal illnesses are associated with prolonged stimulation from the vagus nerve, which suppress the SA node. Atropine's primary pharmacologic effect is to block the effects of vagal stimulation. Answer **a** is incorrect because atropine is relatively contraindicated in patients with acute ischemic events. An acute increase in heart rate from giving atropine in ischemic patients can increase the demand on the myocardium and worsen ischemia or increase the zone of infarction. Answer **b** is incorrect because atropine is seldom effective in the treatment of bradycardia from AV block at the His-Purkinje level (type II AV block and third-degree block and new wide-QRS complexes). The cause of these blocks is not affected by atropine. A vagolytic agent cannot affect a conduction block at the AV node. Answer **c** is incorrect because atropine, which works through blocking the effects of the vagus nerve, will have no effects on a denervated heart that has no vagus nerve. Treatment of bradycardia in patients with heart transplants includes pacing, catecholamine infusion, or both.

Read more about it in the ECC Guidelines 2000, *page 121: "Atropine"; pages 155-157: Figure 6: Bradycardia Algorithm and notes*

Case 8: Unstable Tachycardia

1. You are working in the ED when a 34-year-old woman arrives with a complaint of palpitations. She has a history of mitral valve prolapse and a heart rate of 165 bpm, a respiratory rate of 14 breaths/min, and blood pressure of 118/82 mm Hg. Her lungs are clear to auscultation, she has no hepatomegaly, and she denies any shortness of breath. She is placed on an ECG monitor, which indicates that a narrow-complex regular tachycardia is present. Which of the following phrases best characterizes this patient's condition?

a. stable tachycardia

b. unstable tachycardia

c. heart rate appropriate for clinical condition

d. tachycardia with poor cardiovascular function

The correct answer is a.

To identify patients with unstable tachycardia, the ACLS provider must be able to identify stable patients. This patient is tachycardic but has no signs of congestive heart failure (no tachypnea or shortness of breath, no rales, no hepatomegaly) and has an adequate blood pressure. Answer **b** is incorrect because the unstable patient would demonstrate congestive heart failure, chest pain, hypotension, or other signs of inadequate cardiac output and systemic perfusion. Answer **c** is incorrect because a heart rate of 165 bpm is extremely rapid and does not appear to be appropriate for a patient with no signs of congestive heart failure or shock. Answer **d** is incorrect because the patient has no signs of poor cardiovascular function (no hypotension, no apparent compromise in systemic perfusion, no pulmonary congestion, no CHF, no chest pain, no altered level of consciousness).

Read more about it in the ECC Guidelines 2000, *page 117: "Paroxysmal Supraventricular Tachycardia"; and page 118: "Atrial Tachycardia and Atrial Fibrillation/Flutter"*

2. You are working in a clinic when a 58-year-old man walks in complaining of chest pain. He is diaphoretic and complains of dizziness. He sits in a chair at the triage desk while you check his pulse, which is rapid. As you prepare to attach a cardiac monitor to the patient, he suddenly slumps over unresponsive. Which of the following best describes this man's condition?

a. stable tachycardia

b. unstable tachycardia, possible cardiac arrest

c. heart rate appropriate for clinical condition

d. tachycardia with adequate cardiovascular function

The correct answer is b.

Unlike the previous patient, this patient complains of chest pain and dizziness and is diaphoretic. He has unstable tachycardia. When he slumps over and is unresponsive, you must consider the possibility that the patient is in cardiac arrest and begin BLS. Answer **a** is incorrect because the man is unstable. Chest pain, diaphoresis, and dizziness in the presence of a rapid pulse indicates symptomatic tachycardia. Once the man becomes unresponsive, he absolutely cannot be considered stable. Answer **c** is incorrect because you have no indication that there is a legitimate cause of the tachycardia. It is more logical to interpret the patient's clinical condition as caused by the tachycardia. Answer **d** is incorrect because cardiac output is poor. By the end of the scenario cardiac arrest may be present.

Read more about it in the ECC Guidelines 2000, *page 115: "New Concerns From the International Guidelines 2000 Conference: Impaired Hearts and 'Proarrhythmic Antiarrhythmics'"; "Summary: Treatment of Hemodynamically Stable, Wide-Complex Tachycardias"; and "Hemodynamically Stable (Monomorphic) VT"; page 116: "Polymorphic VT and VF/Pulseless VT"; and pages 117-120: "Paroxysmal Supraventricular Tachycardia, Atrial Tachycardia, Atrial Fibrillation/ Flutter, and Junctional Tachycardia"*

3. For which of the following patients would immediate cardioversion be indicated?

a. a 62-year-old man with rheumatic mitral and aortic valve disease, an irregularly irregular heart rate of 153 bpm, and a blood pressure of 88/70 mm Hg

b. a 78-year-old woman with fever, pneumonia, mild chronic congestive heart failure, and sinus tachycardia of 133 bpm

c. a 55-year-old man with multifocal atrial tachycardia, a respiratory rate of 12 breaths per minute, and a blood pressure of 134/86 mm Hg

d. a 69-year-old with a history of coronary artery disease who presents with chest pain, a heart rate of 118 bpm, and ST-segment elevation

The correct answer is a.

A 62-year-old man with rheumatic mitral and aortic valve disease, an irregularly irregular heart rate of 153 bpm, and a blood pressure of 88/70 mm Hg clearly has *unstable* tachycardia with hypotension and a history suggestive of compromised ventricular function. This patient has serious signs and symptoms and should be considered for immediate cardioversion. Answer **b** is incorrect because this patient appears to have a sinus tachycardia caused by fever and pneumonia and possibly contributed to by mild congestive heart failure. Tachycardia should be treated if it appears to be the cause of the patient's symptoms; in this case the tachycardia appears to be caused *by* rather than the cause *of* the patient's other conditions. In addition, cardioversion is not indicated for sinus tachycardia. Answer **c** is incorrect because, although the patient has a tachycardia, he is not tachypneic and is not hypotensive. Thus the patient does not appear to have serious signs and symptoms caused by the tachycardia. Answer **d** is incorrect because it appears to describe a patient with acute coronary syndromes and a tachycardia caused by the chest pain and coronary ischemia. This mild tachycardia does not appear to be the cause of the patient's signs and symptoms and does not require cardioversion.

Read more about it in the ECC Guidelines 2000, *page 117: "Paroxysmal Supraventricular Tachycardia"; page 118: "Atrial Tachycardia and Atrial Fibrillation/Flutter"; and pages 91-92: "Cardioversion"*

4. Which of the following groups of signs would *not* be consistent with evidence of *unstable* tachycardia?

a. heart rate of 140 bpm, tachypnea, wheezing, and pneumonia in a patient receiving albuterol

b. heart rate of 140 bpm with rapid atrial flutter in a patient with aortic stenosis and AMI, blood pressure of 90/55 mm Hg, faint peripheral pulses, diaphoresis, tachypnea, and rales

c. VT in a man complaining of chest pain, shortness of breath, and palpitations

d. heart rate of 155 bpm in a 55-year-old woman with severe chest pain, difficulty breathing, extreme weakness and dizziness, and a blood pressure of 88/54 mm Hg

The correct answer is a.

The tachycardia demonstrated by this patient appears to be caused by the patient's clinical problems and therapy. Tachycardia is a known potential complication of albuterol therapy. In addition, the patient has wheezing and pneumonia, with likely respiratory distress that will probably contribute to tachycardia. Answer **b** is incorrect because this patient is unstable. The patient has heart disease that will likely cause myocardial dysfunction, hypotension and other signs of shock (faint peripheral pulses), and pulmonary congestion. Answer **c** is incorrect because VT, chest pain, and shortness of breath are all potential signs of unstable tachycardia. Answer **d** is incorrect because hypotension, chest pain, respiratory distress, weakness, and dizziness are all signs of unstable tachycardia.

Read more about it in the ECC Guidelines 2000, *page 115: "New Concerns From the International Guidelines 2000 Conference: Impaired Hearts" and 'Proarrhythmic Antiarrhythmics,'" "Summary: Treatment of Hemodynamically Stable, Wide-Complex Tachycardias," and "Hemodynamically Stable (Monomorphic) VT"; page 116: "Polymorphic VT and VF/Pulseless VT"; and pages 117-120: "Paroxysmal Supraventricular Tachycardia, Atrial Tachycardia, Atrial Fibrillation/Flutter, and Junctional Tachycardia"*

5. You decide to convert an unstable, symptomatic tachycardia. You place the cardioverter/defibrillator in synchronization mode and administer a sedative and an analgesic to the patient. Suddenly the patient becomes unresponsive and pulseless, and the ECG rhythm becomes highly irregular, resembling VF. When you attempt to deliver the shock, nothing happens: no shock is delivered and there is no energy transfer. What is the explanation for the failure to deliver a shock?

- **a.** the defibrillator/cardioverter battery has failed
- **b.** the SYNC switch is not functioning properly
- **c.** the patient has developed VF and the defibrillator will not deliver a charge because it is attempting to synchronize shock delivery with an R wave
- **d.** the monitor cannot synchronize the cardioversion shock because a lead has come loose

The correct answer is c.

The patient has become unresponsive and pulseless, so pulseless cardiac arrest is present. The potential rhythms are pulseless VT, VF, PEA, or asystole. The "highly irregular" rhythm "resembling VF" is most likely VF. The defibrillator will not deliver a shock while the SYNCHRONIZE button is activated because it will "wait" until the shock can be synchronized with an R wave. Answers **a** and **b** are incorrect because there is no evidence that the battery or SYNCHRONIZE button has failed. In fact the failure of the unit to deliver a shock suggests that the SYNCHRONIZE button is working well. Answer **d** is incorrect. The statement itself is accurate: a monitor cannot synchronize delivery of a shock if a lead is loose. This patient, however, is in VF, and attempts to synchronize a VF patient are inappropriate. Consider the context. You cannot synchronize to VF.

Read more about it in the ECC Guidelines 2000, *pages 92-93: "Synchronized Cardioversion"; and page 164: Synchronized Cardioversion Algorithm*

Case 9: Stable Tachycardia

Questions 1 to 5 are basic. Questions 6 to 10 require a bit more sophistication than the others and are included primarily for more experienced providers.

1. A 75-year-old man presents to the ED complaining of having lightheadedness and palpitations for 1 week. His heart rate is 160 bpm and irregular; his blood pressure is 100/70 mm Hg. The physical examination is normal with no evidence of cardiac or circulatory failure. The 12-lead ECG shows rapid atrial fibrillation but is otherwise normal. Which of the following should be included in your initial orders for this patient?

- **a.** oxygen–IV–monitor
- **b.** immediate defibrillation
- **c.** no therapy is indicated
- **d.** epinephrine 1 mg IV every 3 to 5 minutes

The correct answer is a.

This patient is symptomatic and has a potentially serious tachycardia. Therefore, oxygen, an IV, and cardiac monitoring should be instituted promptly. Once oximetry is available, the patient's inspired oxygen concentration can be titrated based on the oxygen saturation. This is the first of a 2-part question continued in question 2. Answer **b** is incorrect because defibrillation is not indicated for treatment of atrial fibrillation. It is indicated for VF. Answer **c** is incorrect because the patient is clearly symptomatic. Although the patient is not in hypotensive shock, he is lightheaded, with a blood pressure of 100/70 mm Hg. Answer **d** is incorrect because there is no indication for epinephrine in this patient. Although he is mildly hypotensive, he is tachycardic, not bradycardic or pulseless.

Read more about it in the ECC Guidelines 2000, *page 118: "Atrial Fibrillation/Flutter"; pages 120-124: "Antiarrhythmic Drugs and the Arrhythmias They Treat"; and pages 158-165: "The Tachycardia Algorithms"*

2. You continue to manage the patient in question 1. You conclude that he has been in atrial fibrillation for at least 1 week. His vital signs remain unchanged. Which of the following would be the most appropriate treatment for atrial fibrillation?

- **a.** IV digoxin to slow ventricular response
- **b.** IV diltiazem to slow ventricular response
- **c.** IV amiodarone in an attempt to convert atrial fibrillation to a sinus rhythm
- **d.** synchronized cardioversion

The correct answer is b.

The patient, an elderly man, has been in atrial fibrillation for at least 1 week. Therefore, although you want to treat his tachycardia, you must be aware of the possibility that he has developed an atrial thrombus or thrombi in the more than 48 hours this arrhythmia has been present. Diltiazem is the correct answer because this agent, a calcium channel blocker, has a rapid onset of action, is likely to slow the ventricular rate (which is desirable and is the therapeutic goal), and is *not* likely to convert the patient to a sinus rhythm (which would be undesirable because of the risk of dislodging an atrial thrombus and causing an embolic event such as a stroke. (IV verapamil, another calcium channel blocker, would also be an acceptable choice.) Answer **a** is incorrect because digoxin has a slow onset of action and would take several hours to slow the ventricular rate. This patient is too sick for that—he is elderly, lightheaded, and has a heart rate of 160. His ventricular rate should be lowered over a period of minutes, not hours. Answer **c** is incorrect because amiodarone will frequently convert atrial fibrillation to a sinus rhythm, which would carry the risk of embolization. Answer **d** is incorrect because of the risk of embolization if this patient is converted to a sinus rhythm.

Read more about it in the ECC Guidelines 2000, *page 118: "Atrial Fibrillation/Flutter"; pages 120-124: "Antiarrhythmic Drugs and the Arrhythmias They Treat"; and pages 158-165: "The Tachycardia Algorithms"*

3. A 55-year-old man with known heart failure develops sustained wide-complex tachycardia after an episode of chest pain relieved by nitroglycerin. Currently HR = 150 bpm, BP = 100/60 mm Hg; ECG before the tachycardia = old left bundle branch block, which prevents determination of the wide-complex tachycardia as ventricular or supraventricular in origin. Which of the following is the *most appropriate* initial medication?

a. IV lidocaine

b. IV adenosine

c. IV amiodarone

d. IV verapamil

The correct answer is c.

This patient has a wide-complex tachycardia of uncertain type. The currently recommended treatment strategy for this condition is to select a drug that is effective for both supraventricular and ventricular tachycardias. Answer **a** is incorrect because lidocaine is effective only for VTs. This drug is no longer considered particularly effective even for VT; it is no longer considered the drug of choice in this setting. Answer **b** is incorrect because adenosine is effective only for paroxysmal supraventricular tachycardia and would not cover VT in this case (which is the most likely diagnosis because about 90% of wide-complex tachycardia is VT). Answer **d** is incorrect for at least 2 reasons. First, verapamil is effective only for supraventricular tachycardias, not VT. Second, verapamil is specifically contraindicated in wide-complex tachycardias because it can cause hemodynamic deterioration if the rhythm is VT or paradoxical acceleration of the heart rate if there is a pre-excitation syndrome such as Wolff-Parkinson-White syndrome, which has not been ruled out in this patient.

Read more about it in the ECC Guidelines 2000, *page 118: "Atrial Fibrillation/Flutter"; pages 120-124: "Antiarrhythmic Drugs and the Arrhythmias They Treat"; and pages 158-165: "The Tachycardia Algorithms"*

4. A 25-year-old woman presents to the ED saying, "I'm having another episode of *PSVT!*" Her prior medical history includes an electrophysiologic stimulation study that confirmed a reentry tachycardia, no WPW, and no pre-excitation. Her heart rate is 180 bpm; she reports palpitations and mild shortness of breath. Vagal maneuvers with carotid sinus massage have no effect on heart rate or rhythm. Which would be the most appropriate *next* intervention?

a. DC cardioversion

b. IV diltiazem

c. IV propranolol

d. IV adenosine

The correct answer is d.

This is a classic case of paroxysmal supraventricular tachycardia. Adenosine is very safe and effective in this setting. For that reason it is the first drug in the algorithm for narrow-complex tachycardias. Answer **a** is incorrect because DC cardioversion would probably be unnecessary in this case and because it is generally not the first intervention for routine PSVT. Answers **b** and **c** are incorrect—or at least *less* correct—because diltiazem and propranolol are not considered the *best* initial drugs for PSVT. This should be obvious from a review of the algorithm, which places adenosine in a box at the top of the page, reflecting its status as the usual first drug of choice.

Read more about it in the ECC Guidelines 2000, *page 118: "Atrial Fibrillation/Flutter"; pages 120-124: "Antiarrhythmic Drugs and the Arrhythmias They Treat"; and pages 158-165: "The Tachycardia Algorithms"*

5. Your patient is an 80-year-old woman who complains of palpitations and lightheadedness. Her physical exam is unremarkable. The initial ECG shows a regular, narrow-complex tachycardia with a heart rate of 150 bpm. The Valsalva maneuver does not produce conversion, but the ventricular rate slows to reveal classic atrial flutter waves. Which of the following would an acceptable next intervention?

a. IV diltiazem to slow ventricular rate

b. IV metoprolol to slow ventricular rate

c. DC cardioversion

d. any of the above

The correct answer is d.

The patient is a symptomatic elderly woman with atrial flutter of 150 bpm. Any of the 3 listed interventions would be appropriate. Either IV diltiazem (a calcium channel blocker) or IV metoprolol (a β-blocker) are recommended agents to slow ventricular response with atrial fibrillation or atrial flutter. Synchronized cardioversion would be a reasonable alternative to pharmacologic therapy, given the patient's age, symptoms, and heart rate. Atrial flutter is particularly sensitive to electrical cardioversion, often converting with energies as low as 5 to 10 J, making it a reasonable first intervention in this particular case (in part because it would avoid the potential side effects of an IV calcium or IV β-blocker in this elderly patient).

Read more about it in the ECC Guidelines 2000, *page 118: "Atrial Fibrillation/Flutter"; pages 120-124: "Antiarrhythmic Drugs and the Arrhythmias They Treat"; and pages 158-165: "The Tachycardia Algorithms"*

6. An elderly male patient complains of chest tightness, palpitations, and dizziness. His heart rate is 170 bpm; his blood pressure is 90/60 mm Hg. The ECG shows multifocal atrial tachyardia. Which of the following treatments would be *inappropriate?*

a. DC cardioversion

b. IV metoprolol

c. IV diltiazem

d. IV amiodarone

The correct answer is a.

The patient has multifocal atrial tachycardia—an *automatic* tachycardia, not a reentry rhythm; therefore, DC cardioverson is ineffective. The key teaching point here is that automatic tachycardias do not respond to electrical cardioversion. This is an important fundamental principle that is reflected in the algorithm for narrow-complex tachycardias. Answer **a** is correct because it is ineffective and inappropriate for this patient. The other agents—metoprolol, diltiazem, and amiodarone—are listed as acceptable medications in the algorithm.

Read more about it in the ECC Guidelines 2000, *page 118: "Atrial Fibrillation/Flutter"; pages 120-124: "Antiarrhythmic Drugs and the Arrhythmias They Treat"; and pages 158-165: "The Tachycardia Algorithms"*

7. A 66-year-old homeless man with a history of chronic alcoholism presents with polymorphic tachycardia. He is tolerating the tachycardia well. You correctly diagnose torsades de pointes; HR = 160 bpm; BP = 90/60 mm Hg. On physical examination you find a malnourished man with no evidence of heart failure. Which of the following treatments would be *most appropriate* at this time?

a. amiodarone

b. IV magnesium

c. IV lidocaine

d. IV procainamide

The correct answer is b.

This patient has torsades de pointes, a form of polymorphic VT usually associated with a long QT interval. Treatment of torsades is quite different from treatment of monomorphic VT. Moreover, torsades is often due to an underlying metabolic disorder or drug toxicity. In this case the patient is malnourished and has a history of alcoholism, so it is likely that hypomagnesemia is present and is the cause of torsades. Answer **a** is incorrect because amiodarone will prolong the QT interval and may make torsades worse. Answer **c** is incorrect because lidocaine is considered less effective than overdrive pacing or magnesium for treatment of torsades de pointes. Lidocaine can be administered, but it is not the most appropriate drug to administer at this time. Answer **d** is incorrect because procainamide and other drugs in the same pharmacologic family (including quinidine, which this patient is taking) can prolong the QT interval and worsen or cause torsades.

Read more about it in the ECC Guidelines 2000, *page 118: "Atrial Fibrillation/Flutter"; pages 120-124: "Antiarrhythmic Drugs and the Arrhythmias They Treat"; and pages 158-165: "The Tachycardia Algorithms"*

8. You have just evaluated a 60-year-old woman with known Wolff-Parkinson-White syndrome. Her chief complaint is palpitations and mild chest discomfort that started 1 hour ago. Her ECG shows rapid atrial fibrillation at a rate of 175 bpm. Which of the following drugs is contraindicated?

a. IV diltiazem

b. IV propranolol

c. IV digoxin

d. all of the above

The correct answer is d.

Wolff-Parkinson-White syndrome is a type of pre-excitation syndrome associated with an accessory conduction pathway. This patient's heart rate is dangerously rapid at 175 bpm. The point of the question is to see if the clinician knows which drugs are contraindicated in the presence of a pre-excitation syndrome because they selectively block the AV node but not the accessory pathway and can therefore cause a paradoxical acceleration of heart rate. All of the drugs listed—diltiazem, propranolol, and digoxin—can have this undesirable and potentially fatal effect. This is a 2-part question, continued in question 9.

Read more about it in the ECC Guidelines 2000, *page 118: "Atrial Fibrillation/Flutter"; pages 120-124: "Antiarrhythmic Drugs and the Arrhythmias They Treat"; and pages 158-165: "The Tachycardia Algorithms"*

9. Which of the following treatments would also be *contraindicated* in the patient in question 8?

a. IV adenosine

b. IV procainamide

c. IV amiodarone

d. synchronized electrical cardioversion

The correct answer is a.

This is a continuation of the same case in question 8. Answer **a** is correct because adenosine is also relatively contraindicated in patients with WPW. This issue is covered in a separate question to underscore the point that until recently adenosine was considered safe and effective for treating patients with WPW. There is now mounting evidence that adenosine, because it selectively blocks the AV node but not accessory pathways, is less safe than previously believed, despite its short half-life. It is no longer recommended in the *ECC Guidelines*.

Answers **b, c,** and **d** are incorrect because procainamide, amiodarone, and electrical cardioversion are treatments of choice for WPW, depending on the specific clinical situation.

Read more about it in the ECC Guidelines 2000, *page 118: "Atrial Fibrillation/Flutter"; pages 120-124: "Antiarrhythmic Drugs and the Arrhythmias They Treat"; and pages 158-165: "The Tachycardia Algorithm"*

10. A 50-year-old man presents to the ED. His chief complaint is that he is "feeling weak and dizzy" since getting up this morning. His previous medical history includes an extensive AMI 1 year ago, known left ventricular dysfunction, and an ejection fraction less than 40%. He is doing well clinically, with only mild exercise intolerance. On physical examination you note fine bibasilar rales that have been documented on every physical exam the patient has had since the AMI. The ECG shows monomorphic VT; his heart rate is 150 bpm; and his blood pressure is 90/60 mm Hg. Which of the following would be the most appropriate treatment sequence for this patient?

a. IV amiodarone, then synchronized cardioversion if the rhythm does not convert

b. IV procainamide, then synchronized cardioversion if the rhythm does not convert

c. IV magnesium, then synchronized cardioversion if the rhythm does not convert

d. immediate synchronized DC cardioversion

The correct answer is a.

The patient in this scenario has monomorphic VT and impaired ventricular function, as evidenced by chronic rales and low ejection fraction. This question is designed to remind experienced providers that cardiac function should be considered in treating patients with virtually pathologic tachycardia, either ventricular or supraventricular (VT is used to illustrate this question). One key point is to avoid drugs with negative inotropic effects that can reduce contractility and worsen pump function. Another key point is to select only 1 agent and if that doesn't work, then proceed to synchronized cardioversion. The use of multiple antiarrhythmics increases the chance that the patient will experience proarrhythmic side effects, another important concept in the *ECC Guidelines*. Answer **a** is correct because it lists the recommended sequence for stable monomorphic VT as presented in the algorithm: first amiodarone and if that doesn't work, then cardioversion. Answer **b** is incorrect because procainamide has negative inotropic effects and should be avoided in patients with impaired ventricular function. Answer **c** is incorrect because magnesium has not been shown to be effective in this setting. Answer **d** is not quite correct because the patient is essentially "stable"—or at least "more good than bad"—and the *ECC Guidelines* recommend that stable patients with tachycardia be treated with medication before attempting DC cardioversion. (Note that the question asks which is the most appropriate therapy.)

Read more about it in the ECC Guidelines 2000, *page 118: "Atrial Fibrillation/Flutter"; pages 120-124: "Antiarrhythmic Drugs and the Arrhythmias They Treat"; and pages 158-165: "The Tachycardia Algorithms"*

Case 10: Acute Ischemic Stroke

1. You are walking through a shopping mall when you encounter a 65-year-old woman who stumbled and fell as she walked out of a store. She complains of a severe headache, has a facial droop, and slurs her words. She also complains of numbness in her right arm and leg. She has difficulty raising her right arm, although her left arm moves freely. When you ask if she takes medications, she says that she has "high blood pressure." Which of the following actions would be most appropriate to take at this time?

a. phone 911 immediately and tell the dispatcher that you are with a conscious woman who may be demonstrating signs of a stroke

b. suggest that the woman sit down for a few minutes and see if the symptoms disappear

c. offer to drive the woman to the ED of the local hospital

d. suggest that the woman contact her physician immediately

The correct answer is a.

Phone 911 immediately and tell the dispatcher that you are with a conscious woman who may be demonstrating signs of a stroke. The 3 major warning signs of a stroke include unilateral limb weakness, facial droop, and speech abnormalities. Once you observe signs of a stroke, you should phone 911 immediately. Answer **b** is incorrect because you should not delay phoning 911 if you suspect signs of a stroke. Answers **c** and **d** are incorrect because both of these options will delay EMS involvement and support during transport and will delay the patient's arrival at and evaluation in a hospital capable of providing acute stroke care. EMS involvement is needed as soon as possible for several reasons. First, EMS personnel will perform a stroke screen or scale exam to identify the patient as a potential stroke victim and communicate this to the dispatcher and receiving hospital. In addition, EMS personnel will know where to transport the patient to ensure that the patient can receive acute stroke care (including the potential to receive fibrinolytic therapy). Finally, EMS personnel can provide prearrival notification to the hospital to ensure that diagnostic interventions can be accomplished swiftly. If the patient demonstrates acute ischemic stroke signs with no contraindications to fibrinolytic therapy, EMS rapid transport and prearrival notification will increase the likelihood that the patient will be eligible to receive the therapy within 3 hours of the onset of stroke symptoms.

Read more about it in the ECC Guidelines 2000, *page 204: "Early Recognition and Role of EMS in Stroke Care"*

2. A 70-year-old woman presents to the ED with acute onset of garbled speech and weakness in her right arm and leg, which started 15 minutes ago. Which of the following neurologic evaluation sequences should be performed for this patient over the next 45 minutes?

a. obtain a patient history, perform a physical and neurologic examination, obtain a noncontrast CT scan, and ensure that it is read within 45 minutes of the patient's arrival in the ED

b. obtain a noncontrast CT scan of the head, and if the scan is positive for a stroke, begin fibrinolytic treatment

c. obtain a targeted history and perform a physical exam and immediate lumbar puncture to rule out meningitis; obtain a noncontrast CT scan of the head

d. obtain a noncontrast CT scan of the head, wait until the neurologic symptoms start to improve, then begin fibrinolytic treatment

The correct answer is a.

Obtain a patient history, perform a physical and neurologic examination, obtain a noncontrast CT scan, and ensure that it is read within 45 minutes of ED arrival. Answer **a** includes the best combination of actions that will help determine if this patient is eligible for fibrinolytic therapy within the narrow window of time in which these drugs can be administered. The neurologic exam should include a stroke exam. The CT scan must be negative for hemorrhage.

Answer **b** is incorrect because it misrepresents the purpose of the CT scan and its role in identification of patients eligible for fibrinolytic therapy. Most CT scans of patients with acute ischemic stroke will be normal. Therefore, eligibility for thrombolytic therapy does not require a scan that is "positive for stroke." In fact, the CT scan is performed to rule out *hemorrhagic* stroke, a form of stroke that is likely to be visible on CT scan. If the CT scan is positive for hemorrhagic stroke, the patient will be ineligible for fibrinolytic therapy.

Answer **c** is incorrect because the lumbar puncture is not a routine part of the evaluation of patients who present with signs of stroke. The LP is performed *only* if there is a high suspicion of subarachnoid hemorrhage (hemorrhagic stroke) despite a negative CT scan. Fibrinolytic therapy is then contraindicated following a LP.

Answer **d** is incorrect because you do not wait until symptoms start improving before administering fibrinolytic therapy. This therapy is recommended only if the patient can be screened, eligibility determined, and the drug administered within 3 hours of the onset of symptoms. In addition, the patient with mild stroke symptoms or rapidly improving stroke signs may not be eligible for fibrinolytic therapy because in such patients the potential risk of hemorrhage may outweigh the potential benefit of improved outcome.

Read more about it in the ECC Guidelines 2000, *page 206: "Brief Emergency Neurological Evaluation"; page 208: "Emergency Diagnostic Studies"; and page 209: Table 7: NINDS-Recommended Stroke Evaluation Targets for Potential Fibrinolytic Candidates*

3. Which of the following conditions can mimic the signs and symptoms of an acute stroke?

a. hypoglycemia

b. cardiac arrest

c. pneumothorax

d. Wolff-Parkinson-White syndrome

The correct answer is a.

Hypoglycemia is included in a table of differential diagnoses of stroke contained in the *ECC Guidelines 2000*. Because hypoglycemia can cause signs and symptoms similar to those of stroke, a normal blood glucose between 60 and 400 is required in the Los Angeles Prehospital Stroke Screen. In addition, determination of blood glucose and treatment of hypoglycemia is part of the initial management of the patient with signs of acute stroke.

Answer **b** is incorrect because the signs of cardiac arrest (unresponsiveness, no breathing, no pulse or other signs of circulation) are not the same as signs of stroke (facial droop, unilateral weakness of extremities, speech difficulty). Answer **c** is incorrect because a pneumothorax is likely to produce difficulty in breathing, with decreased breath sounds and chest expansion on the involved side and not the signs of a stroke. Answer **d** is incorrect because although atrial fibrillation and flutter may increase the risk of stroke, the signs of supraventricular tachycardia such as Wolff-Parkinson-White syndrome will likely include signs of cardiovascular compromise (palpitations, congestive heart failure, etc) rather than signs of a stroke.

Read more about it in the ECC Guidelines 2000, *page 206: "Stroke Screen or Scale"; and page 208: "Differential Diagnosis" and Table 6: Differential Diagnosis of Stroke*

4. The following patients were given a diagnosis of an acute ischemic stroke. Which of the patients as described has no apparent contraindications to IV fibrinolytic therapy?

a. an 80-year-old man presenting within 2 hours of onset of symptoms

b. a 65-year-old woman who lives alone and was found unresponsive by a relative

c. a 54-year-old man presenting within 4 hours of onset of symptoms

d. a 40-year-old woman diagnosed with bleeding ulcers 2 weeks before onset of stroke symptoms

The correct answer is a.

With this simple statement the patient appears to be within the "window of therapy," provided that all appropriate assessment and diagnostic studies can be performed and evaluated within 60 minutes. Answer **b** is incorrect because patients who are found to present with stroke symptoms upon awakening are not eligible for fibrinolytic therapy because the time of onset of symptoms cannot be determined. Because this woman lives alone, it is unlikely that someone was present who could document the last time she was observed without stroke symptoms. Answer **c** is incorrect because this patient has presented beyond the 3-hour therapeutic window for fibrinolytic therapy (administration 3 to 6 hours after onset of symptoms is a Class Indeterminate recommendation: there is not sufficient evidence to support it at this time). Answer **d** is incorrect because bleeding ulcers in the past 2 weeks would be a contraindication to fibrinolytic therapy.

Read more about it in the ECC Guidelines 2000, *page 211: "Fibrinolytic Therapy" and Table 10: Contraindications to tPA Therapy for Acute Ischemic Stroke. Also see the* ECC Handbook: *"Fibrinolytic Therapy Checklist for Ischemic Stroke"*

5. A 56-year-old woman arrives at the ED with new onset of facial droop when she smiles, arm drift when she holds both arms out, and inability to speak clearly. Before beginning fibrinolytic therapy, the *most* important question you need to answer is

a. have her vital signs remained stable?

b. when exactly did the neurologic signs begin?

c. does she have a history of heart attack?

d. does she have any medication allergies?

The correct answer is b.

The reason that most patients are ineligible for fibrinolytic therapy is that they present more than 3 hours after the onset of stroke signs and symptoms. Answer **a** is incorrect because stable vital signs are not required for fibrinolytic therapy. Answer **c** is incorrect because a history of heart attack has no effect on acute stroke therapy. Answer **d** is incorrect because this is not the *most* important question to ask the patient and is not a question that will significantly and immediately influence therapy.

Read more about it in the ECC Guidelines 2000, *page 207: "Time of Onset of Symptoms"; and page 211: "Fibrinolytic Therapy"*

ACLS Rhythms for the ACLS Algorithms

The Basics

1. Anatomy of the cardiac conduction system: relationship to the ECG cardiac cycle. **A,** Heart: anatomy of conduction system. **B,** P-QRS-T complex: lines to conduction system. **C,** Normal sinus rhythm.

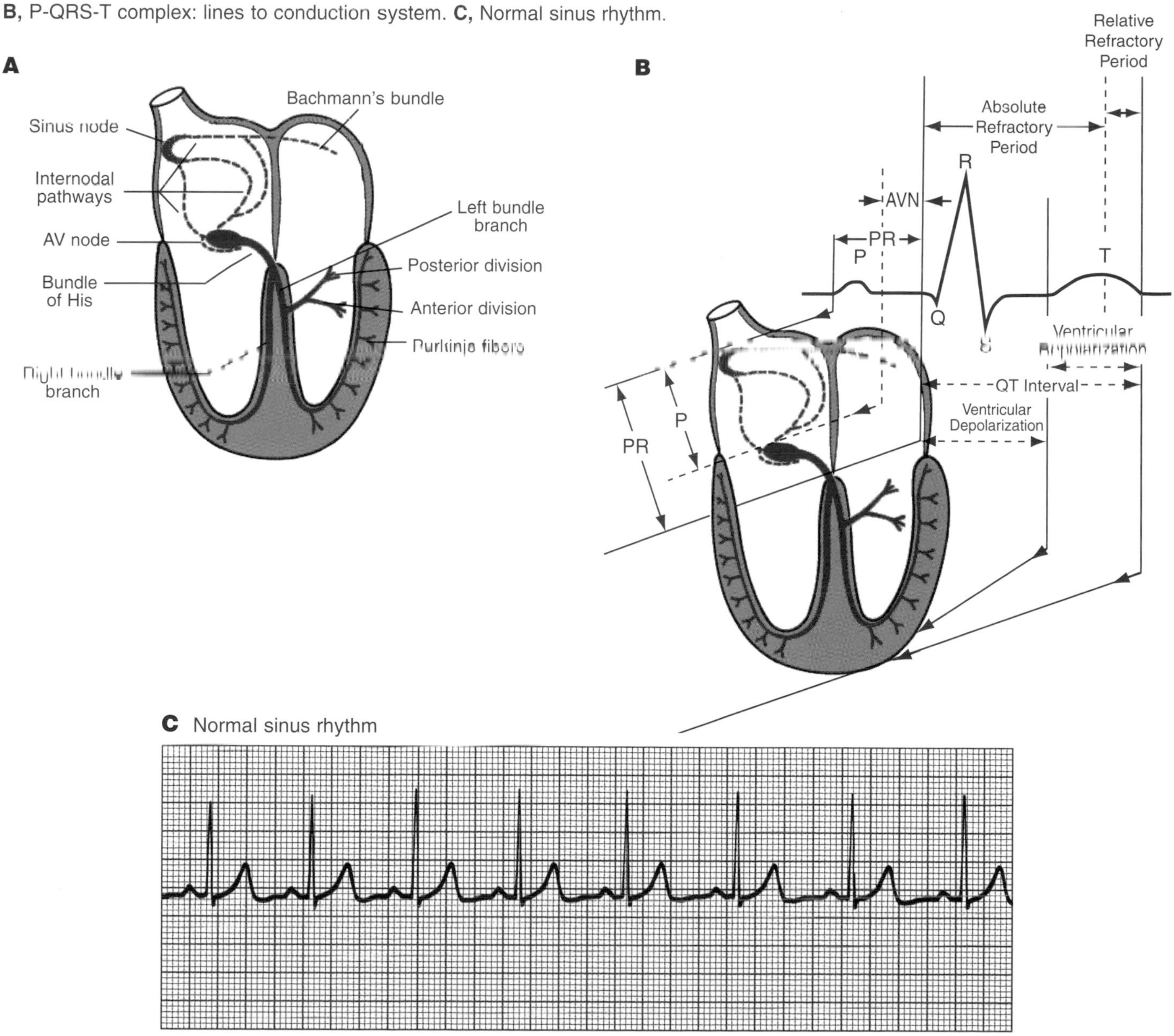

The Cardiac Arrest Rhythms

2. Ventricular Fibrillation/Pulseless Ventricular Tachycardia	
Pathophysiology	■ Ventricles consist of areas of normal myocardium alternating with areas of ischemic, injured, or infarcted myocardium, leading to chaotic pattern of ventricular depolarization
Defining Criteria per ECG	■ **Rate/QRS complex:** unable to determine; no recognizable P, QRS, or T waves ■ **Rhythm:** indeterminate; pattern of sharp up (peak) and down (trough) deflections ■ **Amplitude:** measured from peak-to-trough; often used subjectively to describe VF as *fine* (peak-to-trough 2 to <5 mm), *medium-moderate* (5 to <10 mm), coarse (10 to <15 mm), *very coarse* (>15 mm)
Clinical Manifestations	■ Pulse disappears with onset of VF ■ Collapse, unconsciousness ■ Agonal breaths ➔ apnea in <5 min ■ Onset of *reversible death*
Common Etiologies	■ Acute coronary syndromes leading to ischemic areas of myocardium ■ Stable-to-unstable VT, untreated ■ PVCs with R-on-T phenomenon ■ Multiple drug, electrolyte, or acid-base abnormalities that prolong the relative refractory period ■ Primary or secondary QT prolongation ■ Electrocution, hypoxia, many others
Recommended Therapy *Comprehensive ECC algorithm, page 10; VF/pulseless VT algorithm, page 77*	■ Early defibrillation is essential ■ Agents given to prolong period of reversible death (*oxygen,* CPR, intubation, *epinephrine, vasopressin*) ■ Agents given to prevent refibrillation after a shock causes defibrillation *(lidocaine, amiodarone, procainamide, β-blockers)* ■ Agents given to adjust metabolic milieu *(sodium bicarbonate, magnesium)*

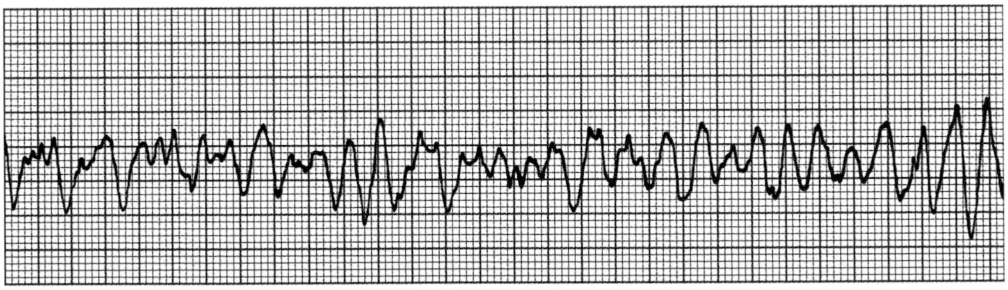

Coarse VF

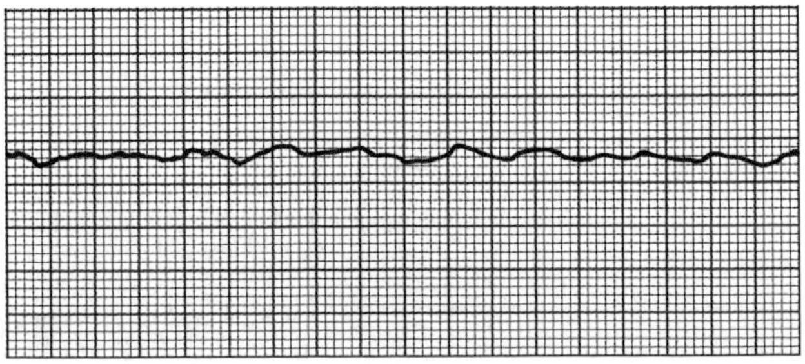

Fine VF

3. PEA (Pulseless Electrical Activity)

Pathophysiology	■ Cardiac conduction impulses occur in organized pattern, but this fails to produce myocardial contraction (former "electromechanical dissociation"); or insufficient ventricular filling during diastole; or ineffective contractions
Defining Criteria per ECG	■ Rhythm displays organized electrical activity (not VF/pulseless VT) ■ Seldom as organized as normal sinus rhythm ■ Can be narrow (QRS <0.10 mm) or wide (QRS >0.12 mm); fast (>100 beats/min) or slow (<60 beats/min) ■ Most frequently: fast and narrow (noncardiac etiology) or slow and wide (cardiac etiology)
Clinical Manifestations	■ Collapse; unconscious ■ Agonal respirations or apnea ■ No pulse detectable by arterial palpation (thus could still be as high as 50-60 mm Hg; in such cases termed *pseudo-PEA*)
Common Etiologies	*Mnemonic of 5 H's and 5 T's aids recall:* ■ Hypovolemia ■ Hypoxia ■ Hydrogen ion—acidosis ■ Hyperkalemia/Hypokalemia ■ Hypothermia ■ "Tablets" (drug OD, ingestions) ■ Tamponade, cardiac ■ Tension pneumothorax ■ Thrombosis, coronary (ACS) ■ Thrombosis, pulmonary (embolism)
Recommended Therapy *Comprehensive ECC Algorithm, page 10; PEA Algorithm, page 100*	■ Per PEA algorithm ■ Primary ABCD (basic CPR) ■ Secondary **AB** (advanced airway and ventilation); **C** (IV, *epinephrine, atropine* if electrical activity <60 complexes per minute); **D** (identify and treat reversible causes) ■ **Key:** identify and treat a reversible cause of the PEA

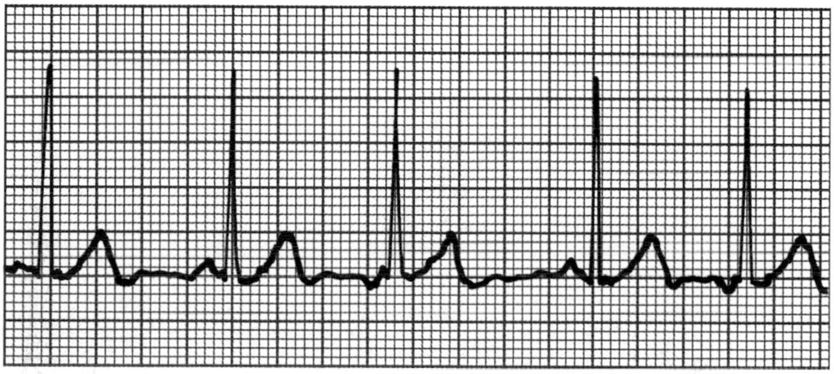

Any **organized rhythm without detectable pulse is "PEA"**

4. Asystole	
Defining Criteria per ECG Classically *asystole* presents as a "flat line"; any defining criteria are virtually nonexistent	■ **Rate:** no ventricular activity seen or ≤6/min; so-called "P-wave asystole" occurs with only atrial impulses present to form P waves ■ **Rhythm:** no ventricular activity seen; or ≤6/min ■ **PR:** cannot be determined; occasionally P wave seen, but by definition R wave must be absent ■ **QRS complex:** no deflections seen that are consistent with a QRS complex
Clinical Manifestations	■ Early may see agonal respirations; unconscious; unresponsive ■ No pulse; no blood pressure ■ Cardiac arrest
Common Etiologies	■ End of life (death) ■ Ischemia/hypoxia from many causes ■ Acute respiratory failure (no oxygen; apnea; asphyxiation) ■ Massive electrical shock: electrocution; lightning strike ■ Postdefibrillatory shocks
Recommended Therapy *Comprehensive ECC Algorithm, page 10; Asystole Algorithm, page 112*	■ Always check for DNAR status ■ Primary ABCD survey (basic CPR) ■ Secondary ABCD survey

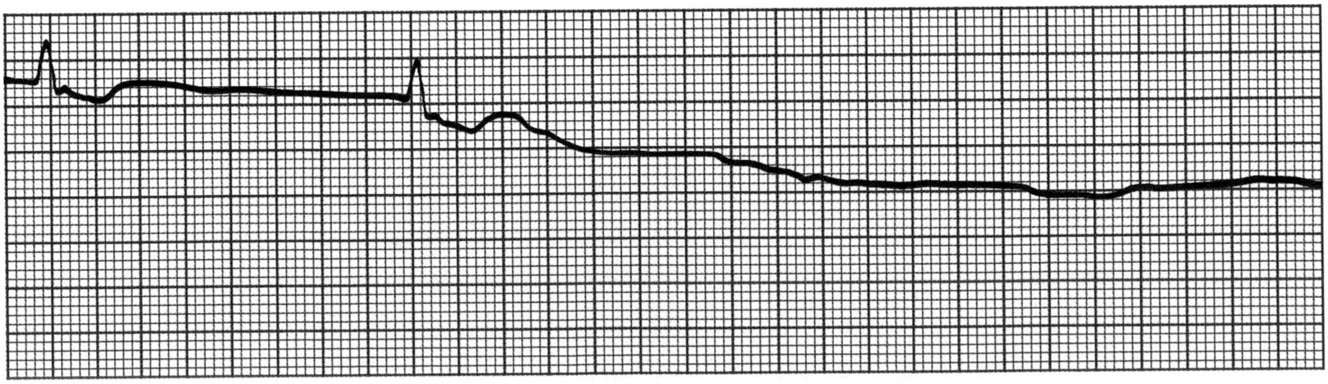

Asystole: agonal complexes too slow to make this rhythm "PEA"

5. Sinus Tachycardia	
Pathophysiology	■ None—more a physical sign than an arrhythmia or pathologic condition ■ Normal impulse formation and conduction
Defining Criteria and ECG Features	■ **Rate:** >100 beats/min ■ **Rhythm:** sinus ■ **PR:** <0.20 sec ■ **QRS complex:** normal
Clinical Manifestations	■ None specific for the tachycardia ■ Symptoms may be present due to the cause of the tachycardia (fever, hypovolemia, etc)
Common Etiologies	■ Normal exercise ■ Fever ■ Hypovolemia ■ Adrenergic stimulation; anxiety ■ Hyperthyroidism
Recommended Therapy No specific treatment for sinus tachycardia	■ Never treat the tachycardia per se ■ Treat only the causes of the tachycardia ■ Never countershock

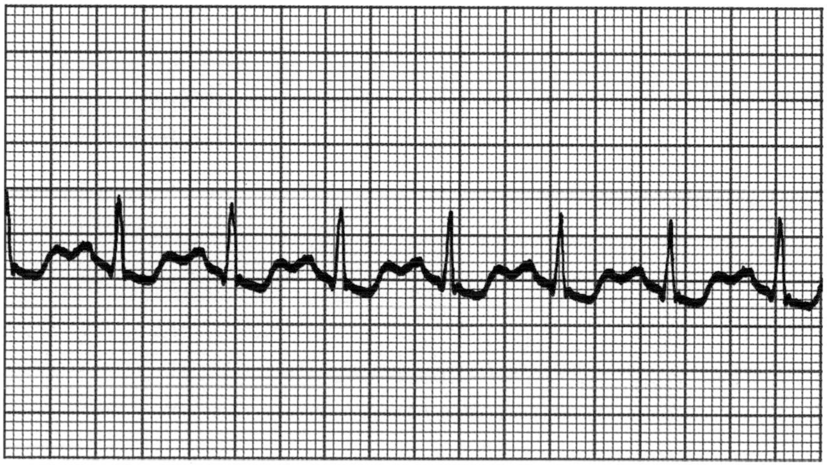

Sinus tachycardia

Rhythmic Algorithm No. 1: Tachycardias Overview

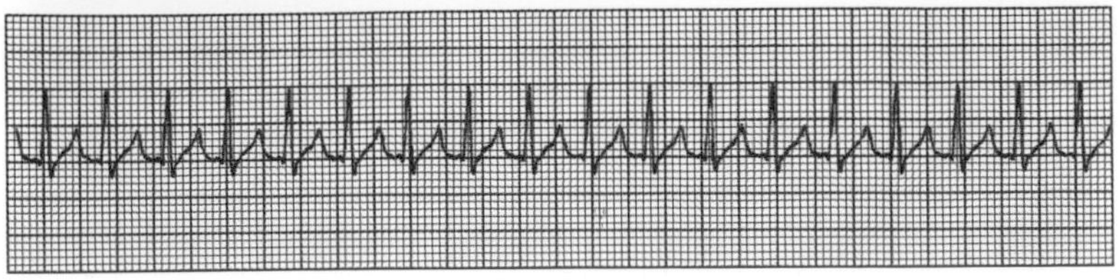

Tachycardia

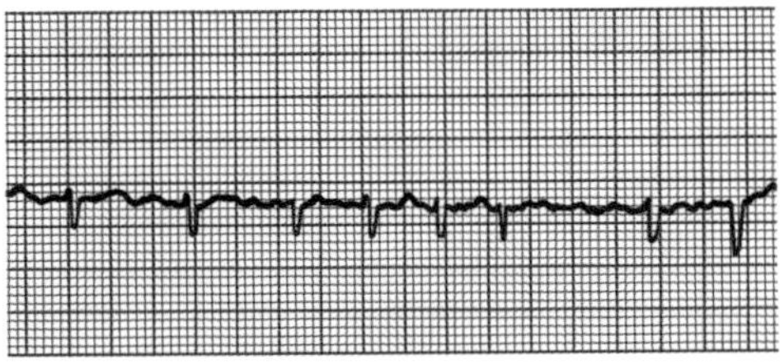

Atrial fibrillation

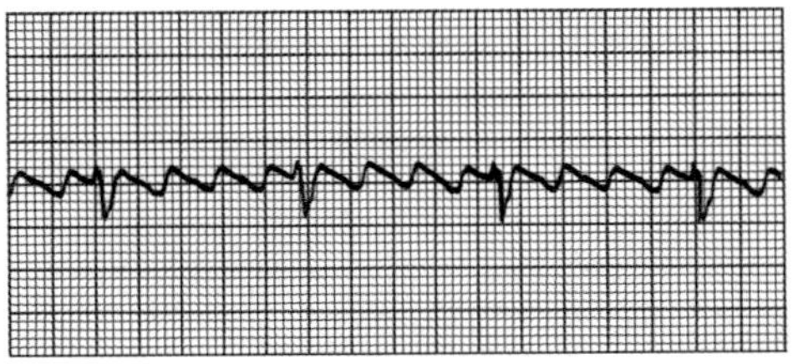

Atrial flutter

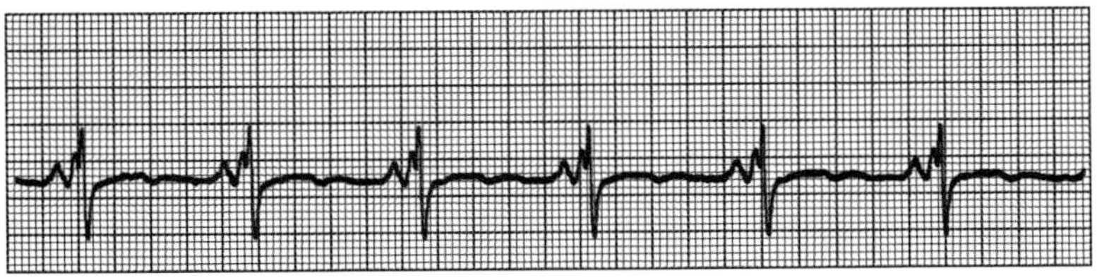

Sinus rhythm with WPW syndrome

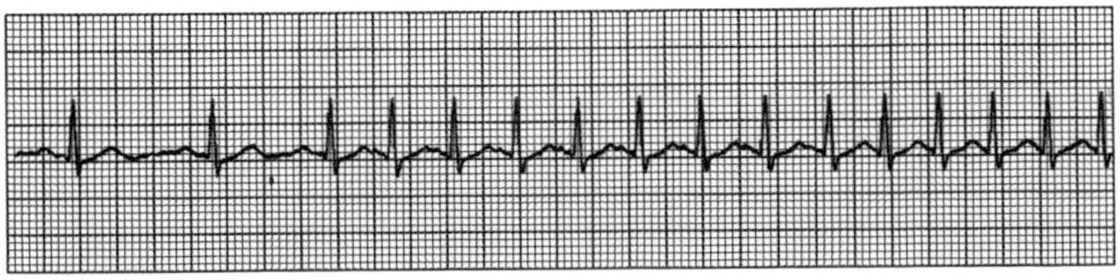

Initial sinus rhythm with paroxysmal onset of supraventricular tachycardia (PSVT)

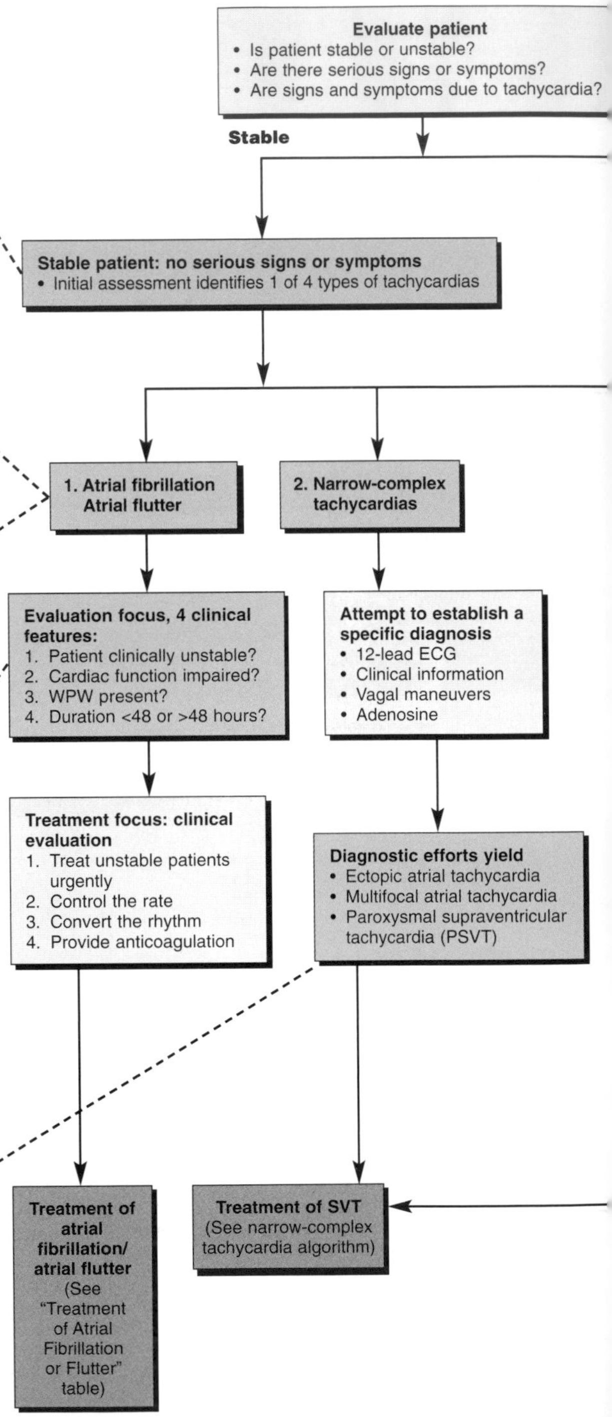
Evaluate patient
• Is patient stable or unstable?
• Are there serious signs or symptoms?
• Are signs and symptoms due to tachycardia?
Stable
Stable patient: no serious signs or symptoms
• Initial assessment identifies 1 of 4 types of tachycardias
1. Atrial fibrillation Atrial flutter
2. Narrow-complex tachycardias
Evaluation focus, 4 clinical features:
1. Patient clinically unstable?
2. Cardiac function impaired?
3. WPW present?
4. Duration <48 or >48 hours?
Attempt to establish a specific diagnosis
• 12-lead ECG
• Clinical information
• Vagal maneuvers
• Adenosine
Treatment focus: clinical evaluation
1. Treat unstable patients urgently
2. Control the rate
3. Convert the rhythm
4. Provide anticoagulation
Diagnostic efforts yield
• Ectopic atrial tachycardia
• Multifocal atrial tachycardia
• Paroxysmal supraventricular tachycardia (PSVT)
Treatment of atrial fibrillation/ atrial flutter (See "Treatment of Atrial Fibrillation or Flutter" table)
Treatment of SVT (See narrow-complex tachycardia algorithm)

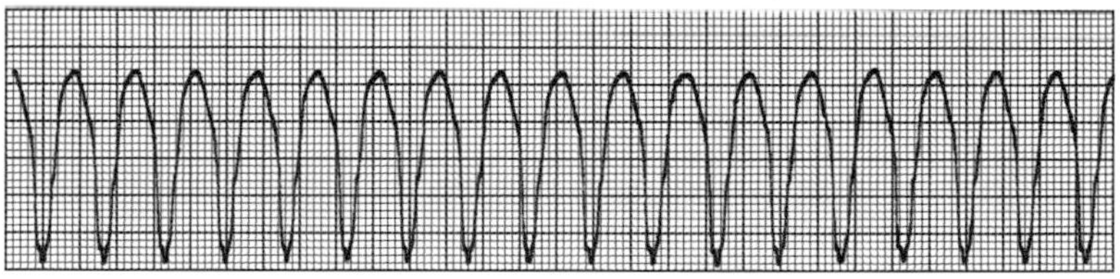

Monomorphic ventricular tachycardia

Unstable

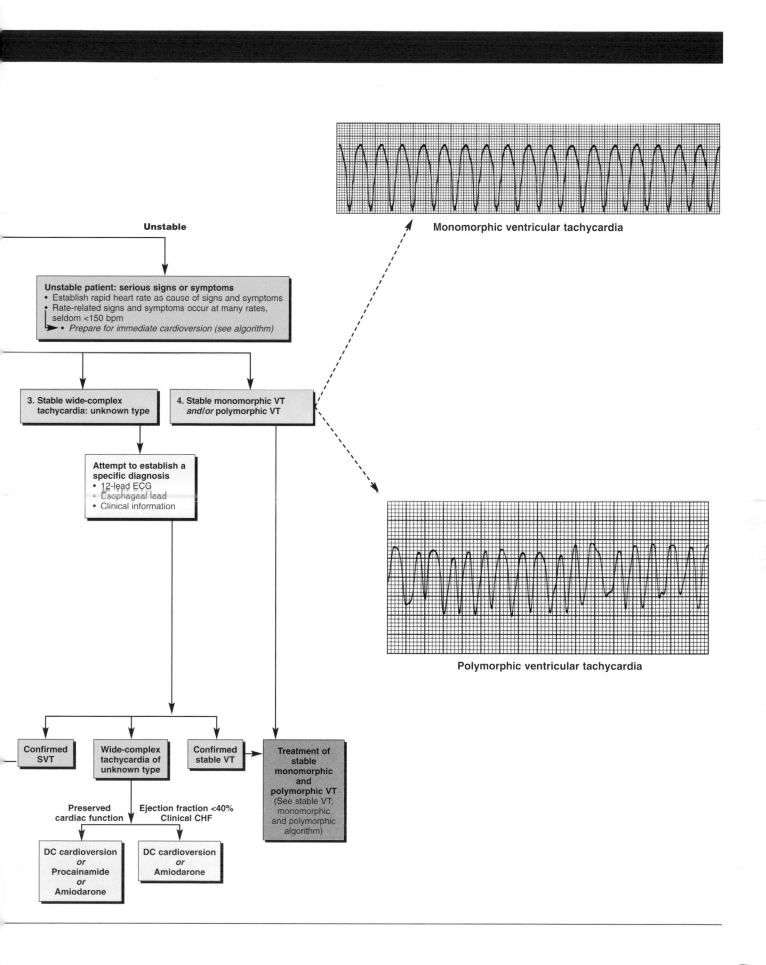

Unstable patient: serious signs or symptoms
- Establish rapid heart rate as cause of signs and symptoms
- Rate-related signs and symptoms occur at many rates, seldom <150 bpm
- *Prepare for immediate cardioversion (see algorithm)*

3. Stable wide-complex tachycardia: unknown type

4. Stable monomorphic VT *and/or* polymorphic VT

Attempt to establish a specific diagnosis
- 12-lead ECG
- Esophageal lead
- Clinical information

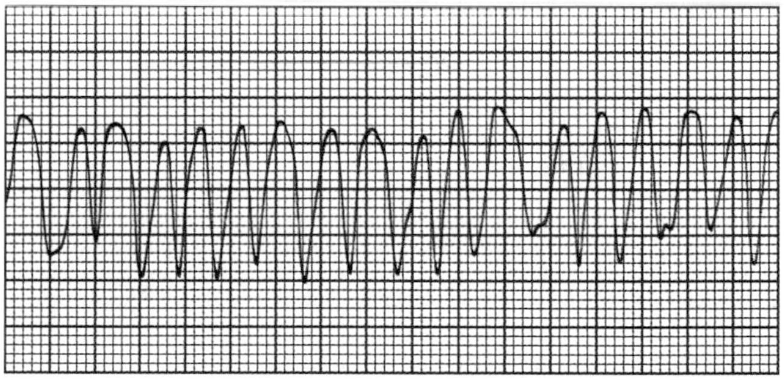

Polymorphic ventricular tachycardia

Confirmed SVT

Wide-complex tachycardia of unknown type

Confirmed stable VT

Treatment of stable monomorphic and polymorphic VT
(See stable VT: monomorphic and polymorphic algorithm)

Preserved cardiac function

DC cardioversion *or* Procainamide *or* Amiodarone

Ejection fraction <40% Clinical CHF

DC cardioversion *or* Amiodarone

6. Reentry Tachycardia Mechanism

A — Normal impulse comes down Purkinje fibers to join muscle fibers.
B — One impulse (B_1) encounters an area of one-way (unidirectional) block (B_2) and stops.
C — Meanwhile, the normally conducted impulse (C_1) has moved down the Purkinje fiber, into the muscle fiber (C_2); and as a retrograde impulse, moves through the area of slow conduction (C_3).
D — The retrograde impulse (D_1) now reenters the Purkinje and muscle fibers (D_2); and keeps this reentry cycle repeating itself multiple times (D_3).

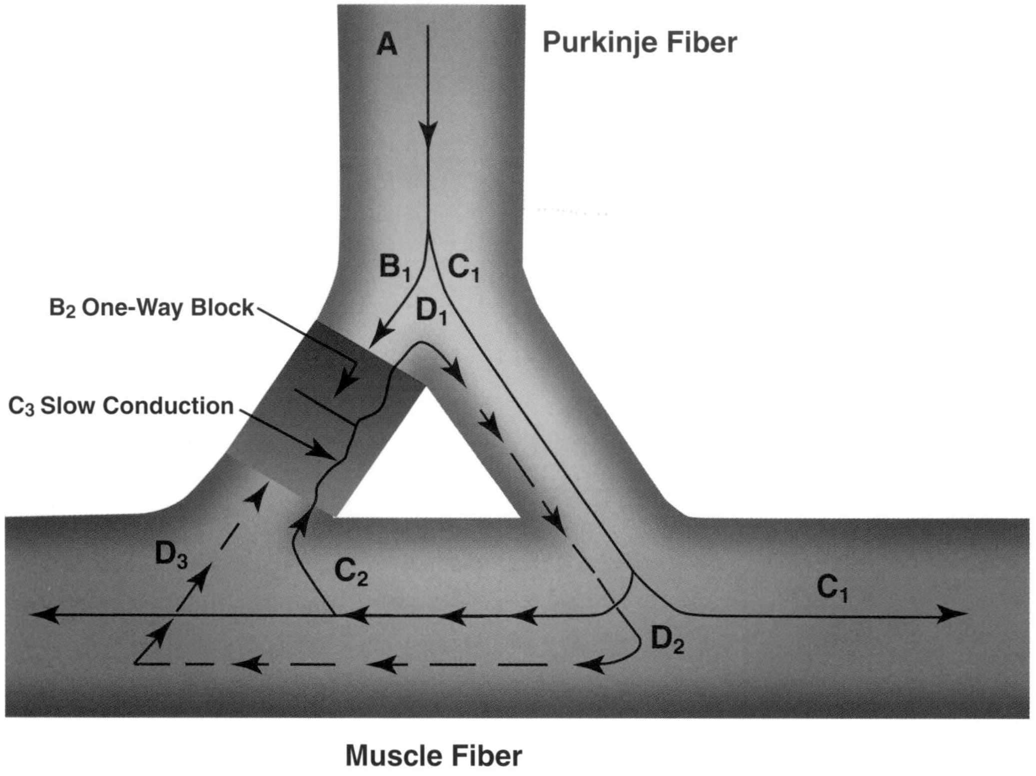

7. Atrial Fibrillation/Atrial Flutter

Pathophysiology	■ Atrial impulses faster than SA node impulses ■ Atrial fibrillation → impulses take multiple, chaotic, random pathways through the atria ■ Atrial flutter → impulses take a circular course around the atria, setting up the flutter waves ■ Mechanism of impulse formation: reentry		
Defining Criteria and ECG Features (Distinctions here between atrial fibrillation vs atrial flutter; all other characteristics are the same) **Atrial Fibrillation Key:** A classic clinical axiom: *"Irregularly irregular rhythm—with variation in both interval and amplitude from R wave to R wave—is always atrial fibrillation."* This one is dependable. **Atrial Flutter Key:** Flutter waves seen in classic "sawtooth pattern"		**Atrial Fibrillation**	**Atrial Flutter**
	Rate	■ Wide-ranging ventricular response to atrial rate of 300-400 beats/min	■ Atrial rate 220-350 beats/min ■ Ventricular response = a function of AV node block or conduction of atrial impulses ■ Ventricular response rarely >150-180 beats because of AV node conduction limits
	Rhythm	■ Irregular (classic "irregularly irregular")	■ Regular (unlike atrial fibrillation) ■ Ventricular rhythm often regular ■ Set ratio to atrial rhythm, eg, 2-to-1 or 3-to-1
	P waves	■ Chaotic atrial fibrillatory waves only ■ Creates disturbed baseline	■ No true P waves seen ■ Flutter waves in "sawtooth pattern" is classic
	PR	■ Cannot be measured	
	QRS	■ Remains ≤0.10-0.12 sec unless QRS complex distorted by fibrillation/flutter waves or by conduction defects through ventricles	
Clinical Manifestations	■ Signs and symptoms are function of the rate of ventricular response to atrial fibrillatory waves; *"atrial fibrillation with rapid ventricular response"* → DOE, SOB, acute pulmonary edema ■ Loss of *"atrial kick"* may lead to drop in cardiac output and decreased coronary perfusion ■ Irregular rhythm often perceived as *"palpitations"* ■ Can be asymptomatic		
Common Etiologies	■ Acute coronary syndromes; CAD; CHF ■ Disease at mitral or tricuspid valve ■ Hypoxia; acute pulmonary embolism ■ Drug-induced: *digoxin* or *quinidine* most common ■ Hyperthyroidism		

<table>
<tr><th colspan="2">7. Atrial Fibrillation/Atrial Flutter (continued)</th><th colspan="2"></th></tr>
<tr><td colspan="2">Recommended Therapy</td><td colspan="2">Control Rate</td></tr>
<tr><td>Evaluation Focus:</td><td>Treatment Focus:</td><td>Normal Heart</td><td>Impaired Heart</td></tr>
<tr><td rowspan="4">1. Patient clinically unstable?
2. Cardiac function impaired?
3. WPW present?
4. Duration ≤48 or >48 hr?

Consider anticoagulants</td><td rowspan="4">1. Treat unstable patients urgently
2. Control the rate
3. Convert the rhythm
4. Provide anticoagulation</td><td>■ Diltiazem or another calcium channel blocker or metoprolol or another β-blocker</td><td>■ Digoxin or diltiazem or amiodarone</td></tr>
<tr><td colspan="2">Convert Rhythm</td></tr>
<tr><td>Impaired Heart</td><td>Normal Heart</td></tr>
<tr><td>■ If ≤48 hours:
— DC cardioversion or amiodarone or others
■ If >48 hours:
— Anticoagulate × 3 wk, then
— DC cardioversion, then
— Anticoagulate × 4 wk
or
■ IV heparin and TEE to rule out atrial clot, then
■ DC cardioversion within 24 hours, then
■ Anticoagulation × 4 more wk</td><td>■ If ≤48 hours:
— DC Cardioversion or amiodarone
■ If >48 hours:
— Anticoagulate × 3 wk, then
— DC cardioversion, then
— Anticoagulate × 4 more wk</td></tr>
</table>

TEE indicates transesophageal echocardiogram.

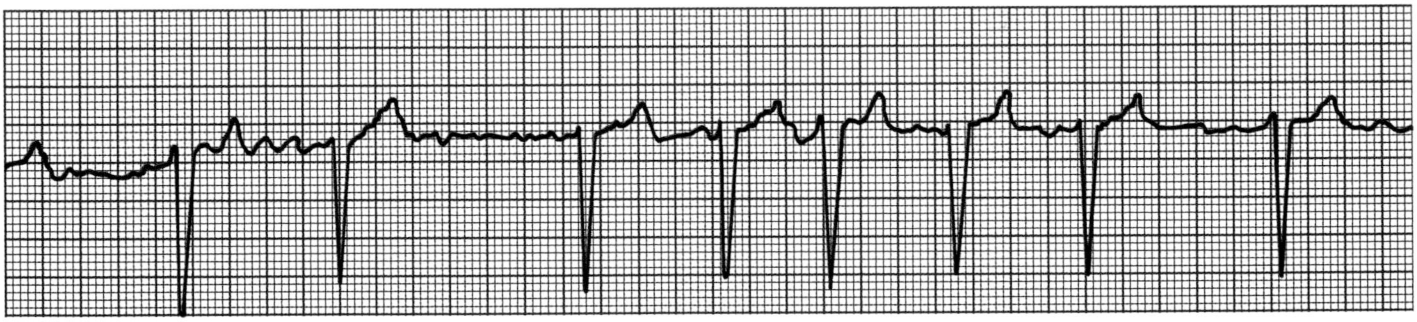

Atrial fibrillation

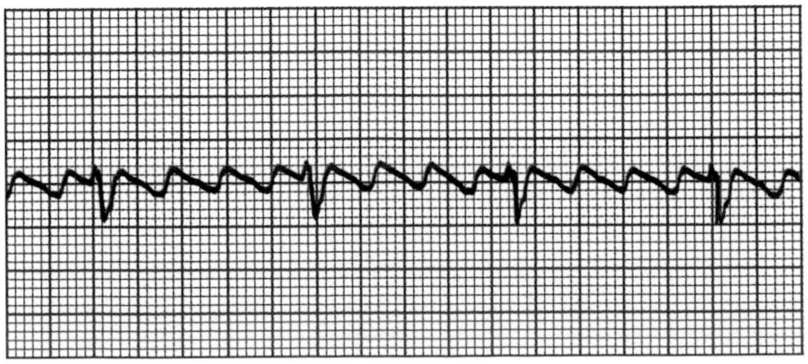

Atrial flutter

8. WPW (Wolff-Parkinson-White) Syndrome	
Pathophysiology	■ The prototypical **pre-excitation syndrome:** congenital malformation; strands of conducting myocardial tissue between atria and ventricles ■ When persistent after birth strands can form an accessory pathway (eg, bundle of Kent)
Defining Criteria and ECG Features **Key: QRS complex** is classically distorted by delta wave (upwards deflection of QRS is slurred)	■ **Rate:** most often 60-100 beats/min as usual rhythm is sinus ■ **Rhythm:** normal sinus except during pre-excitation tachycardia ■ **PR:** shorter since conduction through accessory pathway is faster than through AV node ■ **P waves:** normal conformation ■ **QRS complex:** classically distorted by delta wave (upwards deflection of QRS is slurred)
Clinical Manifestations	■ A person with WPW may never have symptoms ■ People with WPW have same annual incidence of atrial fibrillation as age- and gender-matched population ■ Onset of atrial fibrillation for WPW patients, however, poses risk of rapid ventricular response through the accessory pathway ■ This rapid ventricular response can lead to all signs and symptoms of stable and unstable tachycardias
Common Etiology	■ The accessory pathway in WPW is a congenital malformation

8. WPW (Wolff-Parkinson-White) Syndrome (continued)

Recommended Therapy

Evaluation Focus	Treatment Focus
1. Patient clinically unstable? 2. Cardiac function impaired? 3. WPW present? 4. Duration ≤48 or >48 hr?	1. Treat unstable patients urgently 2. Control the rate 3. Convert the rhythm 4. Provide anticoagulation

Class III (can be harmful) in treating atrial fibrillation with WPW:

- *Adenosine*
- *β-Blockers*
- *Calcium channel blockers*
- *Digoxin*

Wolff-Parkinson-White: Control Rate

Normal Heart	Impaired Heart
■ **Cardioversion or** ■ **Antiarrhythmic (IIb):** *amiodarone* **or** *flecainide* **or** *procainamide* **or** *propafenone* **or** *sotalol*	■ **Cardioversion** **or** ■ ***Amiodarone***

Wolff-Parkinson-White: Convert Rhythm

Duration ≤48 Hours	Duration >48 Hours
■ **Cardioversion or** ■ **Antiarrhythmic (IIb):** *amiodarone* **or** *flecainide* **or** *procainamide* **or** *propafenone* **or** *sotalol* **If impaired heart:** cardioversion **or** *amiodarone*	■ Anticoagulate × 3 wk **then** ■ DC cardioversion **then** ■ Anticoagulate × 4 wk

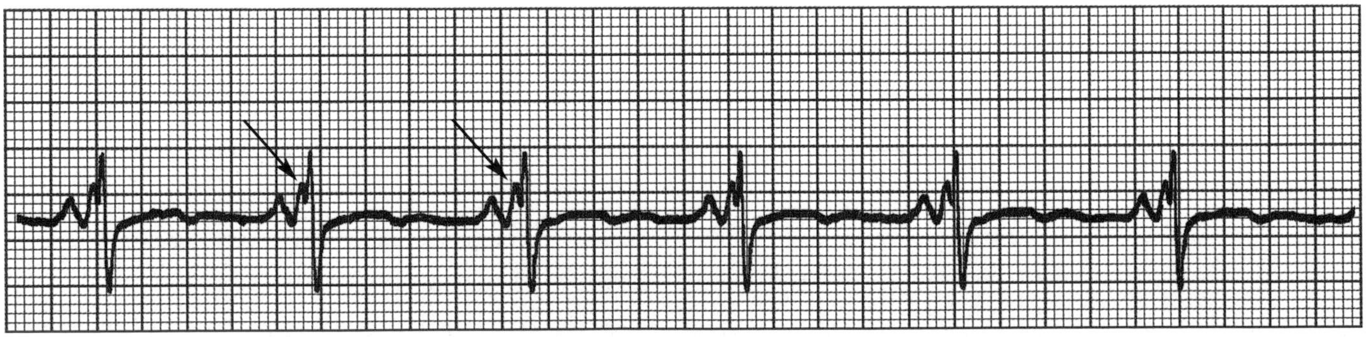

Wolff-Parkinson-White syndrome: normal sinus rhythm with *delta wave* (arrow) notching of positive upstroke of QRS complex

9. Junctional Tachycardia	
Pathophysiology	■ Area of *automaticity* (automatic impulse formation) develops in the AV node ("junction") ■ Both retrograde and antegrade transmission occurs
Defining Criteria and ECG Features ■ **Key:** position of the P wave; may show antegrade or retrograde propagation because origin is at the junction; may arise before, after, or with the QRS	■ **Rate:** 100-180 beats/min ■ **Rhythm:** regular atrial and ventricular firing ■ **PR:** often not measurable unless P wave comes before QRS; then will be short (<0.12 secs) ■ **P waves:** often obscured; may propagate antegrade or retrograde with origin at the junction; may arise before, after, or with the QRS ■ **QRS complex:** narrow; ≤0.10 secs in absence of intraventricular conduction defect
Clinical Manifestations	■ Patients may have clinical signs of a reduced ejection fraction because augmented flow from atrium is lost ■ Symptoms of unstable tachycardia may occur
Common Etiologies	■ Digoxin toxicity ■ Acute sequelae of acute coronary syndromes
Recommended Therapy If specific diagnosis unknown, attempt therapeutic/diagnostic maneuver with ■ Vagal stimulation ■ *Adenosine* . . . THEN →	**Preserved heart function:** ■ *β-Blocker* ■ *Calcium channel blocker* ■ *Amiodarone* ■ **NO DC cardioversion!** **If impaired heart function:** ■ *Amiodarone* ■ **NO DC cardioversion!**

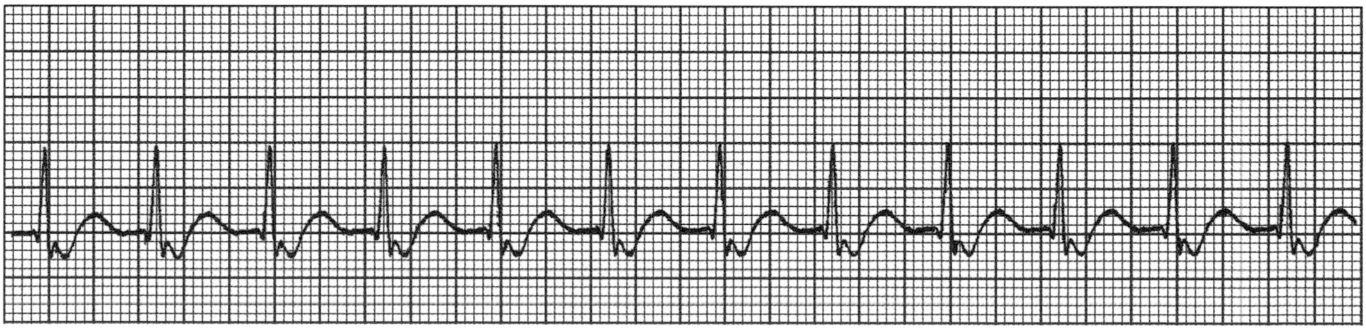

Junctional tachycardia: narrow QRS complexes at 130 bpm; P waves arise with QRS

Rhythmic Algorithm No. 2: Narrow-Complex Tachycardias

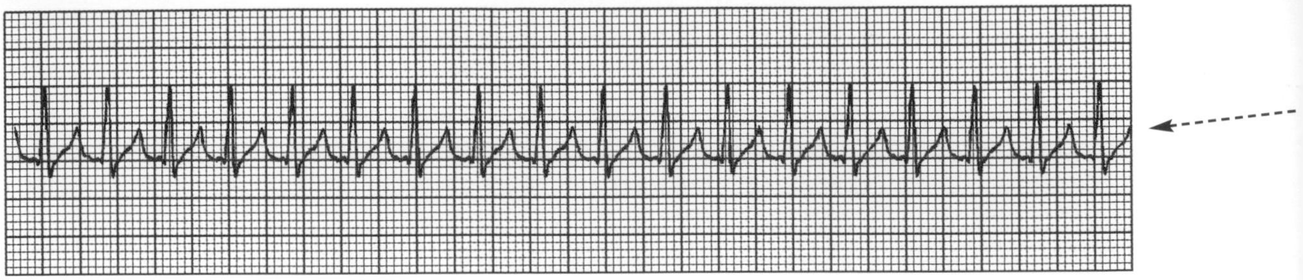

Supraventricular tachycardia

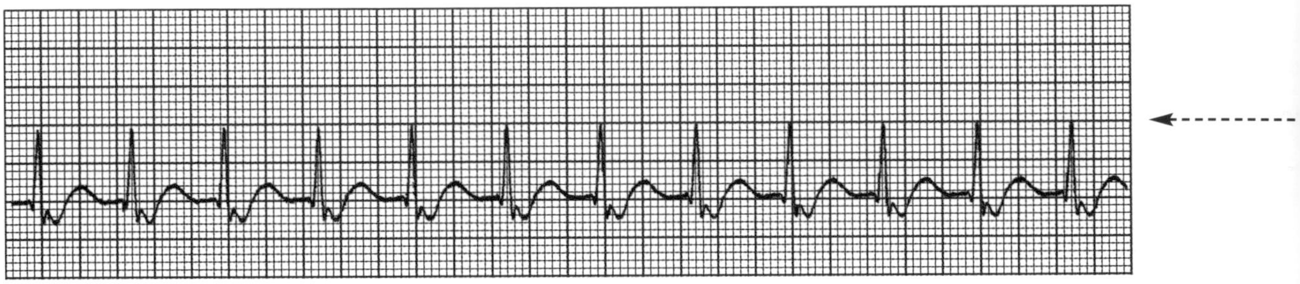

Junctional tachycardia

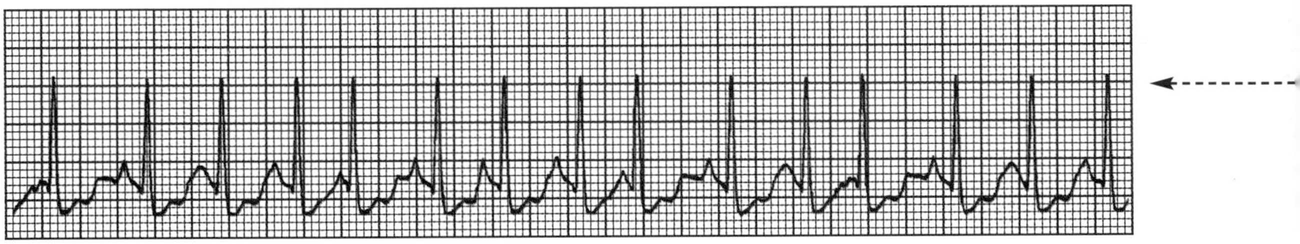

Multifocal atrial tachycardia

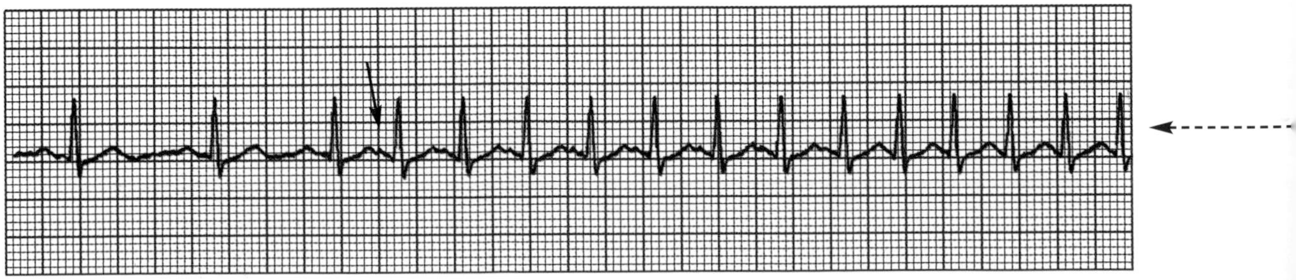

Sinus rhythm (3 complexes) with paroxysmal onset (arrow) of supraventricular tachycardia (PSVT)

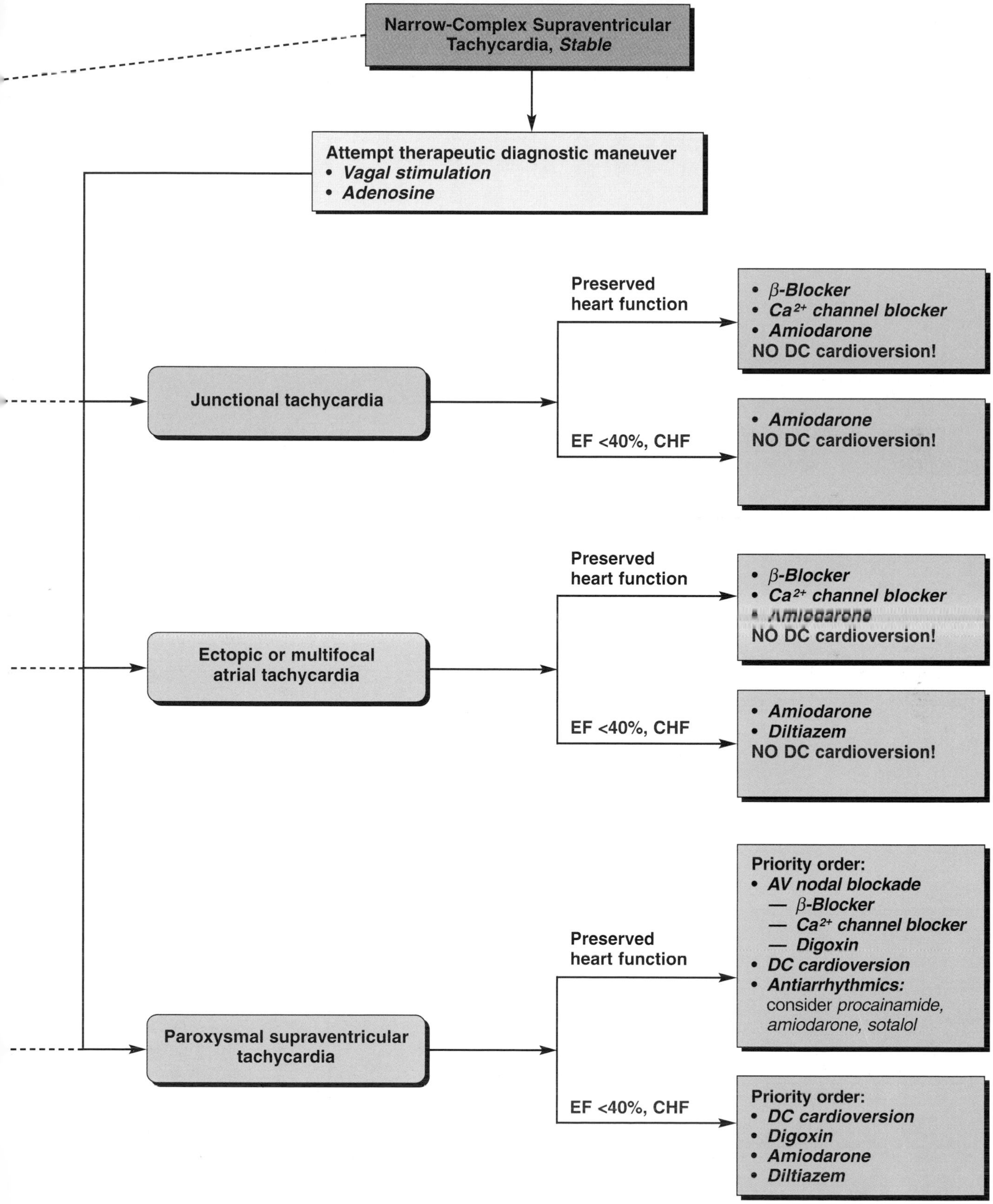
Narrow-Complex Supraventricular Tachycardia, *Stable*
Attempt therapeutic diagnostic maneuver
• *Vagal stimulation*
• *Adenosine*
Junctional tachycardia
Preserved heart function
• *β-Blocker*
• *Ca^{2+} channel blocker*
• *Amiodarone*
NO DC cardioversion!
EF <40%, CHF
• *Amiodarone*
NO DC cardioversion!
Ectopic or multifocal atrial tachycardia
Preserved heart function
• *β-Blocker*
• *Ca^{2+} channel blocker*
• *Amiodarone*
NO DC cardioversion!
EF <40%, CHF
• *Amiodarone*
• *Diltiazem*
NO DC cardioversion!
Paroxysmal supraventricular tachycardia
Preserved heart function
Priority order:
• *AV nodal blockade*
— *β-Blocker*
— *Ca^{2+} channel blocker*
— *Digoxin*
• *DC cardioversion*
• *Antiarrhythmics:* consider *procainamide, amiodarone, sotalol*
EF <40%, CHF
Priority order:
• *DC cardioversion*
• *Digoxin*
• *Amiodarone*
• *Diltiazem*

10. Multifocal Atrial Tachycardia

Pathophysiology	■ Areas of *automaticity* (impulse formation) originate irregularly and rapidly at different points in the atria
Defining Criteria and ECG Features If the rate is <100 beats/min, this rhythm is termed *"wandering atrial pacemaker"* or *"multifocal atrial rhythm"* **Key:** By definition must have 3 or more P waves that differ in polarity (up/down), shape, and size since the atrial impulse is generated from multiple foci.	■ **Rate:** >100 beats/min; usually >130 bpm ■ **Rhythm:** irregular atrial firing ■ **PR:** variable ■ **P waves:** by definition must have 3 or more P waves that differ in polarity (up/down), shape, and size since the atrial impulse is generated from multiple foci ■ **QRS complex:** narrow; ≤0.10 sec in absence of intraventricular conduction defect
Clinical Manifestations	■ Patients may have no clinical signs ■ Symptoms of unstable tachycardia may occur
Common Etiologies	■ Most common cause is COPD *(cor pulmonale)* where pulmonary hypertension places increased strain on the right ventricle and atrium ■ Impaired and hypertrophied atrium gives rise to automaticity ■ Also digoxin toxicity, rheumatic heart disease, acute coronary syndromes
Recommended Therapy If specific diagnosis unknown, attempt therapeutic/diagnostic maneuver with ■ Vagal stimulation ■ *Adenosine* . . . THEN →	**Preserved heart function:** ■ *β-blocker* ■ *Calcium channel blocker* ■ *Amiodarone* ■ **NO DC cardioversion!** **If impaired heart function:** ■ *Amiodarone* ■ *Diltiazem* ■ **NO DC cardioversion!**

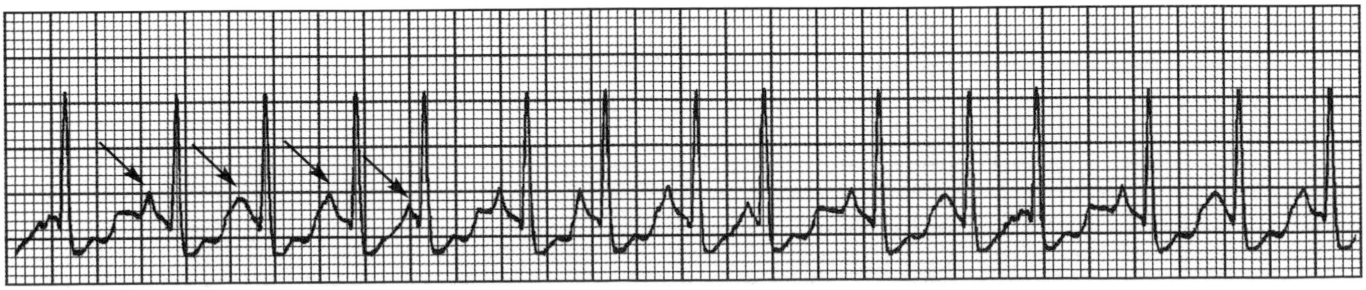

Multifocal atrial tachycardia: narrow-complex tachycardia at 140 to 160 bpm with multiple P-wave morphologies (arrows)

11. PSVT (Paroxysmal Supraventricular Tachycardia)

Pathophysiology	■ **Reentry phenomenon** (see page 260)**:** impulses arise and recycle repeatedly in the AV node because of areas of unidirectional block in the Purkinje fibers
Defining Criteria and ECG Features **Key:** Regular, narrow-complex tachycardia without P-waves, and <u>sudden</u>, *paroxysmal* onset or cessation, or both **Note:** To merit the diagnosis some experts require capture of the paroxysmal onset or cessation on a monitor strip	■ **Rate:** exceeds upper limit of sinus tachycardia (>120 beats/min); seldom <150 beats/min; up to 250 beats/min ■ **Rhythm:** regular ■ **P waves:** seldom seen because rapid rate causes P wave loss in preceding T waves or because the origin is low in the atrium ■ **QRS complex:** normal, narrow (≤0.10 sec usually)
Clinical Manifestations	■ Palpitations felt by patient at the paroxysmal onset; becomes anxious, uncomfortable ■ Exercise tolerance low with very high rates ■ Symptoms of unstable tachycardia may occur
Common Etiologies	■ Accessory conduction pathway in many PSVT patients ■ For such otherwise healthy people many factors can provoke the paroxysm, such as caffeine, hypoxia, cigarettes, stress, anxiety, sleep deprivation, numerous medications ■ Also increased frequency of PSVT in unhealthy patients with CAD, COPD, CHF
Recommended Therapy If specific diagnosis unknown, attempt therapeutic/diagnostic maneuver with ■ Vagal stimulation ■ *Adenosine* . . . THEN→	**Preserved heart function:** ■ AV nodal blockade — *β-Blocker* — *Calcium channel blocker* — *Digoxin* ■ DC cardioversion ■ Parenteral antiarrhythmics: — *Procainamide* — *Amiodarone* — *Sotalol* (not available in the United States) **Impaired heart function:** ■ *DC cardioversion* ■ *Digoxin* ■ *Amiodarone* ■ *Diltiazem*

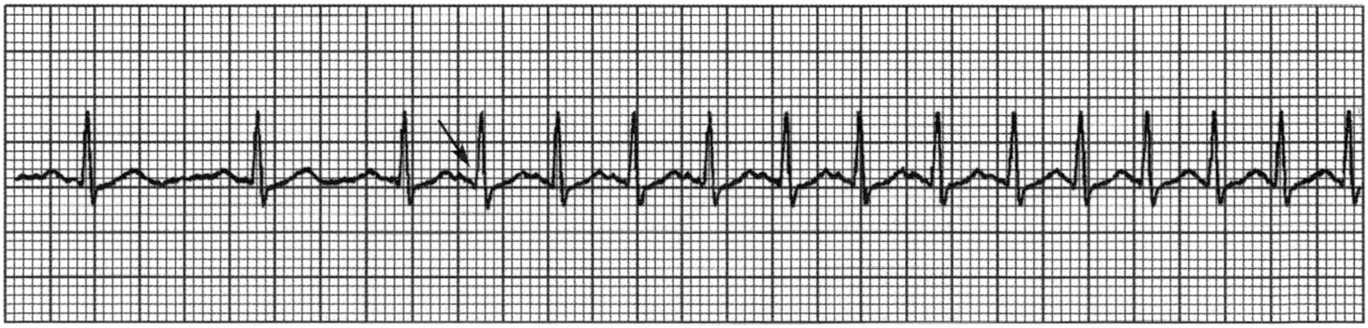

Sinus rhythm (3 complexes) with paroxysmal onset (arrow) of supraventricular tachycardia (PSVT)

Rhythmic Algorithm No. 3: Stable Ventricular Tachycardias

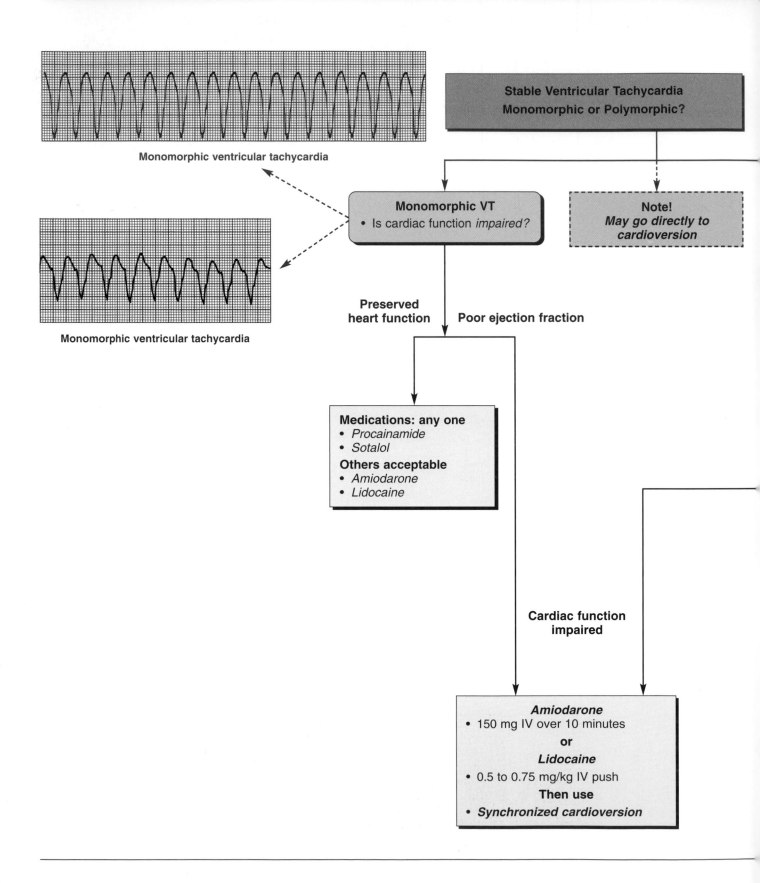

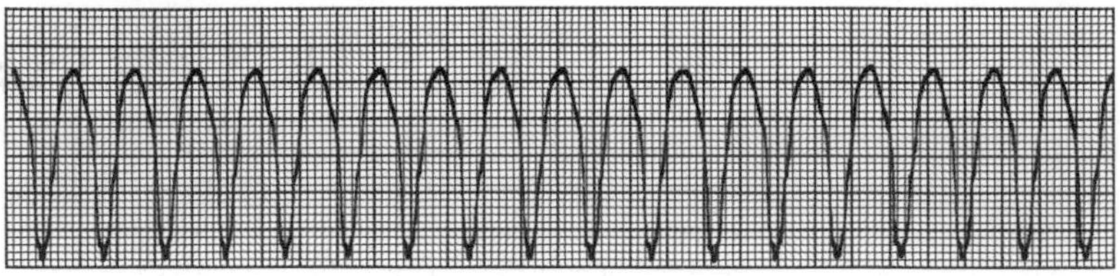

Monomorphic ventricular tachycardia

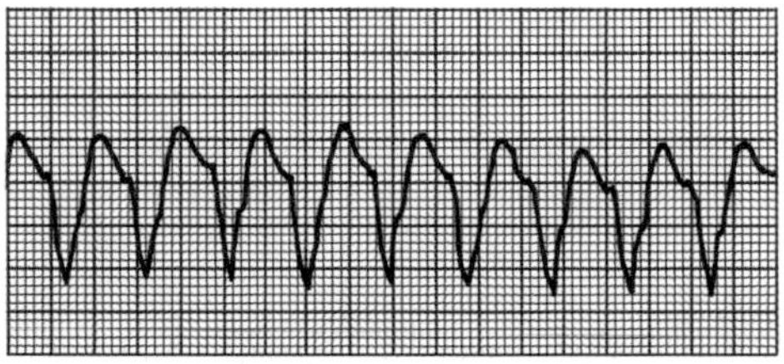

Monomorphic ventricular tachycardia

Stable Ventricular Tachycardia
Monomorphic or Polymorphic?

Note!
May go directly to cardioversion

Monomorphic VT
- Is cardiac function *impaired?*

Preserved heart function

Poor ejection fraction

Medications: any one
- *Procainamide*
- *Sotalol*

Others acceptable
- *Amiodarone*
- *Lidocaine*

Cardiac function impaired

Amiodarone
- 150 mg IV over 10 minutes

or

Lidocaine
- 0.5 to 0.75 mg/kg IV push

Then use
- ***Synchronized cardioversion***

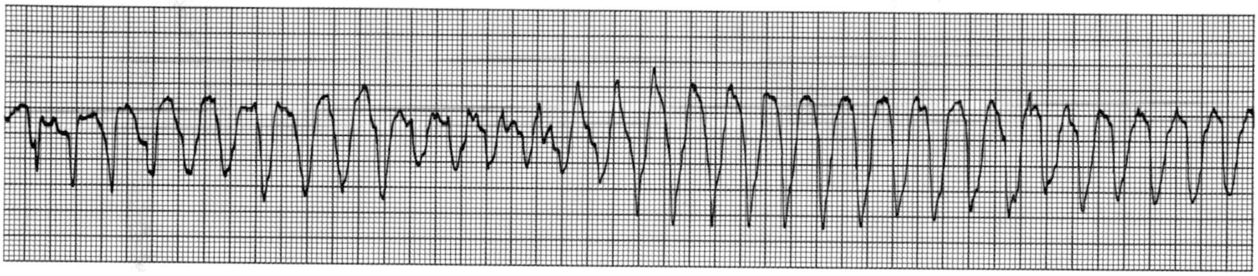

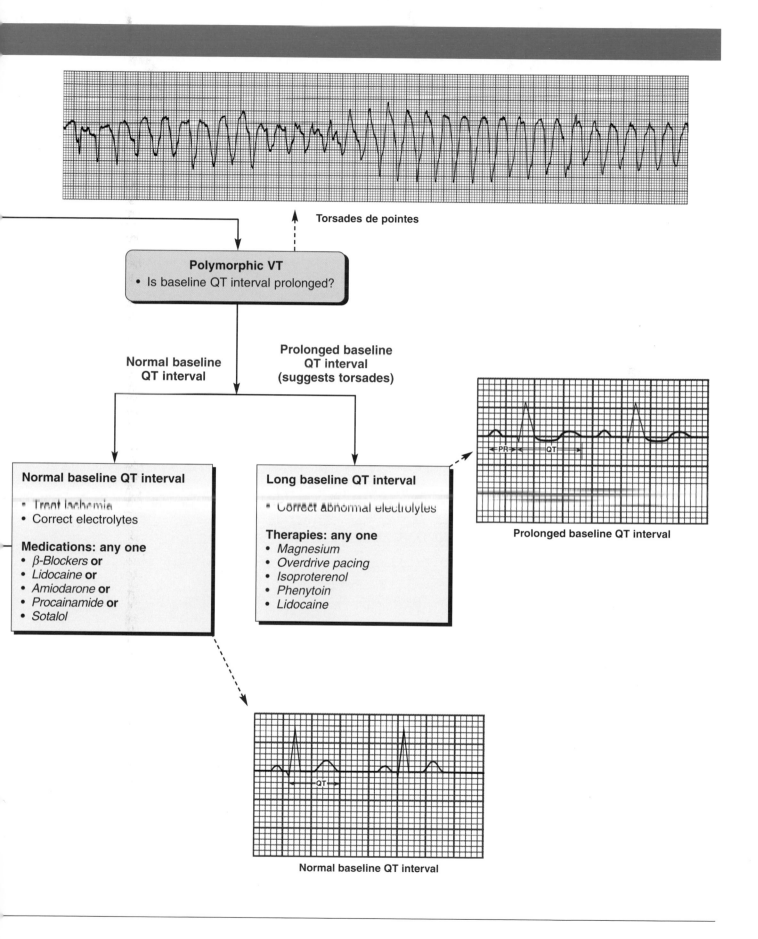

Torsades de pointes

Polymorphic VT

- Is baseline QT interval prolonged?

Normal baseline QT interval

Prolonged baseline QT interval (suggests torsades)

Normal baseline QT interval

- Treat ischemia
- Correct electrolytes

Medications: any one

- *β-Blockers* **or**
- *Lidocaine* **or**
- *Amiodarone* **or**
- *Procainamide* **or**
- *Sotalol*

Long baseline QT interval

- Correct abnormal electrolytes

Therapies: any one

- *Magnesium*
- *Overdrive pacing*
- *Isoproterenol*
- *Phenytoin*
- *Lidocaine*

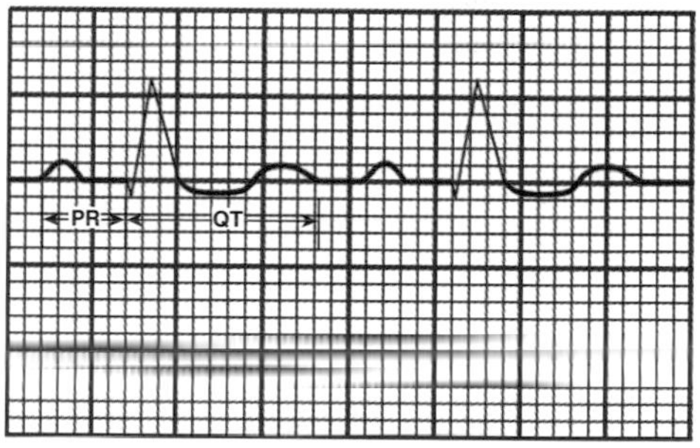

Prolonged baseline QT interval

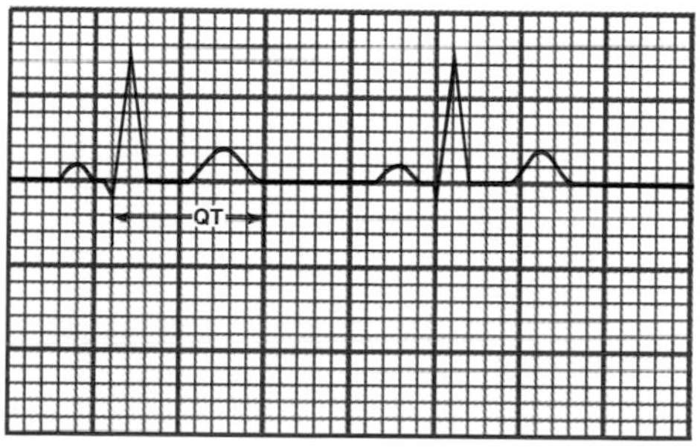

Normal baseline QT interval

12. Monomorphic Ventricular Tachycardia (Stable)

Pathophysiology	■ Impulse conduction is slowed around areas of ventricular injury, infarct, or ischemia ■ These areas also serve as source of ectopic impulses *(irritable foci)* ■ These areas of injury can cause the impulse to take a circular course, leading to the reentry phenomenon and rapid repetitive depolarizations
Defining Criteria per ECG **Key:** The same morphology, or shape, is seen in every QRS complex **Notes:** ■ 3 or more consecutive PVCs: *ventricular tachycardia* ■ VT <30 sec duration ➔ *non-sustained VT* ■ VT >30 sec duration ➔ *sustained VT*	■ **Rate:** ventricular rate >100 bpm; typically 120 to 250 bpm ■ **Rhythm:** no atrial activity seen, only regular ventricular ■ **PR:** nonexistent ■ **P waves:** seldom seen but present; VT is a form of AV dissociation (which is a defining characteristic for wide-complex tachycardias of ventricular origin vs supraventricular tachycardias with aberrant conduction) ■ **QRS complex:** wide and bizarre, "PVC-like" complexes >0.12 sec, with large T wave of opposite polarity from QRS
Clinical Manifestations	■ Monomorphic VT can be asymptomatic, despite the widespread erroneous belief that sustained VT always produces symptoms ■ Majority of times, however, symptoms of decreased cardiac output (orthostasis, hypotension, syncope, exercise limitations, etc) are seen ■ Untreated and sustained will deteriorate to unstable VT, often VF
Common Etiologies	■ An acute ischemic event (see pathophysiology) with areas of "ventricular irritability" leading to PVCs ■ PVCs that occur during the relative refractory period of the cardiac cycle ("R-on-T phenomenon") ■ Drug-induced, prolonged QT interval (tricyclic antidepressants, procainamide, digoxin, some long-acting antihistamines)

Recommended Therapy	**Normal Heart**	**Impaired Heart**
	Any one of following parenteral antiarrhythmics: ■ *Procainamide* ■ *Sotalol* ■ *Amiodarone* ■ *Lidocaine*	■ *Amiodarone* **or** ■ *Lidocaine* **then** ■ *DC cardioversion* if persists

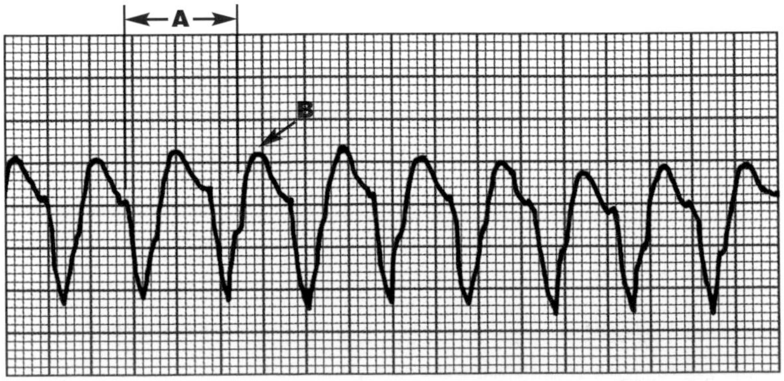

Monomorphic ventricular tachycardia at rate of 150 bpm: wide QRS complexes (arrow A) with opposite polarity T waves (arrow B)

<table>
<tr><th colspan="2">13. Polymorphic Ventricular Tachycardia (Stable)</th></tr>
<tr><td>Pathophysiology</td><td>■ Impulse conduction is slowed around multiple areas of ventricular injury, infarct, or ischemia
■ These areas also serve as the source of ectopic impulses (irritable foci); irritable foci occur in multiple areas of the ventricles, thus “polymorphic”
■ These areas of injury can cause impulses to take a circular course, leading to the reentry phenomenom and rapid repetitive depolarizations</td></tr>
<tr><td>Defining Criteria per ECG
Key: Marked variation and inconsistency seen in the QRS complexes</td><td>■ Rate: ventricular rate >100 bpm; typically 120 to 250 bpm
■ Rhythm: only regular ventricular
■ PR: nonexistent
■ P waves: seldom seen but present; VT is a form of AV dissociation
■ QRS complexes: marked variation and inconsistency seen in the QRS complexes</td></tr>
<tr><td>Clinical Manifestations</td><td>■ Rare: asymptomatic polymorphic VT
■ Majority of times: symptoms of decreased cardiac output (orthostasis, hypotension, syncope, exercise limitations, etc) are seen
■ Seldom → sustained VT; seldom → “stable” VT
■ Tends toward rapid deterioration to pulseless VT or VF</td></tr>
<tr><td>Common Etiologies</td><td>■ An acute ischemic event (see pathophysiology) with areas of “ventricular irritability” leading to PVCs
■ PVCs that occur during the relative refractory period of the cardiac cycle (“R-on-T phenomenon”)
■ Drug-induced prolonged QT interval (tricyclic antidepressants, procainamide, digoxin, some long-acting antihistamines)</td></tr>
<tr><td>Recommended Therapy</td><td>Review most recent 12-lead ECG (baseline)
■ Measure QT interval just prior to onset of the polymorphic tachycardia
■ QT interval prolongation? (if YES go to Torsades de Pointes; if NO see below)
Normal baseline QT interval:
■ Treat ischemia
■ Correct electrolytes if abnormal
Then:
<table>
<tr><th>Normal Heart</th><th>Impaired Heart</th></tr>
<tr><td>Parenteral medications: any one
■ β-Blockers or
■ Lidocaine or
■ Amiodarone or
■ Procainamide or
■ Sotalol</td><td>■ Amiodarone
or
■ Lidocaine
then
■ DC cardioversion if persists</td></tr>
</table></td></tr>
</table>

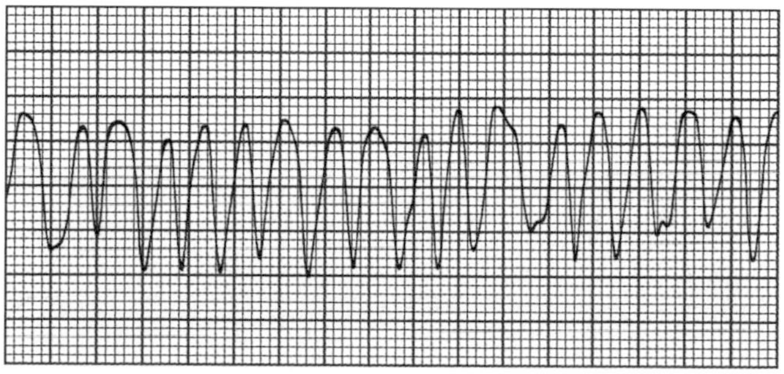

Polymorphic ventricular tachycardia: QRS complexes display multiple morphologies (“polymorphic”)

14. Torsades de Pointes (a Unique Subtype of Polymorphic Ventricular Tachycardia)	
Pathophysiology	Specific pathophysiology for classic torsades: ■ QT interval is abnormally long (see below for etiology of QT prolongation) ■ Leads to increase in the relative refractory period ("vulnerable period") of the cardiac cycle ■ Increases probability that an irritable focus (PVC) will occur on the T-wave ("vulnerable period" or "R-on-T phenomenon") ■ R-on-T phenomenon often induces VT
Defining Criteria per ECG **Key:** QRS complexes display "spindle-node" pattern ➔ VT amplitude increases then decreases in regular pattern (creates the "spindle") ➔ initial deflection at start of one spindle (eg, negative) will be followed by the opposite (eg, positive) deflection at the start of the next spindle (creates the "node")	■ **Atrial Rate:** cannot determine atrial rate ■ **Ventricular rate:** 150-250 complexes/min ■ **Rhythm:** only irregular ventricular rhythm ■ **PR:** nonexistent ■ **P waves:** nonexistent ■ **QRS complexes:** display classic "spindle-node" pattern (see left column: "Key")
Clinical Manifestations	■ Majority of times patients with torsades have symptoms of decreased cardiac output (orthostasis, hypotension, syncope, exercise limitations, etc) ■ Asymptomatic torsades, *sustained* torsades, or *"stable"* torsades is uncommon ■ Tends toward sudden deterioration to pulseless VT or VF
Common Etiologies	Most commonly occurs with prolonged QT interval, from many causes: ■ Drug-induced: tricyclic antidepressants, procainamide, digoxin, some long-acting antihistamines ■ Electrolyte and metabolic alterations (hypomagnesemia is the prototype) ■ Inherited forms of long QT syndrome ■ Acute ischemic events (see pathophysiology)
Recommended Therapy	**Review most recent 12-lead ECG** (baseline): ■ Measure QT interval just before onset of the polymorphic tachycardia ■ QT interval prolongation? (if YES see below; if NO go to the polymorphic VT algorithm) **Long baseline QT interval:** ■ Treat ischemia ■ Correct electrolytes if abnormal **Then therapies (any one):** ■ Magnesium ■ Overdrive pacing ■ Isoproterenol (pharmacologic overdrive pacing) ■ Phenytoin ■ Lidocaine

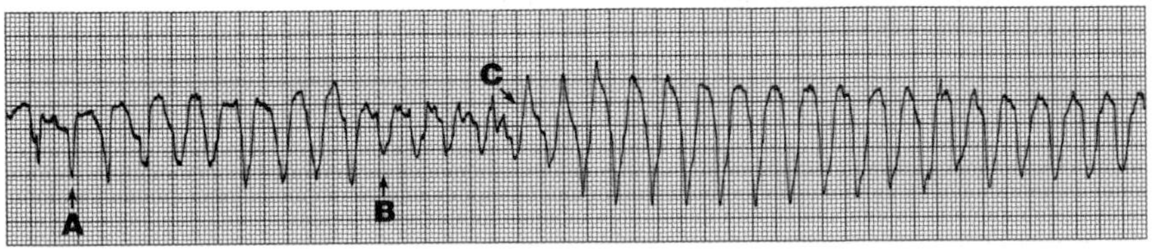

Torsades de pointes (a unique subtype of polymorphic ventricular tachycardia)
Arrows: A — Start of a "spindle"; note negative initial deflection; note increasing QRS amplitude
B — End of "spindle"; start of "node"
C — End of "node"; start of next "spindle"; note positive initial deflection; increase-decrease in QRS amplitude

15. Normal and Prolonged Baseline QT Interval

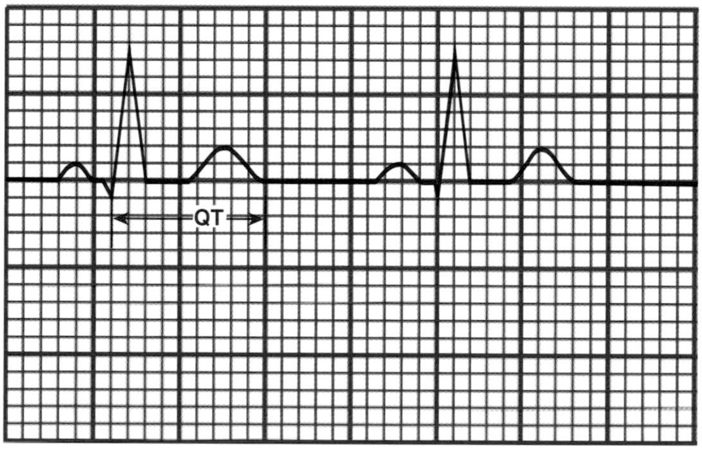

Normal baseline QT interval
Rate: 80 bpm
QT interval: 0.36 sec
(within QT_c range of 0.32 – 0.39 sec
for a heart rate of 80 bpm)

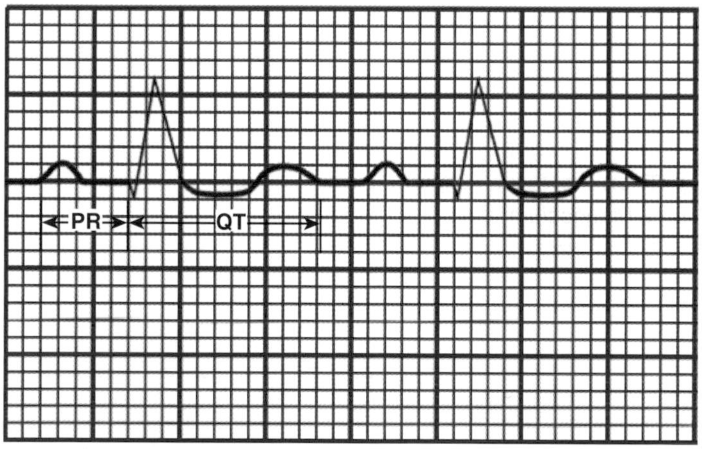

Prolonged baseline QT interval
Due to drug toxicity
PR interval: >0.20 sec
Rate: 80 bpm
QT interval: prolonged, 0.45 sec
(above QT_c range of 0.32 – 0.39 sec
for a heart rate of 80 bpm)
QRS complex: widened, >0.12 sec

Rhythmic Algorithm No. 4: Bradycardias

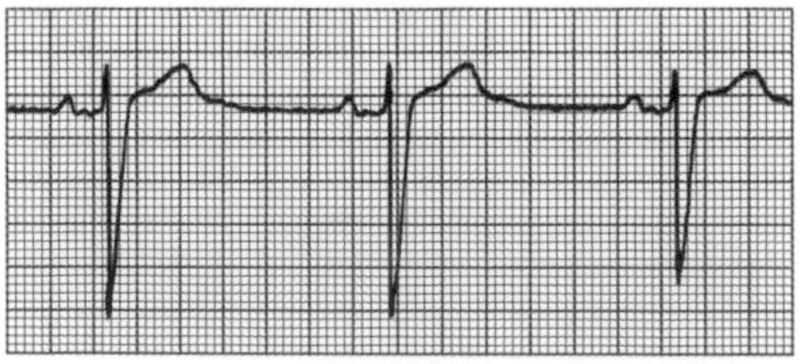

Sinus bradycardia with borderline first-degree AV block

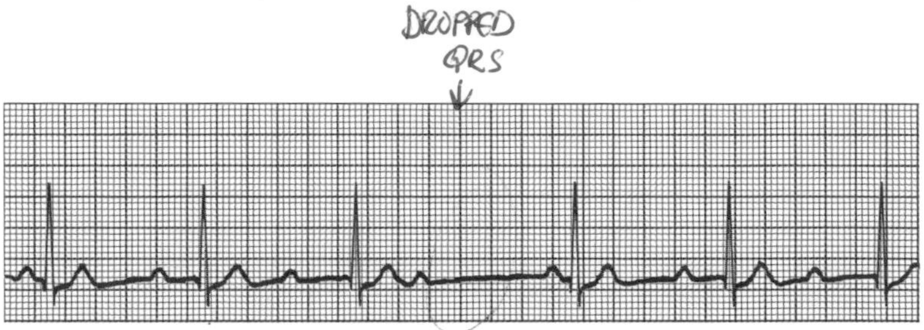

Second-degree AV block type I

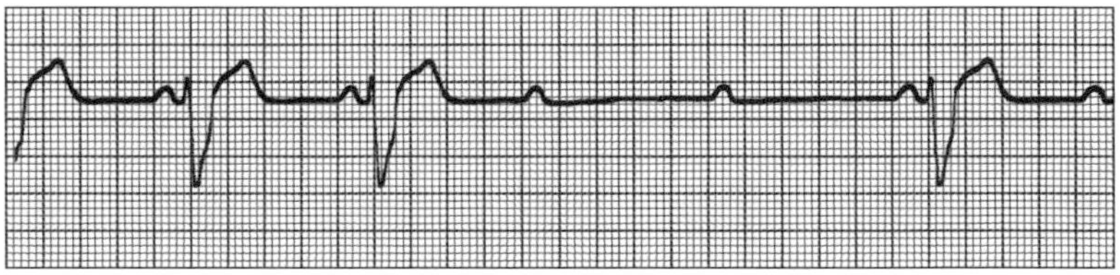

Second-degree AV block type II

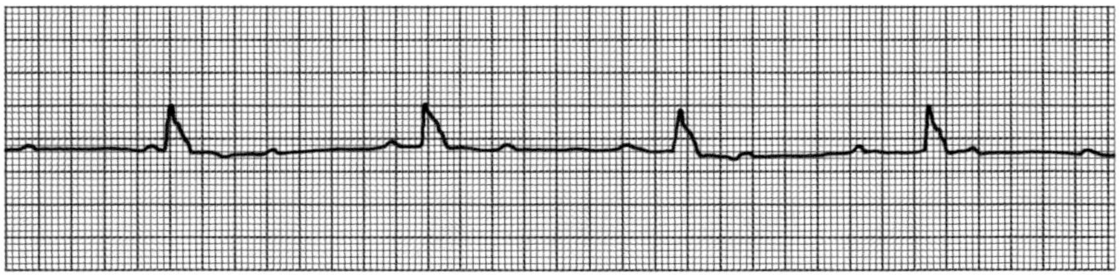

Complete AV block with a ventricular escape pacemaker (wide QRS: 0.12 to 0.14 sec)

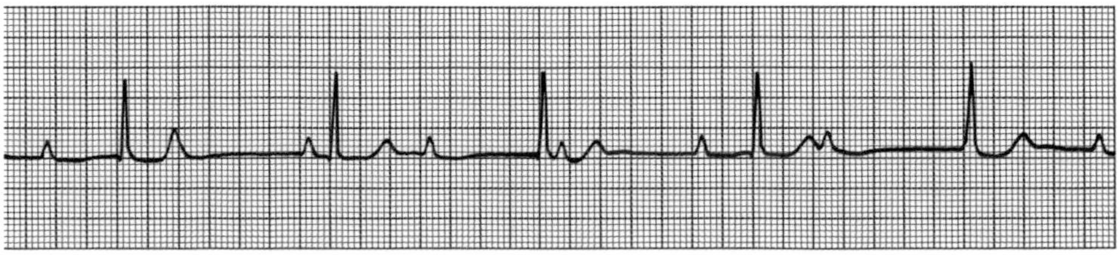

Third-degree AV block with a junctional escape pacemaker (narrow QRS: <0.12)

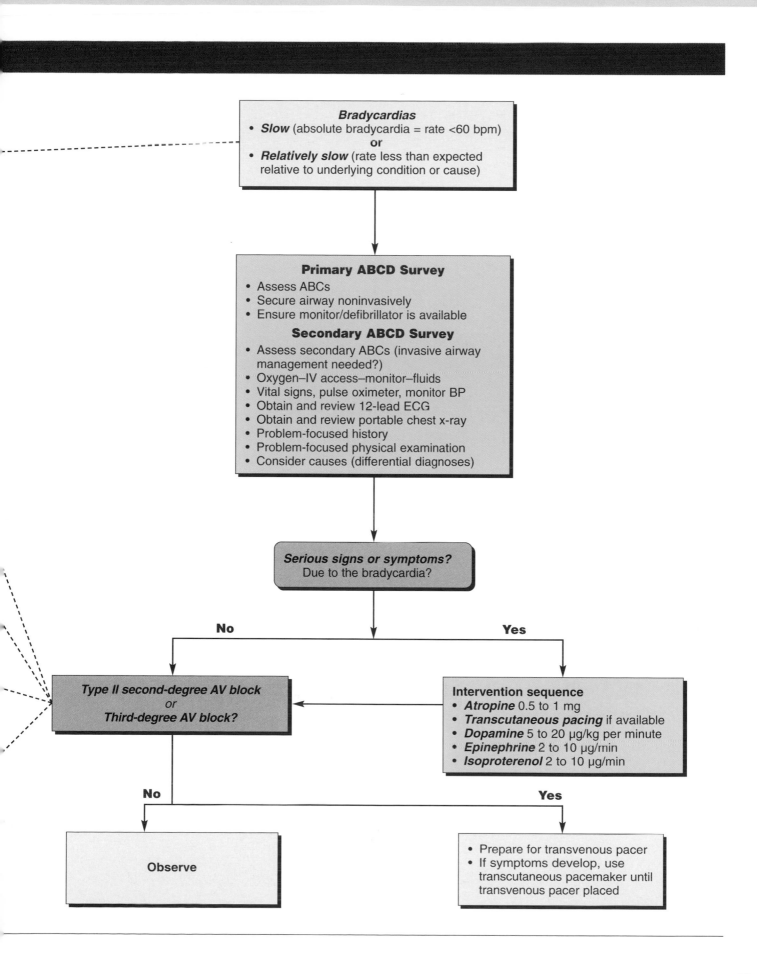

Bradycardias
- ***Slow*** (absolute bradycardia = rate <60 bpm)

or
- ***Relatively slow*** (rate less than expected relative to underlying condition or cause)

Primary ABCD Survey
- Assess ABCs
- Secure airway noninvasively
- Ensure monitor/defibrillator is available

Secondary ABCD Survey
- Assess secondary ABCs (invasive airway management needed?)
- Oxygen–IV access–monitor–fluids
- Vital signs, pulse oximeter, monitor BP
- Obtain and review 12-lead ECG
- Obtain and review portable chest x-ray
- Problem-focused history
- Problem-focused physical examination
- Consider causes (differential diagnoses)

Serious signs or symptoms?
Due to the bradycardia?

No / **Yes**

Type II second-degree AV block
or
Third-degree AV block?

Intervention sequence
- ***Atropine*** 0.5 to 1 mg
- ***Transcutaneous pacing*** if available
- ***Dopamine*** 5 to 20 µg/kg per minute
- ***Epinephrine*** 2 to 10 µg/min
- ***Isoproterenol*** 2 to 10 µg/min

No / **Yes**

Observe

- Prepare for transvenous pacer
- If symptoms develop, use transcutaneous pacemaker until transvenous pacer placed

16. Sinus Bradycardia	
Pathophysiology	■ Impulses originate at SA node at a slow rate ■ Not pathological; not an abnormal arrhythmia ■ More a physical sign
Defining Criteria per ECG **Key:** Regular P waves followed by regular QRS complexes at rate <60 beats/min **Note:** Often a physical sign rather than an abnormal rhythm	■ **Rate:** <60 beats/min ■ **Rhythm:** regular sinus ■ **PR:** regular; <0.20 sec ■ **P waves:** size and shape normal; every P wave is followed by a QRS complex; every QRS complex is preceded by a P wave ■ **QRS complex:** narrow; ≤0.10 sec in absence of intraventricular conduction defect
Clinical Manifestations	■ At rest, usually asymptomatic ■ With increased activity, persistent slow rate will lead to symptoms of easy fatigue, SOB, dizziness or lightheadedness, syncope, hypotension
Common Etiologies	■ Normal for well-conditioned people ■ A vasovagal event such as vomiting, valsalva, rectal stimuli, inadvertent pressure on carotid sinus ("shaver's syncope") ■ Acute MIs that affect circulation to SA node (right coronary artery); most often inferior AMIs ■ Adverse drug effects, eg, blocking agents (β or calcium channel), digoxin, quinidine
Recommended Therapy	■ Treatment rarely indicated ■ Treat only if patient has significant signs or symptoms due to the bradycardia ■ Oxygen is always appropriate **Intervention sequence for bradycardia** ■ *Atropine* 0.5 to 1 mg IV if vagal mechanism ■ *Transcutaneous pacing* if available **If signs and symptoms are severe, consider catecholamine infusions:** ■ *Dopamine* 5 to 20 μg/kg per min ■ *Epinephrine* 2 to 10 μg/min ■ *Isoproterenol* 2 to 10 μg/min

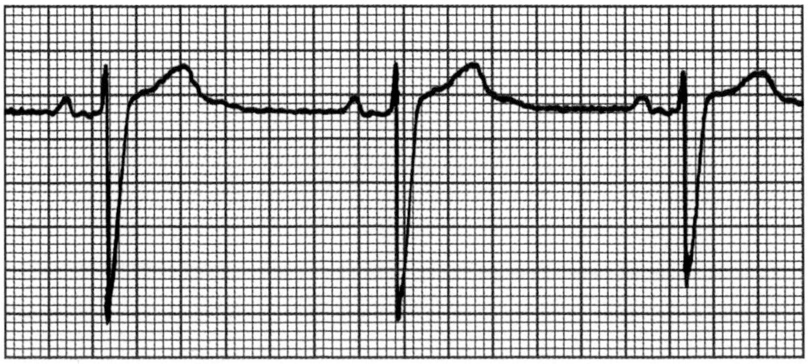

Sinus bradycardia: rate of 45 bpm; with borderline first-degree AV block (PR ≈ 0.20 sec)

17. First-Degree Heart Block	
Pathophysiology	■ Impulse conduction is slowed *(partial block)* at the AV node by a fixed amount ■ Closer to being a physical sign than an abnormal arrhythmia
Defining Criteria per ECG **Key:** PR interval >0.20 sec	■ **Rate:** First-degree heart block can be seen with both sinus bradycardia and sinus tachycardia ■ **Rhythm:** sinus, regular, both atria and ventricles ■ **PR:** prolonged, >0.20 sec, but does not vary *(fixed)* ■ **P waves:** size and shape normal; every P wave is followed by a QRS complex; every QRS complex is preceded by a P wave ■ **QRS complex:** narrow; ≤0.10 sec in absence of intraventricular conduction defect
Clinical Manifestations	■ Usually asymptomatic at rest ■ Rarely, if bradycardia worsens, person may become symptomatic from the slow rate
Common Etiologies	■ Large majority of first-degree heart blocks are due to drugs, usually the AV nodal blockers: β-blockers, calcium channel blockers, and digoxin ■ Any condition that stimulates the parasympathetic nervous system (eg, vasovagal reflex) ■ Acute MIs that affect circulation to AV node (right coronary artery); most often inferior AMIs
Recommended Therapy	■ Treat only when patient has significant signs or symptoms that are due to the bradycardia ■ Be alert to block deteriorating to second-degree, type I or type II block ■ Oxygen is always appropriate **Intervention sequence for symptomatic bradycardia** ■ *Atropine* 0.5 to 1 mg IV if vagal mechanism ■ *Transcutaneous pacing* if available **If signs and symptoms are severe, consider catecholamine infusions:** ■ *Dopamine* 5 to 20 μg/kg per min ■ *Epinephrine* 2 to 10 μg/min ■ *Isoproterenol* 2 to 10 μg/min

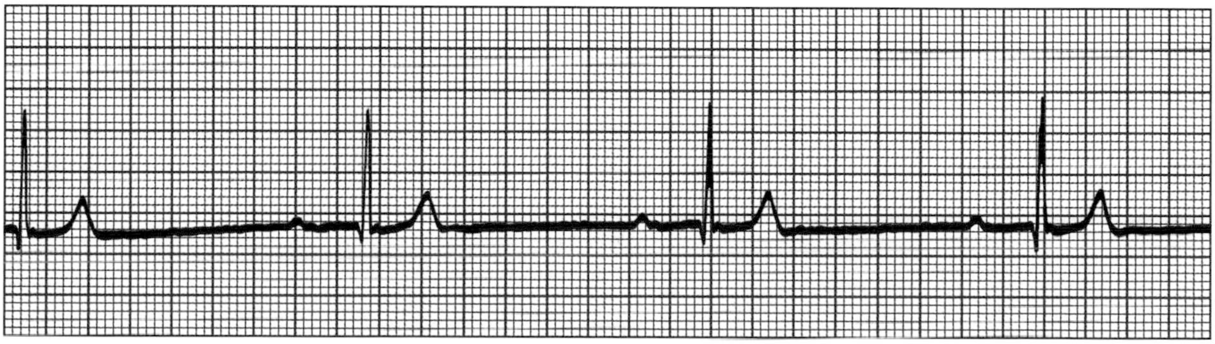

First-degree AV block at rate of 37 bpm; PR interval 0.28 sec

18. Second-Degree Heart Block Type I (Mobitz I–Wenckebach)

Pathophysiology	■ Site of pathology: AV node ■ AV node blood supply comes from branches of the right coronary artery ■ Impulse conduction is increasingly slowed at the AV node (causing increasing PR interval) ■ Until one sinus impulse is completely blocked and a QRS complex fails to follow
Defining Criteria per ECG **Key:** There is progressive lengthening of the PR interval until one P wave is not followed by a QRS complex (the dropped beat)	■ **Rate:** atrial rate just slightly faster than ventricular (because of dropped beats); usually normal range ■ **Rhythm:** regular for atrial beats; irregular for ventricular (because of dropped beats); can show regular P waves marching through irregular QRS ■ **PR:** progressive lengthening of the PR interval occurs from cycle to cycle; then one P wave is not followed by a QRS complex (the "dropped beat") ■ **P waves:** size and shape remain normal; occasional P wave not followed by a QRS complex (the "dropped beat") ■ **QRS complex:** ≤0.10 sec most often, but a QRS "drops out" periodically
Clinical Manifestations—Rate-Related	**Due to bradycardia:** ■ **Symptoms:** chest pain, shortness of breath, decreased level of consciousness ■ **Signs:** hypotension, shock, pulmonary congestion, CHF, angina
Common Etiologies	■ AV nodal blocking agents: β-blockers, calcium channel blockers, digoxin ■ Conditions that stimulate the parasympathetic system ■ An acute coronary syndrome that involves the *right* coronary artery
Recommended Therapy **Key:** Treat only when patient has significant signs or symptoms that are due to the bradycardia	**Intervention sequence for symptomatic bradycardia:** ■ *Atropine* 0.5 to 1 mg IV if vagal mechanism ■ *Transcutaneous pacing* if available **If signs and symptoms are severe, consider catecholamine infusions:** ■ *Dopamine* 5 to 20 μg/kg per min ■ *Epinephrine* 2 to 10 μg/min ■ *Isoproterenol* 2 to 10 μg/min

2° AV Block prolonged P-R interval (varied) c̄ dropped QRS

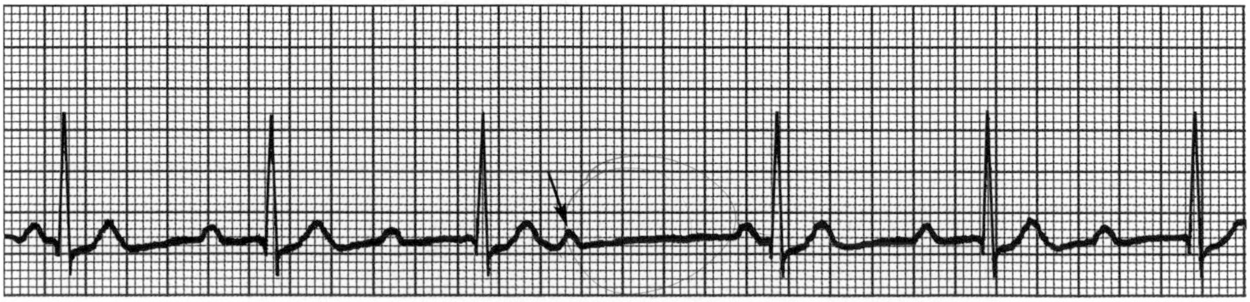

Second-degree heart block type I. Note progressive lengthening of PR interval until one P wave (arrow) is not followed by a QRS.

19. Second-Degree Heart Block Type II (Infranodal) (Mobitz II–Non-Wenckebach)	
Pathophysiology	■ The pathology, ie, the site of the block, is most often *below* the AV node (infranodal); at the bundle of His (infrequent) or at the bundle branches ■ Impulse conduction is normal through the node, thus no first-degree block and no prior PR prolongation
Defining Criteria per ECG	■ **Atrial Rate:** usually 60-100 beats/min ■ **Ventricular rate:** by definition (due to the blocked impulses) slower than atrial rate ■ **Rhythm:** atrial = regular; ventricular = irregular (because of blocked impulses) ■ **PR:** constant and set; no progressive prolongation as with type I—a distinguishing characteristic. ■ **P waves:** typical in size and shape; by definition some P waves will not be followed by a QRS complex ■ **QRS complex:** narrow (≤0.10 sec) implies high block relative to the AV node; wide (>0.12 sec) implies low block relative to the AV node
Clinical Manifestations—Rate-Related	**Due to bradycardia:** ■ **Symptoms:** chest pain, shortness of breath, decreased level of consciousness ■ **Signs:** hypotension, shock, pulmonary congestions, CHF, acute MI
Common Etiologies	■ An acute coronary syndrome that involves branches of the *left* coronary artery
Recommended Therapy **Pearl:** New onset type II second-degree heart block in clinical context of acute coronary syndrome is indication for transvenous pacemaker insertion	**Intervention sequence for bradycardia due to type II second-degree *or* third-degree heart block:** ■ Prepare for *transvenous* pacer ■ Atropine is seldom effective for infranodal block ■ Use *transcutaneous pacing* if available as a bridge to transvenous pacing (verify patient tolerance and mechanical capture. Use sedation and analgesia as needed.) **If signs/symptoms are severe and unresponsive to TCP, and transvenous pacing is delayed, consider catecholamine infusions:** ■ *Dopamine* 5 to 20 μg/kg per min ■ *Epinephrine* 2 to 10 μg/min ■ *Isoproterenol* 2 to 10 μg/min

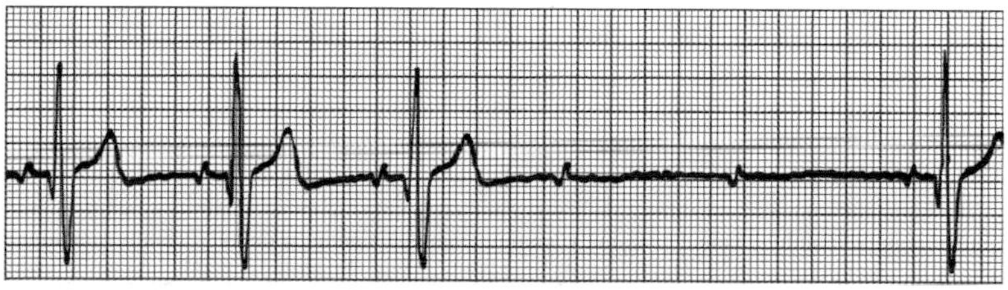

Type II (high block): regular PR-QRS intervals until 2 dropped beats occur; borderline normal QRS complexes indicate high nodal or nodal block

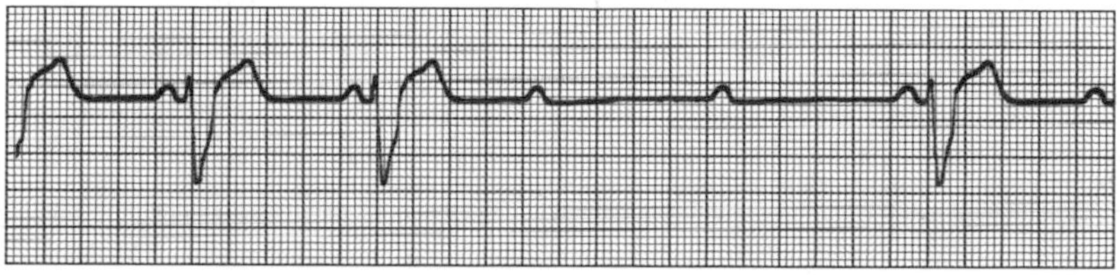

Type II (low block): regular PR-QRS intervals until dropped beats; wide QRS complexes indicate infranodal block

20. Third-Degree Heart Block and AV Dissociation

Pathophysiology **Pearl:** *AV dissociation* is the defining class; *third-degree* or *complete heart block* is one type of AV dissociation. By convention (outdated): if ventricular escape depolarization is faster than atrial rate = *"AV dissociation"*; if slower = "third-degree heart block"	Injury or damage to the cardiac conduction system so that no impulses *(complete block)* pass between atria and ventricles (neither antegrade nor retrograde) This complete block can occur at several different anatomic areas: ■ AV node ("high" or "supra" or "junctional" *nodal block*) ■ Bundle of His ■ Bundle branches ("low-nodal" or "infranodal" block)
Defining Criteria per ECG **Key:** The third-degree block (see pathophysiology) causes the atria and ventricles to depolarize independently, with no relationship between the two (AV dissociation)	■ **Atrial rate:** usually 60-100 beats/min; impulses completely independent ("dissociated") from ventricular rate ■ **Ventricular rate:** depends on rate of the ventricular escape beats that arise: — Ventricular escape beat rate slower than atrial rate = third-degree heart block (20-40 beats/min) — Ventricular escape beat rate faster than atrial rate = AV dissociation (40-55 beats/min) ■ **Rhythm:** both atrial rhythm and ventricular rhythm are regular but independent ("dissociated") ■ **PR:** by definition there is no relationship between P wave and R wave ■ **P waves:** typical in size and shape ■ **QRS complex:** narrow (≤0.10 sec) implies high block relative to the AV node; wide (>0.12 sec) implies low block relative to the AV node
Clinical Manifestations—Rate-Related	**Due to bradycardia:** ■ **Symptoms:** chest pain, shortness of breath, decreased level of consciousness ■ **Signs:** hypotension, shock, pulmonary congestions, CHF, acute MI
Common Etiologies	■ An acute coronary syndrome that involves branches of the *left* coronary artery ■ In particular, the LAD (left anterior descending) and branches to the interventricular septum (supply bundle branches)
Recommended Therapy **Pearl:** New onset third-degree heart block in clinical context of acute coronary syndrome is indication for transvenous pacemaker insertion **Pearl:** *Never treat third-degree heart block plus ventricular escape beats with lidocaine*	**Intervention sequence for bradycardia due to type II second-degree *or* third-degree heart block:** ■ Prepare for *transvenous* pacer ■ Use *transcutaneous pacing* if available as a bridge to transvenous pacing (verify patient tolerance and mechanical capture; use sedation and analgesia as needed) **If signs/symptoms are severe and unresponsive to TCP, and transvenous pacing is delayed, consider catecholamine infusions:** ■ *Dopamine* 5 to 20 µg/kg per min ■ *Epinephrine* 2 to 10 µg/min ■ *Isoproterenol* 2 to 10 µg/min

3° Heart Block Atrial + Ventricular Rhythm are regular but have no correlation c̄ one another

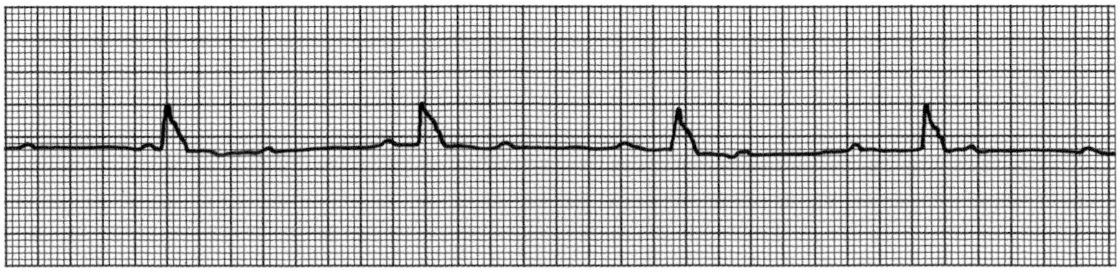

Third-degree heart block: regular P waves at 50 to 55 bpm; regular ventricular "escape beats" at 35 to 40 bpm; no relationship between P waves and escape beats

21. Transcutaneous Pacing	
A. Bradycardia: no pacing **B. Pacing stimulus below threshold: no capture** **C. Pacing stimulus above threshold: capture occurs**	
Rhythm Strip	**Comments**
A. Bradycardia (third-degree heart block): no pacing (**Note:** Rates and intervals slightly altered due to monitor compensation for pacing stimulus)	■ QRS rate = 41 beats/min ■ P waves = 187 beats/min ■ QRS = very wide, 0.24 sec; ventricular escape beats ■ QRS and T wave polarity = both positive ■ Patient: SOB at rest; severe SOB with walking; near syncope
B. Transcutaneous pacing initiated at low current (35 mA) and slow rate (50 beats/min). Below the threshold current needed to stimulate the myocardium	■ With TCP, monitor electrodes are attached in modified lead II position ■ As current (in milliamperes) is gradually increased, the monitor leads detect the pacing stimuli as a squared off, negative marker ■ TC pacemakers incorporate standard ECG monitoring circuitry but incorporate filters to dampen the pacing stimuli ■ A monitor without these filters records "border-to-border" tracings (off the edge of the screen or paper at the top and bottom borders) that cannot be interpreted
C. Pacing current turned up above threshold (60 mA at 71 beats/min) and "captures" the myocardium	■ TCP stimulus does not work through the normal cardiac conduction system but by a direct electrical stimulus of the myocardium ■ Therefore, a "capture," where TCP stimulus results in a myocardial contraction, will resemble a PVC ■ Electrical capture is characterized by a wide QRS complex, with the initial deflection and the terminal deflection *always* in opposite directions ■ A "mechanically captured beat" will produce effective myocardial contraction with production of some blood flow (usually assessed by a palpable carotid pulse)

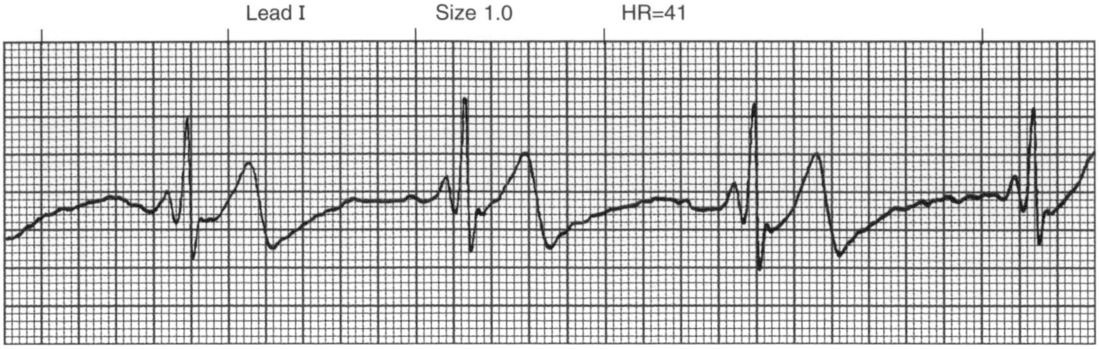

Bradycardia: prepacing attempt

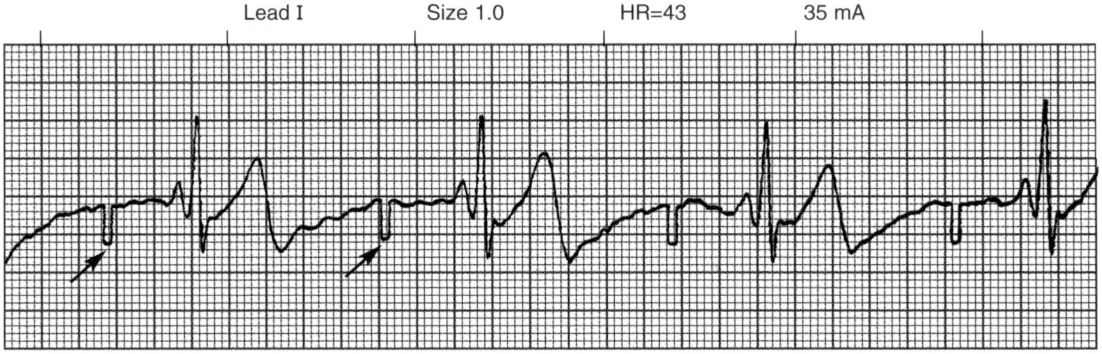

Pacing attempted: note pacing stimulus indicator (arrow) which is below threshold; no capture

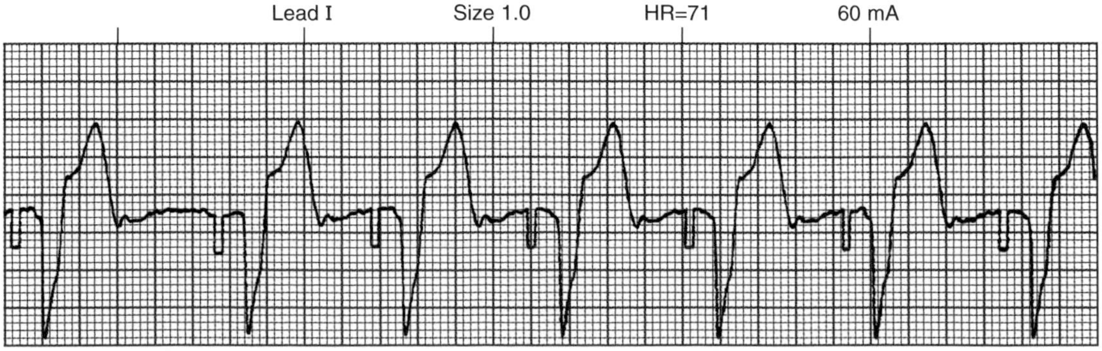

Pacing above threshold (60 mA): with capture (QRS complex broad and ventricular; T wave opposite QRS)

ACLS Drugs, Cardioversion, Defibrillation and Pacing

Drug/Therapy	Indications/Precautions	Adult Dosage
ACE Inhibitors (Angiotensin-Converting Enzyme Inhibitors)	**Indications** ACE inhibitors reduce mortality and improve LV dysfunction in post-AMI patients. They help prevent adverse LV remodeling, delay progression of heart failure, and decrease sudden death and recurrent MI. They are of greatest benefit in patients with the following conditions: • Suspected MI and ST-segment elevation in 2 or more anterior precordial leads. • Hypertension. • Clinical heart failure without hypotension in patients not responding to digitalis or diuretics. • Clinical signs of AMI with LV dysfunction. • LV ejection fraction <40%.	**Approach**: ACE inhibitor therapy should start with low-dose oral administration (with possible IV doses for some preparations) and increase steadily to achieve a full dose within 24 to 48 hours.
Enalapril		**Enalapril (IV = Enalaprilat)** • PO: Start with a single dose of 2.5 mg. Titrate to 20 mg PO BID. • IV: 1.25 mg IV initial dose over 5 minutes, then 1.25 to 5 mg IV every 6 hours.
Captopril		**Captopril** • Start with a single dose of 6.25 mg PO. • Advance to 25 mg TID and then to 50 mg TID as tolerated.
Lisinopril	**Precautions/Contraindications for all ACE inhibitors** • ***Contraindicated*** in pregnancy (may cause fetal injury or death). • Contraindicated in angioedema. • Hypersensitivity to ACE inhibitors. • Reduce dose in renal failure (creatinine >3 mg/dL). Avoid in bilateral renal artery stenosis.	**Lisinopril, AMI Dose** • 5 mg within 24 hours of onset of symptoms, then • 5 mg given after 24 hours, then • 10 mg given after 48 hours, then • 10 mg once daily for 6 weeks
Ramipril	• Avoid hypotension, especially following initial dose and in relative volume depletion. • Generally not started in ED but within first 24 hours after fibrinolytic therapy has been completed and blood pressure has stabilized.	**Ramipril** Start with a single dose of 2.5 mg PO. Titrate to 5 mg PO BID as tolerated.

Drug/Therapy	Indications/Precautions	Adult Dosage
Adenosine	**Indications** • First drug for most forms of narrow-complex PSVT. Effective in terminating those due to reentry involving AV node or sinus node. • Does *not* convert atrial fibrillation, atrial flutter, or VT. **Precautions** • Transient side effects include flushing, chest pain or tightness, brief periods of asystole or bradycardia, ventricular ectopy. • Less effective in patients taking theophyllines; avoid in patients receiving dipyridamole. • If administered for wide-complex tachycardia/VT, may cause deterioration (including hypotension). • Transient periods of sinus bradycardia and ventricular ectopy are common after termination of SVT. • Contraindication: Poison/drug-induced tachycardia.	**IV Rapid Push** • Place patient in mild reverse Trendelenburg position before administration of drug. • Initial bolus of 6 mg given *rapidly* over 1 to 3 seconds followed by normal saline bolus of 20 mL; then elevate the extremity. • Repeat dose of 12 mg in 1 to 2 minutes if needed. • A third dose of 12 mg may be given in 1 to 2 minutes if needed. **Injection Technique** • Record rhythm strip during administration. • Draw up adenosine dose and flush in 2 separate syringes. • Attach both syringes to the IV injection port closest to patient. • Clamp IV tubing above injection port. • Push IV adenosine *as quickly as possible* (1 to 3 seconds). • While maintaining pressure on adenosine plunger, push normal saline flush *as rapidly as possible* after adenosine. • Unclamp IV tubing.
Amiodarone	**Indications** Used in a wide variety of atrial and ventricular tachyarrhythmias and for rate control of rapid atrial arrhythmias in patients with impaired LV function when digoxin has proven ineffective. **Recommended for** • Treatment of shock-refractory VF/pulseless VT. • Treatment of polymorphic VT and wide-complex tachycardia of uncertain origin. • Control of hemodynamically stable VT when cardioversion is unsuccessful. Particularly useful in the presence of LV dysfunction. • Use as adjunct to electrical cardioversion of SVT, PSVT. • Acceptable for termination of ectopic or multifocal atrial tachycardia with preserved LV function. • May be used for rate control in treatment of atrial fibrillation or flutter when other therapies ineffective. **Precautions** • May produce vasodilation and hypotension. • May also have negative inotropic effects. • May prolong QT interval. Be aware of compatibility and interaction with other drugs administered.	**Cardiac Arrest** 300 mg IV push (2000 Guidelines recommend dilution to 20 to 30 mL D_5W). Consider additional 150 mg IV push in 3 to 5 minutes. (Maximum cumulative dose: 2.2 g IV/24 hours.) **Wide-Complex Tachycardia (Stable)** *Maximum cumulative dose:* 2.2 g IV/24 hours. May be administered as follows: • *Rapid infusion:* 150 mg IV over first 10 minutes (15 mg/min). May repeat rapid infusion (150 mg IV) every 10 minutes as needed. • *Slow infusion:* 360 mg IV over 6 hours (1 mg/min). • *Maintenance infusion:* 540 mg IV over 18 hours (0.5 mg/min). **Precautions** • When multiple doses are administered, cumulative doses >2.2 g/24 hours are associated with significant hypotension in clinical trials. • Do not routinely administer with other drugs that prolong QT interval (eg, procainamide). • Terminal elimination is extremely long (half-life lasts up to 40 days).
Amrinone (*Now* Inamrinone)	**Indications** Severe congestive heart failure refractory to diuretics, vasodilators, and conventional inotropic agents. **Precautions** • Do not mix with dextrose solutions or other drugs. • May cause tachyarrhythmias, hypotension, or thrombocytopenia. • Can increase myocardial ischemia.	**IV Loading Dose and Infusion** • 0.75 mg/kg, given over 10 to 15 minutes. • Follow with infusion of 5 to 15 µg/kg per minute titrated to clinical effect. • Optimal use requires hemodynamic monitoring.

Drug/Therapy	Indications/Precautions	Adult Dosage
Aspirin • 160 mg, 325 mg tablets • Chewable tablets more effective in some trials	**Indications** • Administer to all patients with ACS, particularly reperfusion candidates, unless hypersensitive to aspirin. • Blocks formation of thromboxane A_2, which causes platelets to aggregate, arteries to constrict. This reduces overall AMI mortality, reinfarction, nonfatal stroke. • Any person with symptoms ("pressure," "heavy weight," "squeezing," "crushing") suggestive of ischemic pain **Precautions** • Relatively contraindicated in patients with active ulcer disease or asthma. • Contraindicated in patients with known hypersensitivity to aspirin.	• 160 mg to 325 mg tablet taken as soon as possible (chewing is preferable to swallowing) and then daily. • May use rectal suppository for patients who cannot take PO. • Give within minutes of arrival. • Higher doses (1000 mg) interfere with prostacyclin production and may limit positive benefits.
Atropine Sulfate Can be given via tracheal tube push fast	**Indications** • First drug for symptomatic sinus bradycardia (Class I). • May be beneficial in presence of AV block at the nodal level (Class IIa) or ventricular asystole. **Will not be effective when infranodal (Mobitz type II) block is suspected (Class IIb).** NOT CONTRAINDICATED give ATROPINE • Second drug (after epinephrine or vasopressin) for asystole or bradycardic pulseless electrical activity (Class IIb). **Precautions** • Use with caution in presence of myocardial ischemia and hypoxia. Increases myocardial oxygen demand. • Avoid in hypothermic bradycardia. • Will not be effective for infranodal (type II) AV block and new third-degree block with wide QRS complexes. (In these patients may cause paradoxical slowing. Be prepared to pace or give catecholamines.)	**Asystole or Pulseless Electrical Activity** • 1 mg IV push. • Repeat every 3 to 5 minutes (if asystole persists) to a maximum dose of 0.03 to 0.04 mg/kg. ↳ .04 **Bradycardia** • 0.5 to 1 mg IV every 3 to 5 minutes as needed, not to exceed total dose of 0.04 mg/kg. • Use shorter dosing interval (3 minutes) and higher doses (0.04 mg/kg) in severe clinical conditions. **Tracheal Administration** DOSE DOUBLED 2 to 3 mg diluted in 10 mL normal saline.
β-Blockers Metoprolol Atenolol Propranolol Esmolol Labetalol	**Indications** • Administer to all patients with suspected myocardial infarction and unstable angina in the absence of complications. These are effective antianginal agents and can reduce incidence of VF. • Useful as an adjunctive agent with fibrinolytic therapy. May reduce nonfatal reinfarction and recurrent ischemia. • To convert to normal sinus rhythm or to slow ventricular response (or both) in supraventricular tachyarrhythmias (PSVT, atrial fibrillation, or atrial flutter). β-Blockers are second-line agents after adenosine, diltiazem, or digitalis derivative. • To reduce myocardial ischemia and damage in AMI patients with elevated heart rate, blood pressure, or both. • For emergency antihypertensive therapy for hemorrhagic and acute ischemic stroke. **Precautions** Concurrent IV administration with IV calcium channel blocking agents like verapamil or diltiazem can cause severe hypotension. • Avoid in bronchospastic diseases, cardiac failure, or severe abnormalities in cardiac conduction. • Monitor cardiac and pulmonary status during administration. • May cause myocardial depression. • Contraindicated in presence of HR <60 bpm, systolic BP <100 mm Hg, severe LV failure, hypoperfusion, or second- or third-degree AV block.	**Metoprolol** • Initial IV dose: 5 mg slow IV at 5-minute intervals to a total of 15 mg. • Oral regimen to follow IV dose: 50 mg BID for 24 hours, then increase to 100 mg BID. **Atenolol** • 5 mg slow IV (over 5 minutes). • Wait 10 minutes, then give second dose of 5 mg slow IV (over 5 minutes). • In 10 minutes, if tolerated well, may start 50 mg PO; then give 50 mg PO twice a day. **Propranolol** • Total dose: 0.1 mg/kg by slow IV push, divided into 3 equal doses at 2- to 3-minute intervals. Do not exceed 1 mg/min. • Repeat after 2 minutes if necessary. **Esmolol** • 0.5 mg/kg over 1 minute, followed by continuous infusion at 0.05 mg/kg per minute (maximum: 0.3 mg/kg per minute). • Titrate to effect. Esmolol has a short half-life (2 to 9 minutes). **Labetalol** • 10 mg labetalol IV push over 1 to 2 minutes. • May repeat or double labetalol every 10 minutes to a maximum dose of 150 mg, *or* give initial dose as a bolus, then start labetalol infusion at 2 to 8 mg/min.

Drug/Therapy	Indications/Precautions	Adult Dosage
Calcium Chloride 100 mg/mL in 10 mL vial (total = 1 g; a 10% solution)	**Indications** • Known or suspected hyperkalemia (eg, renal failure). • Hypocalcemia (eg, after multiple blood transfusions). • As an antidote for toxic effects (hypotension and arrhythmias) from calcium channel blocker overdose or β-adrenergic blocker overdose. • May be used prophylactically before IV calcium channel blockers to prevent hypotension. **Precautions** • Do not use routinely in cardiac arrest. • Do not mix with sodium bicarbonate.	**IV Slow Push** • 8 to16 mg/kg (usually 5 to 10 mL) IV for hyperkalemia and calcium channel blocker overdose. May be repeated as needed. • 2 to 4 mg/kg (usually 2 mL) IV for prophylaxis before IV calcium channel blockers.
Cardioversion (Synchronized) Administered via remote defibrillation electrodes or handheld paddles from a defibrillator/monitor Place defibrillator/monitor in synchronized (sync) mode Sync mode delivers energy just after the R wave	**Indications** • All tachycardias (rate >150 bpm) with serious signs and symptoms related to the tachycardia. • May give brief trial of medications based on specific arrhythmias. **Precautions** • In critical conditions go to immediate unsynchronized shocks. • Urgent cardioversion is generally not needed if heart rate is ≤150 bpm. • Reactivation of sync mode is required after each attempted cardioversion (defibrillators/cardioverters default to unsynchronized mode). • Prepare to defibrillate immediately if cardioversion causes VF. • Synchronized cardioversion cannot be performed unless the patient is connected to monitor leads; lead select switch must be on lead I, II, or III and not on "paddles." • Contraindication: Poison/drug-induced tachycardia.	**Technique** • See electrical cardioversion algorithm, page 160. • Premedicate whenever possible. • Engage sync mode before each attempt. • Look for sync markers on the R wave. • "Clear" the patient before each shock. • Deliver monophasic shocks in the following sequence: 100 J, 200 J, 300 J, 360 J.* Use this sequence for each of the following: — VT† — PSVT‡ — Atrial flutter‡ — Atrial fibrillation †Treat polymorphic VT (irregular form and rate) with same currents used for VF: 200 J, 200 to 300 J, 360 J. ‡PSVT and atrial flutter often respond to lower energy levels; start with 50 J. • Press "charge" button, "clear" the patient, and press both "shock" buttons simultaneously. *Biphasic waveforms using lower energy are acceptable if documented to be clinically equivalent or superior to reports of monophasic shock success.
Defibrillation Attempt Use conventional monitor/defibrillator Use automated or shock advisory defibrillator Administer shocks via remote adhesive electrodes or handheld paddles	**Indications** First intervention for VF or pulseless VT (Class I). **Precautions** • Always "clear" the patient before discharging a defibrillation shock. • Do not delay defibrillation for VF/VT. • Asystole should not be routinely shocked. • Treat VF/VT in hypothermic cardiac arrest with up to 3 shocks. Repeat shocks for VF/VT only after core temperature rises above 30°C. • If patient in VF/VT has an automatic implantable cardioverter defibrillator (AICD), perform external defibrillation per BLS guidelines. If AICD is delivering shocks, wait 30 to 60 seconds for completion of cycle. • If patient has implanted pacemaker, place paddles and pads several inches from the pacing generator.	**Adult Monophasic Defibrillation Energy Levels*** • 200 J, first shock. • 200 to 300 J, second shock. • 360 J, third shock. • If these shocks fail to convert VF/VT, continue at 360 J for future shocks. • If VF recurs, shock again at the last successful energy level. *Biphasic devices shock at lower energy levels (approximately 150 J). In some clinical settings, initial and repeated shocks at these lower energy levels are acceptable.

Drug/Therapy	Indications/Precautions	Adult Dosage
Digibind (Digoxin-Specific Antibody Therapy) 40 mg vial (each vial binds about 0.6 mg digoxin)	**Indications** Digoxin toxicity with the following: • Life-threatening arrhythmias. • Shock or congestive heart failure. • Hyperkalemia (potassium level >5 mEq/L). • Steady-state serum levels >10 to 15 ng/mL for symptomatic patients. **Precautions** • Serum digoxin levels rise after digibind therapy and should not be used to guide continuing therapy.	**Chronic Intoxication** 3 to 5 vials may be effective. **Acute Overdose** • IV dose varies according to amount of digoxin ingested. • Average dose is 10 vials (400 mg); may require up to 20 vials (800 mg). • See package insert for details.
Digoxin 0.25 mg/mL or 0.1 mg/mL supplied in 1 or 2 mL ampule (totals = 0.1 to 0.5 mg)	**Indications** • To slow ventricular response in atrial fibrillation or atrial flutter. • Alternative drug for PSVT. **Precautions** • Toxic effects are common and are frequently associated with serious arrhythmias. • Avoid electrical cardioversion if patient is receiving digoxin unless condition is life threatening; use lower current settings (10 to 20 J).	**IV Infusion** • Loading doses of 10 to 15 μg/kg lean body weight provide therapeutic effect with minimum risk of toxic effects. • Maintenance dose is affected by body size and renal function.
Diltiazem	**Indications** • To control ventricular rate in atrial fibrillation and atrial flutter. May terminate re-entrant arrhythmias that require AV nodal conduction for their continuation. • Use after adenosine to treat refractory PSVT in patients with narrow QRS complex and adequate blood pressure. **Precautions** • Do not use calcium channel blockers for wide-QRS tachycardias of uncertain origin or for poison/drug-induced tachycardia. • Avoid calcium channel blockers in patients with Wolff-Parkinson-White syndrome plus rapid atrial fibrillation or flutter, in patients with sick sinus syndrome, or in patients with AV block without a pacemaker. • Expect blood pressure drop resulting from peripheral vasodilation (greater drop with verapamil than with diltiazem). • Avoid in patients receiving oral β-blockers. • Concurrent IV administration with IV β-blockers can cause severe hypotension.	**Acute Rate Control** • 15 to 20 mg (0.25 mg/kg) IV over 2 minutes. • May repeat in 15 minutes at 20 to 25 mg (0.35 mg/kg) over 2 minutes. **Maintenance Infusion** 5 to 15 mg/h, titrated to heart rate.
Disopyramide ***(IV dose not approved for use In United States)***	**Indications** Useful for treatment of a wide variety of arrhythmias. It prolongs the effective refractory period, similar to procainamide. **Precautions/Contraindications** Must be infused relatively slowly. It has potent anticholinergic, negative inotropic, and hypotensive effects that limit its use.	**IV Dose** 2 mg/kg over 10 minutes, followed by continuous infusion of 0.4 mg/kg per hour.

Drug/Therapy	Indications/Precautions	Adult Dosage
Dobutamine *IV infusion* Dilute 250 mg (20 mL) in 250 mL normal saline or D_5W	**Indications** Consider for pump problems (congestive heart failure, pulmonary congestion) with systolic blood pressure of 70 to 100 mm Hg and *no* signs of shock. **Precautions** • Avoid with systolic blood pressure <100 mm Hg *and* signs of shock. • May cause tachyarrhythmias, fluctuations in blood pressure, headache, and nausea. • Contraindication: Suspected or known poison/drug-induced shock. • Do not mix with sodium bicarbonate.	**IV Infusion** • Usual infusion rate is 2 to 20 μg/kg per minute. • Titrate so heart rate does not increase by >10% of baseline. • Hemodynamic monitoring is recommended for optimal use.
Dofetilide ***(Not approved for use in United States)***	**Indications** Treatment of atrial fibrillation. **Precautions/Contraindications** Adverse effects include QT prolongation, which can be associated with torsades de pointes. This complication is most likely to occur in patients with a history of congestive heart failure. Its use is limited by its need to be infused relatively slowly, which may be impractical under emergent conditions.	**IV Infusion Dose** Single infusion of 8 μg/kg over 30 minutes.
Dopamine *IV infusion* Mix 400 to 800 mg in 250 mL normal saline, lactated Ringer's solution, or D_5W	**Indications** • Second drug for symptomatic bradycardia (after atropine). • Use for hypotension (systolic blood pressure ≤70 to 100 mm Hg) with signs and symptoms of shock. **Precautions** • May use in patients with hypovolemia but only after volume replacement. • Use with caution in cardiogenic shock with accompanying congestive heart failure. • May cause tachyarrhythmias, excessive vasoconstriction. ↳ leads to ↑O_2 demand • Taper slowly. • Do not mix with sodium bicarbonate. → INACTIVATED DOPAMINE OR (ALKALINE SOLUTIONS)	**Continuous Infusions (titrate to patient response)** **Low Dose** 1 to 5 μg/kg per minute. **Moderate Dose** 5 to 10 μg/kg per minute ("cardiac doses"). **High Dose** 10 to 20 μg/kg per minute ("vasopressor doses"). DOSE RANGE 5 – 20 mg/kg/min
Epinephrine **Note:** Available in 1:10 000 and 1:1000 concentrations. Increases SVR, BP (+) CHRONOTROPE main benefit is peripheral vasoconstriction (so everything is central it only gets blood flow to main compartment)	**Indications** • **Cardiac arrest:** VF, pulseless VT, asystole, pulseless electrical activity. • **Symptomatic bradycardia:** After atropine, dopamine, and transcutaneous pacing. • **Severe hypotension.** • **Anaphylaxis, severe allergic reactions:** Combine with large fluid volumes, corticosteroids, antihistamines. **Precautions** • Raising blood pressure and increasing heart rate may cause myocardial ischemia, angina, and increased myocardial oxygen demand. • High doses do not improve survival or neurologic outcome and may contribute to postresuscitation myocardial dysfunction. • Higher doses *may* be required to treat poison/drug-induced shock.	* **Cardiac Arrest** • **IV Dose:** 1 mg (10 mL of 1:10 000 solution) administered every 3 to 5 minutes during resuscitation. Follow each dose with 20 mL IV flush. • **Higher Dose:** Higher doses (up to 0.2 mg/kg) may be used if 1-mg dose fails. • **Continuous Infusion:** Add 30 mg epinephrine (30 mL of 1:1000 solution) to 250 mL normal saline or 5% dextrose in water; run at 100 mL/h and titrate to response. • **Tracheal Route** 2 to 2.5 mg diluted in 10 mL normal saline. * **Profound Bradycardia or Hypotension** 2 to 10 μg/min infusion (add 1 mg of 1:1000 to 500 mL normal saline; infuse at 1 to 5 mL/min).

Drug/Therapy	Indications/Precautions	Adult Dosage
Fibrinolytic Agents **Alteplase, recombinant *(Activase)*; tissue plasminogen activator (tPA)** 50 and 100 mg vials reconstituted with sterile water to 1 mg/mL For all 5 agents, use 2 peripheral IV lines, *one line exclusively for fibrinolytic administration.*	**Indications** *For AMI in Adults* • ST elevation (≥1 mm in ≥2 contiguous leads) or new or presumably new LBBB; strongly suspicious for injury (BBB obscuring ST analysis). • In context of signs and symptoms of AMI. • Time from onset of symptoms <12 hours. *For Acute Ischemic Stroke* (Alteplase is the only fibrinolytic agent approved for acute ischemic stroke.) • Sudden onset of focal neurologic deficits or alterations in consciousness (eg, language abnormality, motor arm, facial droop). • Absence of intracerebral or subarachnoid hemorrhage or mass effect on CT scan. • Absence of variable or rapidly improving neurologic deficits. • Alteplase can be started in <3 hours from symptom onset. • See Case 10. **Precautions** Specific exclusion criteria: • Active internal bleeding (except menses) within 21 days. • History of cerebrovascular, intracranial, or intraspinal event within 3 months (stroke, arteriovenous malformation, neoplasm, aneurysm, recent trauma, recent surgery). • Major surgery or serious trauma within 14 days. • Aortic dissection. • Severe, uncontrolled hypertension. • Known bleeding disorders. • Prolonged CPR with evidence of thoracic trauma. • Lumbar puncture within 7 days. • Recent arterial puncture at non-compressible site. • During the first 24 hours of fibrinolytic therapy for ischemic stroke, do not administer aspirin or heparin. **Adjuvant Therapy for AMI** • 160 to 325 mg aspirin chewed as soon as possible. • Begin heparin immediately and continue for 48 hours if alteplase or Retavase is used.	**Alteplase, recombinant (tPA)** Recommended total dose is based on patient's weight. For AMI the total dose should not exceed 100 mg; for acute ischemic stroke the total dose should not exceed 90 mg. Note that there are 2 approved dose regimens for AMI patients, and a *different* regimen for acute ischemic stroke. *For AMI:* • Accelerated infusion (1.5 hours) — Give 15 mg IV bolus. — Then 0.75 mg/kg over next 30 minutes (not to exceed 50 mg). — Then 0.50 mg/kg over next 60 minutes (not to exceed 35 mg). • 3-hour infusion — Give 60 mg in first hour (initial 6 to 10 mg is given as a bolus). — Then 20 mg/h for 2 additional hours. *For Acute Ischemic Stroke:* • Give 0.9 mg/kg (maximum 90 mg) infused over 60 minutes. • Give 10% of the total dose as an initial IV bolus over 1 minute. • Give the remaining 90% over the next 60 minutes.
Anistreplase *(Eminase)*; anisoylated plasminogen streptokinase activator complex (APSAC) Reconstitute 30 U in 50 mL sterile water or D_5W		**Anistreplase (APSAC)** 30 IU IV over 2 to 5 minutes.
Reteplase, recombinant *(Retavase)* 10-U vials reconstituted with sterile water to 1 U/mL		**Reteplase, recombinant** • Give first 10-U IV bolus over 2 minutes. • 30 minutes later give second 10-U IV bolus over 2 minutes. (Give NS flush before and after each bolus.)
Streptokinase *(Streptase)* Reconstitute to 1 mg/mL		**Streptokinase** 1.5 million IU in a 1-hour infusion.
Tenecteplase *(TNKase)*		**Tenecteplase** • Bolus: 30 to 50 mg
Flecainide ***(IV form not approved for use in United States)***	**Indications** • Treatment of ventricular arrhythmias. • Treatment of supraventricular arrhythmias in patients without coronary artery disease. • Effective for termination of atrial flutter and fibrillation, ectopic atrial tachycardia, AV nodal reentrant tachycardia, and supraventricular tachycardias associated with an accessory pathway. **Precautions/Contraindications** Should be avoided in patients with impaired LV function because it has significant negative inotropic effects. ***Must be infused slowly.*** Adverse effects include bradycardia, hypotension, and neurologic symptoms such as oral paresthesias and visual blurring.	**IV Dose** Administered at 2 mg/kg body weight at 10 mg/min. ***Must be infused slowly.***

Drug/Therapy	Indications/Precautions	Adult Dosage
Flumazenil	**Indications** Reverse respiratory depression and sedative effects from pure benzodiazepine overdose. **Precautions** • Effects may not outlast effect of benzodiazepines. • Monitor for recurrent respiratory depression. • Do not use in suspected tricyclic overdose. • Do not use in seizure-prone patients. • Do not use in unknown drug overdose or mixed drug overdose with drugs known to cause seizures (tricyclic antidepressants, cocaine, amphetamines, etc)	**First Dose** 0.2 mg IV over 15 seconds. **Second Dose** 0.3 mg IV over 30 seconds. If no adequate response, give third dose. **Third Dose** 0.5 mg IV given over 30 seconds. If no adequate response, repeat once every minute until adequate response or a total of 3 mg is given.
Furosemide	**Indications** • For adjuvant therapy of acute pulmonary edema in patients with systolic blood pressure >90 to 100 mm Hg (without signs and symptoms of shock). • Hypertensive emergencies. • Increased intracranial pressure. **Precautions** • Dehydration, hypovolemia, hypotension, hypokalemia, or other electrolyte imbalance may occur.	**IV Infusion** • 0.5 to 1 mg/kg given over 1 to 2 minutes. • If no response, double dose to 2 mg/kg, slowly over 1 to 2 minutes.
Glucagon Powdered in 1 and 10 mg vials Reconstitute with provided solution	**Indications** Adjuvant treatment of toxic effects of calcium channel blocker or β-blocker. **Precautions** • Do not mix with saline. • May cause vomiting, hyperglycemia.	**IV Infusion** 1 to 5 mg over 2 to 5 minutes.
Glycoprotein IIb/IIIa Inhibitors	**Indications** These drugs inhibit the integrin glycoprotein IIb/IIIa receptor in the membrane of platelets, inhibiting platelet aggregation. Indicated for acute coronary syndromes *without* ST-segment elevation. **Precautions/Contraindications** Active internal bleeding or bleeding disorder in past 30 days, history of intracranial hemorrhage, or other bleeding, surgical procedure or trauma within 1 month, platelet count <150 000/mm³, hypersensitivity and concomitant use of another GP IIb/IIIa inhibitor.	**Note: Check package insert for current indications, doses, and duration of therapy.** Optimal duration of therapy has not been established.
Abciximab (ReoPro®)	**Abciximab Indications** FDA-approved for patients with non–Q-wave MI or unstable angina with planned PCI within 24 hours. **Precautions/Contraindications** Must use with heparin. Binds irreversibly with platelets. Platelet function recovery requires 48 hours (regeneration). Readministration may cause hypersensitivity reaction.	**Abciximab Dose** • *Acute coronary syndromes with planned PCI within 24 hours:* 0.25 mg/kg IV bolus (10 to 60 minutes before procedure), then 0.125 μg/kg per minute IV infusion. • *PCI only:* 0.25 mg/kg IV bolus, then 10 μg/min IV infusion.
Eptifibitide (Integrilin®)	**Eptifibitide Indications** Non–Q-wave MI, unstable angina managed medically, and unstable angina/non–Q-wave MI patients undergoing PCI. **Actions/Precautions** Platelet function recovers within 4 to 8 hours after discontinuation.	**Eptifibitide Dose** • *Acute coronary syndromes:* 180 μg/kg IV bolus, then 2 μg/kg per minute IV infusion. • *PCI:* 135 μg/kg IV bolus, then begin 0.5 μg/kg per minute IV infusion, then repeat bolus in 10 minutes.
Tirofiban (Aggrastat®)	**Tirofiban Indications** Non–Q-wave MI, unstable angina managed medically, and unstable angina/non–Q-wave MI patients undergoing PCI. **Actions/Precautions** Platelet function recovers within 4 to 8 hours after discontinuation.	**Tirofiban Dose** *Acute coronary syndromes or PCI:* 0.4 μg/kg per minute IV for 30 minutes, then 0.1 μg/kg per minute IV infusion.

Drug/Therapy	Indications/Precautions	Adult Dosage
Heparin **Unfractionated (UFH)** Concentrations range from 1000 to 40 000 IU/mL	**Indications** • Adjuvant therapy in AMI. • Begin heparin with fibrin-specific lytics (eg, alteplase). **Precautions** • Same contraindications as for fibrinolytic therapy: active bleeding; recent intracranial, intraspinal, or eye surgery; severe hypertension; bleeding disorders; gastrointestinal bleeding. • Doses and laboratory targets appropriate when used with fibrinolytic therapy. • Heparin reversal: ***Protamine*** 25 mg IV infusion over 10 minutes or longer. (Calculate dose as 1 mg protamine per 100 IU of heparin remaining in patient; heparin plasma half-life is 60 minutes.) • Do not use if platelet count is or falls below <100 000 or with history of heparin-induced thrombocytopenia. For these patients consider direct antithrombins: — ***Desirudin:*** 0.1 mg/kg IV bolus, followed by infusion of 0.1 mg/kg per hour for 72 hours. — ***Leprudin:*** 0.4 mg/kg IV bolus, followed by infusion of 0.15 mg/kg per hour for 72 hours.	**IV Infusion** • Initial bolus 60 IU/kg (maximum bolus: 4000 IU). • Continue12 IU/kg per hour (maximum: 1000 IU/hour for patients >70 kg) (round to the nearest 50 IU). • Adjust to maintain activated partial thromboplastin time (aPTT) 1.5 to 2 times the control values for 48 hours or until angiography. • Target range for aPTT after first 24 hours is between 50 and 70 seconds (may vary with laboratory). • Check aPTT at 6, 12, 18, and 24 hours. • Follow institutional heparin protocol.
Heparin **Low Molecular Weight (LMWH)**	**Indications** For use in acute coronary syndromes, specifically patients with non–Q-wave MI/unstable angina. These drugs inhibit thrombin generation by factor Xa inhibition and also inhibit thrombin indirectly by formation of a complex with antithrombin III. These drugs are **not** neutralized by heparin-binding proteins. **Precautions**	
Dalteparin (Fragmin®) and **Enoxaparin** (Lovenox®)	• Hemorrhage may complicate any therapy with LMWH. Contraindicated in presence of hypersensitivity to heparin or pork products or history of sensitivity to drug. Use **enoxaparin** with extreme caution, if at all, in patients with heparin-induced thrombocytopenia.	**Subcutaneous Dose for Dalteparin and Enoxaparin** 1 mg/kg BID SC for 2 to 8 days, administered with aspirin.
Nadroparin (Fraxiparine®) ***(Not available in United States)***	• Contraindicated if platelet count <100 000. For these patients consider these direct antithrombins: — ***Desirudin:*** 0.1 mg/kg IV bolus, followed by infusion of 0.1 mg/kg per hour for 72 hours. — ***Leprudin:*** 0.4 mg/kg IV bolus, followed by infusion of 0.15 mg/kg per hour for 72 hours.	
Ibutilide	**Indications** Treatment of supraventricular arrhythmias, including atrial fibrillation and atrial flutter. Because it has such a short duration of action, it is most effective for the conversion of atrial fibrillation or flutter of relatively brief duration. **Precautions/Contraindications** Ventricular arrhythmias develop in approximately 2% to 5% of patients (polymorphic ventricular tachycardia, including torsades de pointes, may be observed). *Monitor ECG continuously for arrhythmias during administration and for 4 to 6 hours after administration, with defibrillator nearby.* Patients with significantly impaired LV function are at highest risk for arrhythmias.	**Dose for Adults ≥60 kg:** 1 mg (10 mL) administered IV (diluted or undiluted) over 10 minutes. A second dose may be administered at the same rate 10 minutes later. **Dose for Adults <60 kg:** 0.01 mg/kg initial IV dose.
Inamrinone *See* Amrinone		

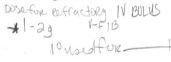

Drug/Therapy	Indications/Precautions	Adult Dosage
Isoproterenol *IV infusion* Mix 1 mg in 250 mL normal saline, lactated Ringer's solution, or D_5W	**Indications** • Use cautiously as *temporizing* measure if *external pacer is not available* for treatment of symptomatic bradycardia. • Refractory torsades de pointes unresponsive to magnesium sulfate. • *Temporary* control of bradycardia in heart transplant patients (denervated heart unresponsive to atropine). • Poisoning from β-adrenergic blockers. **Precautions** • Do not use for treatment of cardiac arrest. • Increases myocardial oxygen requirements, which may increase myocardial ischemia. • Do not give with epinephrine; can cause VF/VT. • Do not administer to patients with poison/drug-induced shock (exception: β-adrenergic blocker poisoning). • Higher doses are Class III (harmful) except for β-adrenergic blocker poisoning.	**IV Infusion** • Infuse at 2 to 10 μg/min. • Titrate to adequate heart rate. • In torsades de pointes titrate to increase heart rate until VT is suppressed.
Lidocaine Can be given via tracheal tube	**Indications** • Cardiac arrest from VF/VT. • Stable VT, wide-complex tachycardias of uncertain type, wide-complex PSVT (Indeterminate). **Precautions** • *Prophylactic* use in AMI patients is *not* recommended. • Reduce maintenance dose (not loading dose) in presence of impaired liver function or left ventricular dysfunction. • Discontinue infusion immediately if signs of toxicity develop. → DEAFNESS >70 y.o. ↓ Blood flow - Chronic Heart failure - Shock	**Cardiac Arrest From VF/VT** • Initial dose: 1 to 1.5 mg/kg IV. • For refractory VF may give additional 0.5 to 0.75 mg/kg IV push, repeat in 5 to 10 minutes; maximum total dose: 3 mg/kg. • A single dose of 1.5 mg/kg IV in cardiac arrest is acceptable. • Tracheal administration: 2 to 4 mg/kg. **Perfusing Arrhythmia** For stable VT, wide-complex tachycardia of uncertain type, significant ectopy, use as follows: • 1 to 1.5 mg/kg IV push. • Repeat 0.5 to 0.75 mg/kg every 5 to 10 minutes; maximum total dose: 3 mg/kg. **Maintenance Infusion** 1 to 4 mg/min (30 to 50 μg/kg per minute).
Magnesium Sulfate Dose for refractory IV BOLUS *1-2g V-FIB 1° used for →	**Indications** • Recommended for use in cardiac arrest only if torsades de pointes or suspected hypomagnesemia is present. • 1° Refractory VF (after lidocaine). • Torsades de pointes with a pulse. • Life-threatening ventricular arrhythmias due to digitalis toxicity. • Prophylactic administration in hospitalized patients with AMI is not recommended. **Precautions** • Occasional fall in blood pressure with rapid administration. • Use with caution if renal failure is present.	**Cardiac Arrest (for hypomagnesemia or torsades de pointes)** * 1 to 2 g (2 to 4 mL of a 50% solution) diluted in 10 mL of D_5W IV push. (BOLUS) **Torsades de Pointes (not in cardiac arrest)** • Loading dose of 1 to 2 g mixed in 50 to 100 mL of D_5W, over 5 to 60 minutes IV. • Follow with 0.5 to 1 g/h IV (titrate dose to control the torsades). **Acute Myocardial Infarction (if indicated)** • Loading dose of 1 to 2 g, mixed in 50 to 100 mL of D_5W, over 5 to 60 minutes IV. • Follow with 0.5 to 1 g/h IV for up to 24 hours.
Mannitol Strengths: 5%, 10%, 15%, 20%, and 25%	**Indications** Increased intracranial pressure in management of neurologic emergencies. **Precautions** • Monitor fluid status and serum osmolality (not to exceed 310 mOsm/kg). • Caution in renal failure because fluid overload may result.	**IV Infusion** • Administer 0.5 to 1 g/kg over 5 to 10 minutes. • Additional doses of 0.25 to 2 g/kg can be given every 4 to 6 hours as needed. • Use with support of oxygenation and ventilation.

Drug/Therapy	Indications/Precautions	Adult Dosage
Morphine Sulfate	**Indications** • Chest pain with ACS unresponsive to nitrates. • Acute cardiogenic pulmonary edema (if blood pressure is adequate). **Precautions** • Administer slowly and titrate to effect. • May compromise respiration; therefore, use with caution in the compromised respiratory state of acute pulmonary edema. • Causes hypotension in volume-depleted patients. • Reverse, if needed, with naloxone (0.4 to 2 mg IV).	**IV Infusion** 2 to 4 mg IV (over 1 to 5 minutes) every 5 to 30 minutes.
Naloxone Hydrochloride	**Indications** Respiratory and neurologic depression due to opiate intoxication unresponsive to O_2 and hyperventilation. **Precautions** • May cause opiate withdrawal. • Effects may not outlast effects of narcotics. • Monitor for recurrent respiratory depression. • Rare anaphylactic reactions have been reported.	**IV Infusion** • 0.4 to 2 mg every 2 minutes. • Use higher doses for complete narcotic reversal. • Can administer up to 10 mg over short period (<10 minutes). • In suspected opiate-addicted patients, titrate dose until ventilations adequate. Begin with 0.2 mg every 2 minutes × 3 doses, then 1.4 mg IV push.
Nitroglycerin Available in IV form, sublingual tablets, and aerosol spray	**Indications** • Initial antianginal for suspected ischemic pain. • For initial 24 to 48 hours in patients with *AMI and CHF*, large anterior wall infarction, persistent or recurrent ischemia, or hypertension. • Continued use (beyond 48 hours) for patients with recurrent angina or persistent pulmonary congestion. • Hypertensive urgency with ACS. **Precautions/Contraindications** • With evidence of AMI, limit systolic blood pressure drop to 10% if patient is normotensive, 30% drop if hypertensive, and avoid drop below 90 mm Hg. • Do not mix with other drugs. • Patient should sit or lie down when receiving this medication. • Do not shake aerosol spray because this affects metered dose. • Contraindications — Hypotension — Severe bradycardia or severe tachycardia — RV infarction — Viagra within 24 hours	**IV Infusion** • IV bolus: 12.5 to 25 μg. • Infuse at 10 to 20 μg/min. • Route of choice for emergencies. • Use appropriate IV sets provided by pharmaceutical companies. • Titrate to effect. **Sublingual Route** 1 tablet (0.3 to 0.4 mg); repeat every 5 minutes. **Aerosol Spray** Spray for 0.5 to 1 second at 5-minute intervals (provides 0.4 mg per dose).

Drug/Therapy	Indications/Precautions	Adult Dosage
Nitroprusside (Sodium Nitroprusside) Mix 50 or 100 mg in 250 mL D_5W only	**Indications** • Hypertensive crisis. • To reduce afterload in heart failure and acute pulmonary edema. • To reduce afterload in acute mitral or aortic valve regurgitation. **Precautions** • Light-sensitive; therefore, wrap drug reservoir in aluminum foil. • May cause hypotension, thiocyanate toxicity, and CO_2 retention. • May reverse hypoxic pulmonary vasoconstriction in patients with pulmonary disease, exacerbating intrapulmonary shunting, resulting in hypoxemia. • Other side effects include headaches, nausea, vomiting, and abdominal cramps.	**IV Infusion** • Begin at 0.1 μg/kg per minute and titrate upward every 3 to 5 minutes to desired effect (up to 5 μg/kg per minute). • Use with an infusion pump; use hemodynamic monitoring for optimal safety. • Action occurs within 1 to 2 minutes. • Cover drug reservoir and tubing with opaque material.
Norepinephrine Mix 4 mg in 250 mL of D_5W or 5% dextrose in normal saline Avoid dilution in normal saline alone	**Indications** • For severe cardiogenic shock and hemodynamically significant hypotension (systolic blood pressure <70 mm Hg) with low total peripheral resistance. • This is an agent of last resort for management of ischemic heart disease and shock. **Precautions** • Increases myocardial oxygen requirements because it raises blood pressure and heart rate. • May induce arrhythmias. Use with caution in patients with acute ischemia; monitor cardiac output. • Extravasation causes tissue necrosis. • If extravasation occurs, administer phentolamine 5 to 10 mg in 10 to 15 mL saline solution, infiltrated into area.	**IV Infusion (Only Route)** • 0.5 to 1 μg/min titrated to improve blood pressure (up to 30 μg/min). • Do not administer in same IV line as alkaline solutions. • Poison/drug-induced hypotension may require higher doses to achieve adequate perfusion.
Oxygen Delivered from portable tanks or installed, wall-mounted sources through delivery devices	**Indications** • Any suspected cardiopulmonary emergency, especially (but *not* limited to) complaints of shortness of breath and suspected ischemic chest pain. • **Note:** Pulse oximetry provides a useful method of titrating oxygen administration to maintain physiologic oxygen saturation (see precautions). **Precautions** • Observe closely when using with pulmonary patients known to be dependent on hypoxic respiratory drive (very rare). • Pulse oximetry inaccurate in low cardiac output states or with vasoconstriction.	See table below

Device	Flow Rate	O_2 (%)
Nasal prongs	1-6 L/min	24-44
Venturi mask	4-8 L/min	24-40
Partial rebreather mask	6-10 L/min	35-60
Bag-mask	15 L/min	up to 100

Drug/Therapy	Indications/Precautions	Adult Dosage
Procainamide	**Indications** • Useful for treatment of a wide variety of arrhythmias. • May use for treatment of PSVT uncontrolled by adenosine and vagal maneuvers if blood pressure stable. • Stable wide-complex tachycardia of unknown origin. • Atrial fibrillation with rapid rate in Wolff-Parkinson-White syndrome. **Precautions** • If cardiac or renal dysfunction is present, reduce maximum total dose to 12 mg/kg and maintenance infusion to 1 to 2 mg/min. • Proarrhythmic, especially in setting of AMI, hypokalemia, or hypomagnesemia. • May induce hypotension in patients with impaired LV function. • Use with caution with other drugs that prolong QT interval (eg, amiodarone, sotalol).	**Recurrent VF/VT** • 20 mg/min IV infusion (maximum total dose: 17 mg/kg). • In urgent situations, up to 50 mg/min may be administered to total dose of 17 mg/kg. **Other Indications** • 20 mg/min IV infusion until one of the following occurs: — Arrhythmia suppression. — Hypotension. — QRS widens by >50%. — Total dose of 17 mg/kg is given. **Maintenance Infusion** 1 to 4 mg/min.
Propafenone ***(IV form not approved for use in United States)***	**Indications** Antiarrhythmic agent used for treatment of ventricular arrhythmias and supraventricular arrhythmias. **Precautions/Contraindications** • Significant negative inotropic effects. *Must be infused slowly.* May increase mortality in patients who have had MI so should be avoided when coronary artery disease is suspected. • Increased plasma concentrations can develop if taken with cimetidine. Digoxin and warfarin levels increase when these drugs are taken with propafenone. • Reported side effects include bradycardia, hypotension, and gastrointestinal upset.	**IV Dose** 1 to 2 mg/kg body weight at 10 mg/min. ***Must be infused slowly.***
Sodium Bicarbonate	**Indications** Specific indications for bicarbonate use are as follows: • **Class I** if known preexisting hyperkalemia. • **Class IIa** if known preexisting bicarbonate-responsive acidosis (eg, diabetic ketoacidosis) or overdose (eg, tricyclic antidepressant overdose, cocaine, diphenhydramine) to alkalinize urine in aspirin or other overdose. • **Class IIb** if prolonged resuscitation with effective ventilation; upon return of spontaneous circulation after long arrest interval. • **Class III** (not useful or effective) in hypercarbic acidosis (eg, cardiac arrest and CPR without intubation). **Precautions** • Adequate ventilation and CPR, not bicarbonate, are the major "buffer agents" in cardiac arrest. • Not recommended for routine use in cardiac arrest patients.	**IV Infusion** • 1 mEq/kg IV bolus. • Repeat half this dose every 10 minutes thereafter. • If rapidly available, use arterial blood gas analysis to guide bicarbonate therapy (calculated base deficits or bicarbonate concentration). **Blood Gas Interpretation** An acute change in $Paco_2$ of 1 mm Hg is associated with an increase or decrease in pH of 0.008 U (relative to normal $Paco_2$ of 40 mm Hg and normal pH of 7.4).

Drug/Therapy	Indications/Precautions	Adult Dosage
Sotalol ***(IV form not approved for use in United States)***	**Indications** In the United States, oral form is approved for treatment of ventricular and atrial arrhythmias. Outside the United States, used for treatment of supraventricular arrhythmias and ventricular arrhythmias in patients without structural heart disease. **Precautions/Contraindications** • Should be avoided in patients with poor perfusion, because of significant negative inotropic effects. ***Must be infused slowly***. • Adverse effects include bradycardia, hypotension, and arrhythmias (torsades de pointes). • Use with caution with other drugs that prolong QT interval (eg, procainamide, amiodarone).	**Dose** Administered as 1 to 1.5 mg/kg body weight, then infused at rate of 10 mg/min. ***Must be infused slowly***.
Thrombolytic Agents *See* Fibrinolytic Agents		
Transcutaneous Pacing External pacemakers have either *fixed* rates (nondemand or asynchronous mode) or *demand* rates (range: 30 to 180 bpm). Current outputs range from 0 to 200 mA.	**Indications** • Class I for hemodynamically unstable bradycardia (eg, blood pressure changes, altered mental status, angina, pulmonary edema). • Class I for pacing readiness in setting of AMI, as follows: — Symptomatic sinus node dysfunction. — Type II second-degree heart block. — Third-degree heart block. — New left, right, or alternating BBB or bifascicular block. • Class IIa for bradycardia with symptomatic ventricular escape rhythms. • Class IIa for overdrive pacing of tachycardias refractory to drug therapy or electrical cardioversion. • Class IIb for bradyasystolic cardiac arrest. Not routinely recommended. If used, use early. **Precautions** • Contraindicated in severe hypothermia or prolonged bradyasystolic cardiac arrest. • Conscious patients may require analgesia for discomfort. • Avoid using carotid pulse to confirm mechanical capture. Electrical stimulation causes muscular jerking that may mimic carotid pulse.	**Technique** • Place pacing electrodes on chest per package instructions. • Turn the pacer ON. • Set demand rate to approximately 80 bpm. • Set current (mA) output as follows: — *Bradycardia:* Increase milliamperes from minimum setting until consistent capture is achieved (characterized by a widening QRS and a broad T wave after each pacer spike). Then add 2 mA for safety margin. — *Asystole:* Begin at full output (mA). If capture occurs, slowly decrease output until capture is lost (threshold). Then add 2 mA for safety margin.
Vasopressin	**Indications** • May be used as an alternative pressor to epinephrine in the treatment of adult shock-refractory VF (Class IIb). • May be useful for hemodynamic support in vasodilatory shock (eg, septic shock). **Precautions/Contraindications** • Potent peripheral vasoconstrictor. Increased peripheral vascular resistance may provoke cardiac ischemia and angina. • Not recommended for responsive patients with coronary artery disease.	**IV, IO, and TT Doses for Cardiac Arrest:** 40 U IV push × 1 is the only route recommended in the AHA *ECC Guidelines 2000.*

Drug/Therapy	Indications/Precautions	Adult Dosage
Verapamil	**Indications** • Alternative drug (after adenosine) to terminate PSVT with narrow QRS complex and adequate blood pressure and *preserved LV function.* • May control ventricular response in patients with atrial fibrillation, flutter, or multifocal atrial tachycardia. **Precautions** • Give *only* to patients with narrow-complex PSVT or arrhythmias known to be of supraventricular origin. Do not use calcium channel blockers for wide-QRS tachycardias of uncertain origin. • Avoid calcium channel blockers in patients with Wolff-Parkinson-White syndrome and atrial fibrillation, sick sinus syndrome, or second- or third-degree AV block without pacemaker. • Expect blood pressure drop caused by peripheral vasodilation. IV calcium is an antagonist that may restore blood pressure in toxic cases. • May decrease myocardial contractility and may exacerbate CHF in patients with LV dysfunction. • Concurrent IV administration with IV β-blockers may produce severe hypotension. • Use with extreme caution in patients receiving oral β-blockers.	**IV Infusion** • 2.5 to 5 mg IV bolus over 2 minutes. • Second dose: 5 to 10 mg, if needed, in 15 to 30 minutes. Maximum dose: 20 mg. • Alternative: 5 mg bolus every 15 minutes to total dose of 30 mg. • Older patients: Administer over 3 minutes.

LIDOCAINE 1-4 mg/min